KT-119-115

Measures of Need and Outcome for Primary Health Care

David Wilkin, Lesley Hallam,
and Marie-Anne Doggett

Centre for Primary Care Research
Rusholme Health Centre
Manchester

OXFORD · NEW YORK · TOKYO
OXFORD UNIVERSITY PRESS

Oxford University Press, Walton Street, Oxford OX2 6DP

Oxford New York Toronto
Delhi Bombay Calcutta Madras Karachi
Kuala Lumpur Singapore Hong Kong Tokyo
Nairobi Dar es Salaam Cape Town
Melbourne Auckland Madrid
and associated companies in
Berlin Ibadan

Oxford is a trade mark of Oxford University Press

Published in the United States by
Oxford University Press Inc., New York

© Crown Copyright, 1992
First published 1992
First published in paperback 1993
(with corrections)
Reprinted 1994

A catalogue record for this book is
available from the British Library

Library of Congress Cataloging in Publication Data
Wilkin, David.
Measures of need and outcome for primary health care / David
Wilkin, Lesley Hallam, and Marie-Anne Doggett.
p. cm.
Includes bibliographical references and index.
1. Health status indicators.   2. Patient satisfaction-
-Measurement. I. Hallam, Lesley. II. Doggett, Marie-Anne.
III. Title.
[DNLM: 1. Health Services Needs and Demand.   2. Outcome and
Process Assessment (Health Care)—methods.   3. Primary Health Care-
-standards. 4. Quality Assurance, Health Care. W . 84.6 W683m]
RA407.W55   1991   362.1'068'5—dc20   91–31914
ISBN 0 19 262420 2 (Pbk)

Printed by Bookcraft (Bath) Ltd., Midsomer Norton, Avon

11731

362.1042 WIL

T

OXFORD MEDI

Measures of Need and Outcome
for Primary Health Care

**This book is to be returned on or before
the last date stamped below.**

11731

Acknowledgements

We are very grateful for all the help we have received from the many researchers and practitioners whose instruments are reviewed in this volume. We are grateful not only for their permission to reproduce schedules and questionnaires, but also for their help in providing us with information about recent developments. We hope that they will consider our comments a fair assessment of their instruments.

The collection and review of the enormous volume of published and unpublished material which was necessary for this book would have been impossible without Janet Candlin. Over a period of more than three years, Janet has devoted many hours to tracking down more than a thousand books and papers. She has coped cheerfully with inaccurate and incomplete references and has usually succeeded. We should like to thank Anne Pearcey for her skill and patience in preparing the final manuscript, and Pat Nix for typing an earlier version. Lastly, we should like to thank other members of the Centre for Primary Care Research who in giving us their support and encouragement have played an important part in bringing this project to fruition.

The work necessary to complete a book such as this imposes burdens on those with whom we share our lives outside of work. We should like to thank our respective partners and families for their support, both practical and emotional, over the past five years since we originally conceived the idea of this review.

Contents

1 Defining need and outcome

Introduction

The emphasis placed on controlling health care costs over the past decade or so in all western nations has created a powerful stimulus for research into the effectiveness and efficiency of health services. This in turn has generated a wide range of measures designed in varying degrees to estimate the needs for, and outcomes of, health care. It was the existence of this plethora of measures which prompted us to write this book in the hope of offering the intending researcher and the practitioner a guide through the jungle.

Our particular focus is on the needs of practitioners, managers, and academics working in the field of primary health care. Research into the provision of primary health care, and general medical practice in particular, has developed more slowly than in most other specialties. Although there have been considerable developments in primary health care research in the past decade, the absence of strong traditions has resulted in much of this work being concerned with basic description of the structure and process of care, rather than with identifying needs for services or measuring the outcomes of interventions. To the extent that the problems of measuring outcomes have been addressed, this has tended to be in terms of the predominant biomedical model, rather than adopting a broad range of outcome criteria.

The following chapters are addressed primarily to those whose want to measure needs and/or outcomes using non-clinical instruments, but who do not have the time, resources, and/or expertise to evaluate the full range of available instruments. Despite the low level of development of primary health care research, many instruments for measuring needs and outcomes are already available, some of these come from other specialties, but by far the majority have been developed in the USA, where the pressure to demonstrate effectiveness and efficiency has been much stronger. The task of assembling, reviewing, and evaluating the mountain of books, reports, and papers dealing with the development and use of measures is daunting. Even professional researchers are unlikely to have the time or resources to adequately survey all of the potentially useful instruments. The practitioner, whose research has to compete with the demands of professional practice, stands little chance of undertaking such a task. Indeed the sheer volume of published material and the large number of available measures is itself partly a reflection of the difficulties encountered in carrying out a review of available methods. Too often intending researchers develop their own measures, rather than embark on a systematic review of already developed instruments to find one suitable for the purpose in hand. In doing so, they add to the number of instruments and the volume of publications. We hope that the present guide will both help researchers and practitioners to use the best available measures and discourage the unnecessary proliferation of new measures which add little to existing techniques. We hope that it will provide managers and policy makers with a knowledge of the strengths and limitations of current measurement techniques which will aid both their commissioning of new research and their ability to assess the value of research findings.

The core of the book in Chapters 4–10 is a guide to 40 measures of need and outcome suitable in varying degrees for use in primary health care research and practice, divided according to subject matter. Although these chapters are likely to constitute the most useful reference section, we urge readers to devote some time to the introductory chapters. It is essential that users of the instruments we have reviewed should have at least a basic understanding of the theoretical and methodological issues relevant to the measurement of needs and outcomes in health care. What are we trying to measure and why? What makes a good measure? What are the limitations on its use and interpretation? These and similar questions are addressed in Chapters 2 and 3. Chapter 2 deals with the basic concepts relevant to need and outcomes with respect to health care. Chapter 3 deals with issues of measurement, the development of measures, their reliability and validity, and the problems of selecting a measure for a particular purpose. Although these chapters are intended particularly for the reader who has relatively little prior knowledge of these issues, the more experienced reader may also find them a useful reminder of the problems and pitfalls of measurement in health care.

It is important first to devote some space to what we mean by needs and outcomes. In what sense can the instruments which are presented in this book be considered to be measures of need for, or outcomes of, health care? What questions should be asked when planning research into needs and outcomes?

The concept of need

The concept of need is central to the provision of health care since it defines the objectives of care. To speak of a need is to imply a goal, a measurable deficiency from the goal, and a means of achieving the goal. Thus, for example, a goal may be freedom from pain. A person suffering from a headache has a measurable deficiency from the goal. Taking an analgesic is a means of achieving the goal. But even such an apparently straightforward example contains certain problematic assumptions. Complete freedom from pain may be undesirable, since it is a necessary indicator of malfunction. How are we to decide what level of deficiency constitutes a need? Perhaps most problematic: is the taking of an analgesic the most appropriate method of meeting the need?

It is important when considering needs to recognize that these can be defined in a variety of different ways and from a variety of perspectives. Measures of need are, therefore, not neutral objective descriptions of people. They incorporate value judgements about what should be accepted as appropriate goals and what constitutes deficiency from these goals. Although a detailed discussion of the concept of need is beyond the scope of this book, it is desirable that anyone intending to measure needs using any of the instruments included in later chapters should have a basic understanding of different approaches. All measures of need incorporate judgements about what constitute desirable goals and how deficiencies from these goals should be assessed, but these judgements are rarely made explicit. They concern two related areas; the standard against which deficiency or need is to be assessed and who should decide what constitutes a need. There are three broad approaches to defining the criteria against which to assess the existence of need. Firstly, needs can be assessed against some ideal standard. Secondly, they can be defined in terms of a minimum level below which people should not fall, and thirdly, they can be assessed by reference to comparisons with standards achieved by other groups or individuals. The choice of who should decide what constitutes need lies between the individual, a professional group, or society at large.

Ideal standards against which to measure needs are extremely difficult to define in ways which do not make them meaningless for practical purposes. Thus, the WHO definition of health as a state of complete physical, mental, and social well-being can be seen as setting an ideal standard, but it is of little practical value in defining needs for health care. Apart from the fact that everyone could be defined as having needs by this criterion, it begs the fundamental question of how to define such a state. As soon as one attempts to provide a definition which might be capable of being measured, it rapidly loses its universality and becomes specific to a particular culture or even subgroups within a culture. Thus, for example, in a culture which values athleticism, inability to participate in sports may be regarded as an indication of need for health care, but in a culture which values sedentary occupation, obesity may be a sign of well-being. Similarly, in our own society, homosexuality may be regarded by the majority as less than ideal health, but is the culturally accepted norm within the minority of homosexual people.

Social and health policy has tended to rely more heavily on minimum standards against which to measure need. Thus, there have been numerous attempts to define minimum standards of nutrition, income, housing, etc. In the field of measurements specific to health and health care, measures of basic physical function have the character of minimum standards, in so far as they define basic functions (e.g. walking, dressing, working) which all adult human beings should be able to perform for themselves. However, it is clear that such approaches to the definition of need are extremely limited. By focusing on what is easily measurable they tend to ignore all but a very small part of what most people would regard as legitimate needs.

Comparative approaches to the assessment of need are an extension of minimum standards, but rather than attempting to define absolutes, they rely on comparisons with the average for the population as a whole or sub-groups within it. In practical terms, the comparative approach offers a compromise between largely undefinable ideals and highly restrictive minimum standards. Thus, needs for health can be defined in terms of the standards known to be achieved by comparable groups (e.g. adults of the same age and sex living in the same area) or those achieved by the most privileged in the same society.

In selecting an appropriate measure of need for a particular purpose the user should give some thought to the question of whose perspective and definition of need is important. Some measures rely on the individual's own perception of need, a sense of discrepancy between what is and what ought to be. It might be argued that such felt needs are particularly relevant in primary medical care, because it is the expression of these needs that brings people to the doctor to seek care. The disadvantages of relying on the individual's experience of need are on the one hand that low expectations may result in a very low perception of need, and on the other that it is difficult to see how needs can be distinguished from wants.

Traditionally, judgements about needs in the realm of health and illness have been regarded as the province of the medical profession. However, professional judgements tend to avoid the problem of defining goals and standards, preferring instead to define needs in terms of the specific techniques within their sphere of competence. Thus, for example, needs for mobility and freedom from pain become needs for hip replacement operations or non-steroidal anti-inflammatory drugs. The problems with such an approach are that it rules out alternative ways of meeting the need and inhibits the formation of an overall picture in which there may be a variety of needs to be met in different ways.

Some of the more sophisticated measures of need in the field of health and illness attempt to go beyond individual and professional judgements by explicitly incorporating the values of society as a whole through techniques of using lay people as judges. In this way the needs of the individual can be assessed against the norms considered acceptable by other people. The main disadvantage of this approach seems to be that the averaging of a large number of possibly diverse judgements may yield standards which bear little relationship to any individual experience.

None of the different approaches to the definition, and therefore measurement, of need is superior to the others. Each will be appropriate to particular circumstances. What is important is that anyone setting out to determine need should be aware of the variety of ways of defining it and should consider which will be most appropriate to a particular set of circumstances.

The concept of outcome

The dictionary definition of outcome is 'result or visible effect'. To be concerned with outcomes is simply to be concerned with the causal relationships between antecedent and subsequent conditions or events. But in the context of health and illness, outcome is usually defined in terms of the achievement of or failure to achieve desired goals. Relative to these goals, from a defined starting point, outcomes can be either positive or negative, ranging from complete health to death (or worse). This definition in terms of goals or objectives when used in the context of the provision of health care, is common to both outcome and need. Indeed outcome and need can be viewed as different sides of the same coin. Thus, it should not be surprising that most of the measures in this book can be employed as measures of either needs for, or outcomes of, health care. It is not so much the content of the measures, as the uses to which they are put, which is important in drawing a distinction. Thus, for example, an instrument which measures pain can be used to assess the need for pain relief and the outcome of administering an analgesic.

Just as research into need must address the questions of what to measure, from whose perspective, and according to which criteria, so anyone considering research on outcomes should consider a variety of issues in addition to selecting an appropriate measure. The researcher will normally be concerned with the impact of health care on a disease process, so the first task should be to describe its natural history. Secondly, it is essential to define the objectives of health care interventions against which outcomes are to be measured. Thirdly, it will be necessary to ensure that the potentially wide range of inputs can be adequately described. Fourthly, the researcher needs to specify the hypothesized relationship between inputs and outcomes, and lastly select an appropriate research design. These tasks will not necessarily be completed in the order in which they are presented here, but all will need some attention.

Describing the natural history

Whatever the problem under study, (commonly, although not always, defined in terms of disease categories), it should be possible to describe its natural history. If it is possible to determine the course taken by a given problem without health care intervention, this will provide a baseline against which outcomes can be measured. Thus, it is possible to measure the effectiveness of health care for acute appendicitis in terms of case fatality, since we know the natural history of untreated appendicitis. Where there is no known effective treatment, such as for the common cold, it is difficult to see how the effectiveness of a new treatment could be evaluated without reference to its natural history. Unfortunately, it is rare that such information is available in a systematic form. An alternative to plotting the natural history where new patterns of care are being evaluated is to use as a baseline the history of the condition or problem under existing patterns of care. Thus, the efficacy of new drugs is usually assessed against the standard set by drugs already available, rather than in terms of the natural history of the condition without treatment.

Defining the objectives of health care

At the most general level, the objective of health care could be said to be the improvement of health or a reduction in the level of ill health, but this is scarcely very helpful when it comes to attempts to evaluate the effectiveness of specific health care interventions. The general objective provides only a starting point from which to begin to elaborate a wide variety of levels and perspectives. Objectives can be stated at different levels of aggregation, from the individual to the family to the community to the society as a whole. They may refer to different time periods (the present, the immediate future, a lifetime) and they will reflect the differing values of interested parties. In some instances there will be a clear and overriding immediate objective agreed by all parties (e.g. to keep the patient alive following a heart attack), but such instances are rare, and often agreement is only transitory. Explicitly defined objectives are much less common in primary medical care than in many other specialties. For most problems there is a wide range of possible objectives which will be awarded different values and priorities by different interested parties (doctor, nurse, patient, relatives, friends, neighbours, etc.). In the individual encounter between patient and professional, objectives may be assumed or may become the subject of negotiation between patient and professionals. However, the individual encounter excludes other potentially interested parties from any negotiation, and this is not a negotiation between equals. Thus, for example, the consultation between patient and doctor excludes the patient's family, friends, and neighbours. When looking at the outcomes of medical care, it is important to ask who is defining the objectives which determine the selection of outcome criteria. If this is not done, there is a danger that the measures selected will reflect primarily the objectives of professionals. Thus, for example, many studies of cancer treatments have focused solely on survival rates, regardless of the quality of life experienced by patients and their relatives.

Describing inputs

There is little point in attempting to measure outcomes without being able to provide a precise description of inputs, since to use the term 'outcome' implies the existence of a causal model which relates certain structures and/or processes to end results. These inputs can be subdivided into those provided by the health care system and those provided by other agencies, the individual, family, friends, and community. Structural service inputs, such as the number of doctors, nurses, receptionists, etc. may be relatively straightforward to describe, but precise descriptions of the process of care can be extremely problematic, particularly in primary health care. Even apparently straightforward descriptions, such as whether or not a drug was prescribed, can become complicated. Was the drug dispensed, and if it was dispensed did the patient take it as advised? When one is attempting to describe such inputs as diagnosis, counselling, reassurance, monitoring, etc. the problems become infinitely more complex. Indeed finding appropriate methods of measuring inputs can be more difficult than identifying suitable outcome measures. In most instances the attempt to measure inputs ends with a description of a relatively small range of service inputs. But inputs from other agencies and from informal sources can be at least as important. Whilst it would be impossible to take account of all possible inputs, any well planned study of the outcomes of health care should consider the likelihood that systematic variations in the pattern of inputs which are outside the control of the particular service under study will have a direct bearing on outcomes. Thus, for example, the allocation of many supportive services for elderly people is systematically related to their home circumstances. In this situation a straightforward comparison of people receiving the service and those not receiving the service would fail to take account of systematic and important differences between the two groups.

Specifying the relationship between inputs and outcomes

Although it is possible to examine the relationship between inputs and outcomes without clearly specifying the nature of that relationship, this is likely to leave important questions unanswered. For example, evidence might be produced to support the hypothesis that routine follow-up of patients suffering from asthma results in fewer symptoms. Whilst such a finding might be useful, it is difficult to interpret. Does follow-up achieve better outcomes because the medication is reviewed and modified as appropriate, or because patient compliance is improved? If it is compliance that is important, this might be a function of increased knowledge or a fear of being reprimanded. In either case it may be that follow-up is not the best method of achieving the desired outcome. Research into the outcomes of health care will be of much greater value if it can go beyond the crude demonstration of statistical associations between particular patterns of care and outcomes. In order to do this, it is necessary to devote more attention at the planning stage to the clear formulation of questions or hypotheses which attempt to specify the intermediate steps between inputs and outcomes, in ways that make it possible to identify the strengths and weaknesses of the causal model.

Research design

Since it is impossible to accurately measure, or even be aware of, all potentially confounding variables when examining the relationship between the provision of health care and the outcomes of that care, the selection of an appropriate research design is an important way of minimizing their effects. Unfortunately, the use of the classic double-blind, randomized, controlled trial as a research design is only rarely possible in a complex system of health care. Nevertheless, the standards imposed in this model should serve as a guide for studies of the outcomes of health care. Where the research focuses on discrete and easily identifiable categories of problem which are amenable to relatively simple preventive or therapeutic measures it may be possible, with ingenuity, to adopt variants of the randomized control trial in a primary health care setting. However, many studies will be concerned with multidimensional problems and complex patterns of health care. In such circumstances it will be necessary to use either non-randomized trials or observational studies. Comparisons of populations exposed and not exposed to defined patterns of care (prospective cohort studies) and those with and without the desired outcome (retrospective case-control studies) are the two principal analytical approaches. The choice of research design will depend on many factors peculiar to the particular research problem. However, the importance of selecting an appropriate design should not be underestimated. The value of the work done on objective setting, selection of appropriate outcome measures, measurement of inputs, etc., will only be fully realized if these are employed in an appropriate research design.

In this introductory chapter we have identified the sorts of issues which should be addressed when selecting measures of need or outcome and designing research. Our intention is not to discourage the reader, but to help to obtain the best from the measures presented in later chapters. We cannot overemphasize the point that time and effort spent at the planning and design stage will be amply rewarded when it comes to analysing and presenting results.

2 Concepts

In order to begin to make a selection of a measure suited to a particular purpose, the practitioner or researcher must have a clear idea about what it is relevant to measure and in what sense this can be said to represent needs for, or outcomes of, health care. At the most general level, most of the readers of this book will be interested in measuring health or some aspect of health. This, however, begs the question of what is meant by health, and thus how deviations from it might be measured. There are many alternative approaches to the problem of definition, ranging from the narrowly medical to the all embracing. It is beyond the scope of this book to embark on a detailed discussion of the philosophical arguments. However, it is important that users of measures should be aware of the underlying conceptual bases of measures included in later chapters. For each measure, we have tried to identify the conceptual focus, although instruments are all too often presented by their authors without an adequate account of what they are designed to measure, except in the most general terms.

In this chapter, we provide a broad overview of the main approaches to the measurement of needs for, and outcomes of, health care. Firstly, we examine the usefulness of the traditional medical model, in which health is defined as the absence of disease. Secondly, we outline the components of a model based on the consequences of disease for individuals and society. Thirdly, we explore the concept of positive health and its relevance to the definition of needs for, and outcomes of, health care. The final section of the chapter deals with the concept of patient satisfaction and its value as an alternative to health or disease in outcome evaluation of health services.

Disease and the medical model

The task of medicine, and therefore the outcomes against which success or failure are measured, has traditionally been defined in terms of the presence or absence of disease. The medical model views disease within the following framework:

$$\text{Aetiology} \longrightarrow \text{Pathology} \longrightarrow \text{Manifestations.}$$

Diseases are identified and classified in terms of organs and/or bodily systems, and it is assumed that there are direct and unambiguous causal relationships between the different elements of the model. The task of medicine is to identify and classify disease (diagnosis) and to eliminate it through preventive measures or curative treatments. The outcome of treatment is defined in terms of a simple dichotomy, the presence or absence of disease. Organs or individuals are either diseased or well, and there is little scope for intermediate states. At the level of populations, health is measured in terms of morbidity, the incidence or prevalence of disease entities in defined groups. The traditional medical model makes little direct appeal to the consequences of disease as criteria for assessing either needs for, or outcomes of, treatment, except in so far as survival is a successful outcome and death the final negative outcome. Thus, at the population level, somewhat perversely, one of the most commonly used measures of health is the death rate.

A fundamental problem with the medical model as a definition of health is that to define health as the absence of disease simply substitutes one definitional problem for another. 'What is health?' becomes 'What is disease?'. In an attempt to resolve the problem, Boorse lists seven major themes that pervade the literature on health and disease: value (health is desirable, disease is undesirable); treatment by physicians (diseases are undesirable conditions that doctors happen to treat); statistical normality (health conditions are normal, disease is abnormal); pain or discomfort (health contrasts with the pain or discomfort of disease); disability (any disease must at some stage cause disability); adaptation (disease is the absence of appropriate adaptation to environment); homeostasis (disease processes are disruptions of the equilibrium or homeostatic failures).[1] A cursory consideration of each of these themes, will reveal that, in all of them, disease is definable only through reference to its consequences for the organ, the organism or the person. Even Boorse's own definition of disease as 'a type of internal state which impairs health, i.e. reduces one or more functional abilities below typical efficiency' suffers the same problem. Implicit in any definition of disease is the notion that it has negative consequences. In terms of both the need for, and outcomes of, health care it is more useful to think in terms of the consequences of disease rather than its presence or absence.

Such philosophical issues may, however, be considered somewhat irrelevant to the practical concerns of doctors and other health care professionals. It could be argued that it is only at the margins of medical care that there is likely to be any real disagreement between patients and professionals as to what is or is not disease. Whilst the question of whether or not homosexuality should be treated as a disease might engender fierce debate, there can be no doubt that measles, cancer, diabetes, bronchitis, or duodenal ulcer constitute disease. For many of the problems which people present to doctors, the simple presence of disease will be sufficient to establish a need for medical care, whilst the absence of disease and survival will be adequate criteria for the assessment of outcome. In so far as medicine deals with acute illness this is true. Both at the level of the individual patient and at the level of populations, needs can be defined in terms of the presence or absence of given conditions which are amenable to preventive measures or treatment. Outcomes can be defined in terms of cure and/or survival. The disease entity can be separated from the individual in whom it occurs, and any short-term variations in the consequences of disease for different individuals can be largely ignored, since cure will restore all those affected to 'normal' functioning in a relatively short space of time. Thus in an outbreak of meningitis, needs for medical care can be defined in terms of the number of individuals affected. The outcomes of treatment can be measured in terms of the number who are cured and the number who died.

So long as the major health problems facing both individuals and society are predominantly acute, the disease model of health provides an adequate framework for determining needs for, and outcomes of, medical care. However, as living standards and medical techniques have advanced in western society during this century, many of the major life-threatening acute disorders have been all but eliminated in the younger age groups. As more and more people are surviving into middle and old age, the pattern of disease is changing. The newly prevalent diseases may be amenable to medical treatment, but on the whole the underlying causes cannot be eliminated, and thus patients cannot be cured. This shift of emphasis from acute life-threatening conditions to chronic incurable illness necessitates a different approach to the measurement of need and outcome. For chronic illnesses such as diabetes, arthritis, or asthma, cure and survival are no longer appropriate criteria for the evaluation of medical intervention. Most patients will survive, but very few will be cured. Neither is the presence or absence of the condition a suitable basis for assessing needs for care. Any two patients suffering from arthritis will have widely differing needs because of the particular manifestation of the disease and its severity at a point in time. Where medicine is unable to offer a cure, but is able to alleviate the impact of the disease, the notion of severity becomes crucial, both in terms of needs and outcomes. But once we have introduced the idea of severity, we have moved beyond the traditional medical model to explicitly incorporate the consequences of disease for the person.

Consequences of disease

Those medical specialties which focus on the care of patients suffering from chronic illnesses, for example rheumatology, geriatric medicine, cardiology, and oncology, have long recognized the inadequacy of the traditional medical model as a means of evaluating their activity. As a result they have been responsible for the initial development of many of the measures included in later chapters, which are in the main designed to measure the consequences of disease on various aspects of life. These same specialties have played an important role in introducing into the practice of medicine alternative concepts to those central to the traditional model. Over the years a variety of terms has been developed to provide a framework for describing the consequences of disease; impairment, disability, functional limitation, handicap, dependency, etc. As might be expected with a set of concepts derived from practice across diverse specialties, there has been a lack of consistency in the meanings attached to different terms and the uses to which they have been put. This has resulted at times in considerable confusion and calls from both researchers and practitioners for an agreed and consistent terminology.

In recent years a number of attempts have been made to overcome the confusion of terminology and offer a conceptual framework acceptable to both practitioners and researchers. No single model is likely to resolve all problems at the first attempt, but it can provide a framework which is broadly acceptable and thus encourage consistency and aid communication. The conceptual scheme developed by Wood, which forms the basis of the WHO *International classification of impairments, disabilities and handicaps* (ICIDH) seems to us to be preferable to alternatives on offer for two main reasons.[4] Firstly, it provides a clear distinction between the consequences of disease at three different levels; the organ, individual performance, and societal response. Secondly, the very fact that the ICIDH is built around this conceptual scheme suggests that it is likely to attain wider acceptance and application than alternatives.

The ICIDH offers a unifying framework based on planes of experience within which to set the consequences of disease. Table 2.1 identifies the principal events in the development of illness. First, something abnormal occurs within the individual. A chain of causal circumstances gives rise to changes in the structure or functioning of the body, i.e. pathology. These changes may or may not make themselves evident. This first stage can be seen as the intrinsic situation and its features are the components of the traditional medical model. At the second level, someone becomes aware of the occurrence of change. The pathological state is exteriorized. The individual becomes, or is made aware, that he or she is unhealthy and this awareness heralds the recognition of impairments, i.e. abnormalities of body structure and appearance, and of organ or system function resulting from any cause. Impairments represent disturbances at the organ level. The third level is represented by alterations in the performance or behaviour of the individual. Common experience is objectified. These experiences represent disabilities, i.e. the consequences of impairments in terms of functional performance and

Table 2.1   WHO conceptual scheme

Disease or disorder	Impairment	Disability	Handicap
Intrinsic situation	Experience exteriorized	Experience objectified	Experience socialized

activity by the individual. Disabilities represent disturbances at the level of the person. At the fourth and final level, impairment or disability may place the individual at a disadvantage to others, thus socializing the experience. This experience of disadvantage represents handicap.

The definitions and characteristics of impairment, disability, and handicap used in the WHO classification are summarized in Table 2.2. The manual of the ICIDH goes on to present a detailed classification system for impair-

Table 2.2 Definitions and characteristics of impairment, disability and handicap.
(Reproduced with permission from World Health Organization (1980). *International classification of impairments, disabilities and handicaps*. World Health Organization, Geneva).

Impairment

Definition
In the context of health experience, an impairment is any loss or abnormality of psychological, physiological, or anatomical structure or function. (**Note:** 'Impairment' is more inclusive than 'disorder' in that it covers losses — e.g. the loss of a leg is an impairment, but not a disorder)

Characteristics
Impairment is characterized by losses or abnormalities that may be temporary or permanent, and that include the existence or occurrence of an anomaly, defect, or loss in a limb, organ, tissue, or other structure of the body, including the systems of mental function. Impairment represents exteriorization of a pathological state, and in principle it reflects disturbances at the level of the organ.

Disability

Definition
In the context of health experience, a disability is any restriction or lack (resulting from an impairment) of ability to perform an activity in the manner or within the range considered normal for a human being.

Characteristics
Disability is characterized by excesses or deficiencies of customarily expected activity performance and behaviour, and these may be temporary or permanent, reversible or irreversible, and progressive or regressive. Disabilities may arise as a direct consequence of impairment or as a response by the individual, particularly psychologically, to a physical, sensory, or other impairment. Disability represents objectification of an impairment, and as such it reflects disturbances at the level of the person.

Disability is concerned with abilities, in the form of composite activities and behaviours, that are generally accepted as essential components of everyday life. Examples include disturbances in behaving in an appropriate manner, in personal care (such as excretory control and the ability to wash and feed oneself), in the performance of other activities of daily living, and in locomotor activities (such as the ability to walk).

Table 2.2 *cont'd.*

Handicap

Definition
In the context of health experience, a handicap is a disadvantage for a given individual, resulting from an impairment or a disability, that limits or prevents the fulfilment of a role that is normal (depending on age, sex, and social and cultural factors) for that individual.

Characteristics
Handicap is concerned with the value attached to an individual's situation or experience when it departs from the norm. It is characterized by a discordance between the individual's performance or status and the expectations of the individual himself or of the particular group of which he is a member. Handicap thus represents socialization of an impairment or disability, and as such it reflects the consequences for the individual — cultural, social, economic, and environmental — that stem from the presence of impairment and disability.

Disadvantage arises from failure or inability to conform to the expectations or norms of the individual's universe. Handicap thus occurs when there is interference with the ability to sustain what might be designated as 'survival roles'.

---

ments, disabilities, and handicaps. A consideration of this is beyond the scope of the present discussion, but it is worth noting that it provides a useful and comprehensive framework, not only for classifying the consequences of disease for individuals, but also for describing the experience of populations and evaluating the coverage of measures of need and outcomes for particular categories of patients.

The ICIDH is intended as a working basis for classification rather than as a complete and finished system. It will no doubt evolve over time in response to the experience of users. Nevertheless, it constitutes an important step in the direction of greater consistency in the application of concepts relating to the consequences of disease. One of its applications should be in the area of achieving greater conceptual clarity and consistency in the formulation of measures of need and outcome.

Positive health

To the extent that the discussion so far in this chapter has addressed the problem of defining what is meant by the term health, it has focused exclusively on negative conceptions, the absence of disease, and the absence of impairments, disabilities, and handicaps. The idea that health should be seen as something more than the absence of disease and its negative consequences has grown increasingly popular over recent decades. The WHO's declaration in 1958 that health should be defined as 'a state of complete physical, mental and social well-being and not merely the absence of disease or infirmity', was a statement of political commitment as much as a conscious attempt at definition. It has, nevertheless, provided a focus over three decades for debates about the meaning of health, the legitimate concerns of health care providers, and the measurement of needs and outcomes. Despite the fact that it has been repeatedly dismissed as being incapable of meaningful application, it continues to be the most widely quoted definition. More importantly, it has played a part in changing public and professional attitudes towards health, with consequent changes in health-related behaviour and the role of health services.

As far as attempts to measure needs for, and outcomes of, health care are concerned, many of the authors of measurement instruments have tried to respond to the concept of positive health. Attention has shifted from symptoms, function, and disability, to health, quality of life, and well-being, or so it would seem from the titles of more recent instruments. However, as will become apparent in later chapters, the actual content of measures has changed rather less than might be suggested by their titles. Although there has clearly been a widening of scope to include mental and social aspects of health, there is less evidence that measurement has come to grips with the concept of positive health. Indeed it might be argued that the changes in titles are more a reflection of prevailing political pressures than any real change in content. The titles of papers sometimes seem to owe more to the designated subject of the conference or book to which the authors are contributing, than to the content and conceptual foundations of the measures presented.

To understand the reasons for the relative scarcity of measures which truly tap a concept of positive health it is necessary to examine the validity of the concept itself. As numerous authors have remarked, common usage of the term health implies more than the absence of disease. If we conceive of health as a continuum, at one end of the spectrum lies death and at the other a state of complete well-being. The problem for conceptual analysis lies in defining the components of this state of well-being or health. There seems to be general agreement that it includes maximizing one's quality of life through developing full human potential. Positive health can thus be seen as achieving functional excellence. Boorse suggests three ways in which this might be interpreted: individual potential, species potential, and the unlimited view.[1] The individual potential view of positive health asserts that ideal health is achieved by developing individual functional capacities to the highest that one's natural gifts will allow. According to the species potential view, target levels of functioning for ideal health are defined in terms of the highest level of performance achieved by humans. Thus, Olympic athletes might be said to represent functional performance targets for physical health. Lastly, the unlimited view imposes no constraints on performance goals. Any improvement in performance represents an increment to health.

Boorse offers a critique of the notion of positive health, arguing that it is not analogous to the more familiar negative conception of health. Firstly, taking health to be functional excellence changes it from a limited to an unlimited ideal. From the point of view of measurement, it is difficult to see how deviation from an undefinable state might be assessed. The individual potential view may overcome this problem, but health would then need to be defined for each individual. Secondly, and more importantly, Boorse argues that there can be no fixed direction of advance, in that, beyond the elimination of disease and its consequences, one cannot simultaneously advance in all possible areas of performance. This point is illustrated if we consider the choices which face an athlete. It is impossible to maximize one's potential as a weight lifter, sprinter, marathon runner, and discus thrower all at the same time. Maximizing performance in one area of function will impose restrictions on other areas, and may even have negative consequences. Lastly, and related to the previous point, the necessity of making choices between different areas of function requires an evaluative decision about which goals are worthy of pursuit. In contrast to a negative conception of health, the ideals of positive health are not capable of being described, only of being advocated. There are potentially as many different views of what constitutes ideal positive health as there are people.

This discussion of the concept of positive health has important implications for attempts at measurement. Whilst we would not wish to deny the importance and validity of the notion of positive health, its application in instruments designed to measure needs for, and outcomes of, health care must be limited to those which aim to tap subjective experiences. Any attempt to incorporate positive health into objective measures risks imposing a particular set of value judgements about what is and is not desirable. However, even in subjective measures, the problem is not entirely overcome. By their very nature, they are limited to conceptualizing health in terms of the respondents' own definitions. The notion of positive health has little meaning if the expectations of respondents do not extend beyond, or even as far as, the absence of disease and its negative consequences.

Patient satisfaction

Patients' subjective evaluations of their health, disabilities, handicaps, quality of life, etc. are very much within the realms of needs for health care and final outcomes. The conceptual focus is the same whether measurement is made against supposedly universal criteria or in terms of the individual's own particular frame of reference. But the complexities of the relationships between needs, health care provision, and outcomes has led both researchers and practitioners to seek to evaluate health care through the intermediate outcome of patient satisfaction. Firstly, it is argued that satisfaction with care will be directly related to the final outcomes of that care, and secondly, that the satisfaction of consumers should be a legitimate objective of the providers of a health service, just as it is for the providers of any other service. However, health care is clearly not like other services in certain important respects. In a competitive market, consumers can express their dissatisfaction by simply taking their custom elsewhere. Even in a private health care system there is likely to be relatively little choice of providers, but this lack of alternatives is particularly evident in a monolithic service like the National Health Service. More importantly, the nature of consumers' needs for health care and the complex nature of the service provided make it very difficult to apply the same sorts of criteria as might be applied in the choice of a restaurant or a hairdresser. For these reasons, it is necessary to devise ways of measuring satisfaction more directly. In conceptual terms there seem to be three basic problems in any attempt to measure satisfaction. What is satisfaction? What is the relationship between satisfaction values and expectations? What aspects of health care should be assessed in terms of satisfaction, i.e. what are the appropriate objects of satisfaction?

The dictionary offers a number of alternative definitions, the most appropriate of which seem to be 'fulfilment of desire or need' and 'ample provision for desire or need'. If the patient feels that his or her desires or needs have been met, this implies a good outcome. However, common usage of the term is more complex than this. It carries associations with the term 'satisfactory', meaning adequate or acceptable. Thus satisfaction may imply only the achievement of a basic minimum standard.

It is surprising how little attention has been paid in the research literature to developing a theoretical and conceptual model of satisfaction. This is in marked contrast to the extensive reporting of empirical findings which purport to measure satisfaction. One of the few attempts to address these issues is an excellent review paper on patient satisfaction in primary health care by Pascoe, which also tackles the problem of the relationship between expectations, values, and satisfaction.[2] Pascoe defines patient satisfaction as 'health care recipients' reaction to salient aspects of the context, process and result of their experience'. Experience is related to a subjective standard or set of values and expectations. This standard may be one, or a combination, of the following: a subjective ideal, a subjective sense of what one deserves, a subjective average of past experience in similar situations, or some minimally acceptable level. The relationship between the individual's subjective standard and declarations of satisfaction and dissatisfaction is complex. Pascoe suggests that there may be quite a wide latitude of acceptance around the subjective standard, so that most experiences of care would fall within these broad limits, thus eliciting a satisfied response. Exceptions would occur only if there was a gross discrepancy between experience and expectation, or where a negative standard existed, so that care which fell within the expected range was judged unsatisfactory.

Apart from the problem of developing a conceptual model which incorporates the relationship between expectations and satisfaction, it is also necessary to specify what are the objects of satisfaction/dissatisfaction which it is appropriate to measure. It is meaningless to know that patients are satisfied without knowing what they are satisfied with. Theoretically, the objects of satisfaction can be divided into those concerned with the actual provision of care and those concerned with the outcomes for the patient. In practice, virtually all research has concentrated on the former. Although different measures of patient satisfaction have identified a number of dimensions, the American literature suggests that there are only a small number of independent dimensions. Ware and Snyder suggest four dimensions: physician conduct, availability of care, continuity/convenience of care, and access mechanisms.[3] However, other analyses have suggested only two broad categories which account for a large part of the variance in scores on commonly used measures: provider conduct and accessibility/availability.

The concept of patient satisfaction can play an important role in health care evaluation, but it should not be seen as providing an easy alternative to measuring final outcomes. Without an adequate theoretical and conceptual foundation, measures are likely to generate results which are extremely difficult to interpret. In Britain in particular, too little attention has been devoted to developing an understanding of the meaning of patient satisfaction, its potential uses, and its limitations.

Conclusions

In this chapter we have done no more than skate over the fundamental theoretical and conceptual problems encountered in attempts to measure needs for, and outcomes of, health care. Some of the issues will be dealt with in more detail in later chapters where they are relevant to the discussion of particular types of measure.

The pragmatism of clinical practice discourages many health care professionals from grappling with seemingly abstract philosophical debates about the meaning of health, disease, disability, etc. One of the consequences of this is that many of the measures derived from experience in clinical practice make no reference to the concepts that they are trying to measure. They arise from, and are justified primarily in terms of, practical experience. But if such measures are to be useful to others, and the results capable of interpretation in the context of other available measures, more serious attention to concepts and theoretical foundations is essential. Without this it is difficult to assess the validity of one measure as compared with others. It is rather like possessing a thermometer and knowing that it is intended to identify patients with fever, but not knowing that what it actually measures is temperature.

In addition to the need to specify the concepts measured it is also important to work towards common understandings of these. As we noted earlier, research into the consequences of disease has been bedevilled by confusion over terminology and this inevitably places barriers in the way of effective communication.

References

1. Boorse, C. (1977). Health as a theoretical concept. *Philosophy of Science*, **44**, 542–73.
2. Pascoe, G. C. (1983). Patient satisfaction in primary health care. *Evaluation and Program Planning*, **6**, 185–210.
3. Ware, J. E. and Snyder, M. K. (1975). Dimensions of patient attitudes regarding doctors and medical care services. *Medical Care*, **13**, 669–82.
4. World Health Organization (1980). *International classification of impairments, disabilities and handicaps.* World Health Organization, Geneva.

3 Methods of measurement

Introduction

In making a choice of measure it is essential to have an understanding of the principles of measurement and thus to know what to look for in terms of the development and testing of an instrument. Measurement consists of the application of a set of rules for assigning values (usually numerical) to objects or events so as to represent quantities, qualities, or categories of attributes. The fact that rules are explicit and unambiguous implies an ability to standardize, so that the same results will be obtained by different people using the same instrument. Moreover, it is clearly essential that the instrument should actually measure what it is intended to measure. Whilst these conditions may be unproblematic for many everyday measurements in the physical world, this is far from being the case for events and objects in the social world. In this chapter we describe, briefly and as straightforwardly as possible, the different levels of measurement, the process of constructing measures in the field of health and illness, criteria for establishing reliability and validity, the problems of responsiveness, and the practical considerations that must be borne in mind when selecting a measure. First, however, it is necessary to devote some attention to the purposes for which measures will be required, since these will have an important bearing on what criteria should be applied in selecting appropriate tools for the job.

Purposes for which measures are required

The uses of health-related measures can be divided into three broad categories: discrimination, prediction, and evaluation.[11] There will often be more than one purpose in a particular study, but it will be helpful in making a selection to distinguish between different purposes.

Discrimination between individuals or groups on some underlying health-related dimension is commonly required, both as a means of describing differences in health experience and as a means of identifying areas of need. Thus, for example, if we want to know whether people in different social classes have different levels of health, we require a measure which is capable of detecting differences between groups. More practically, a policy of selective allocation of resources will require data collected using a discriminative index in order to be able to target those groups or areas where needs are greatest.

Measures are commonly employed in medicine as means of identifying groups or individuals who have or will develop some target condition or outcome. They are used to *predict future needs*. Prediction is the purpose of screening tests such as cervical smears or developmental tests for children. These measures are used to identify problems at an earlier stage than they would otherwise manifest themselves. Other predictive measures are used because they are less uncomfortable or less costly than alternatives. Thus, for example, simple functional assessments may be used as indicators of needs for services by elderly people in the community, because they are predictive of more detailed assessments by health and social care professionals, or of successful outcomes, such as continued independent living.

The attention of researchers, practitioners, and policy makers has increasingly turned to the use of measures for purpose of *evaluation* or monitoring. For these purposes a measure of the magnitude of longitudinal change in individuals or groups on the dimension of interest is required. Whether or not the measure discriminates between individuals or groups, or is able to predict future outcomes, is less important. Attention is focused on changes between point A and point B which are attributable to particular interventions, i.e. outcomes. This is the purpose of clinical trials and of more broadly based service evaluation. Survival rates and cure rates are classic measures of medical outcome for evaluative research, but many measures of health and quality of life are also intended for use as evaluative criteria.

Within these broad categories of purpose there will be a variety of sub-categories which will also have a bearing on measurement criteria. The most important of these are whether one is concerned with individuals or groups and the magnitude of the differences/outcomes that are the focus of interest. The clinician or practitioner will be primarily concerned with individuals and will thus require measures capable of detecting differences at this level. The researcher, on the other hand, will often require a lower level of precision, being interested in group differences. A less precise measure will be required to detect a real difference between two groups of 100 people than between two individuals. But the level of precision required will also be determined by the expected magnitude of differences. Thus, for example, to identify people who need walking aids may require a relatively low level of precision, simply distinguishing between those who have mobility problems and those who do not. But to assess the effectiveness of such aids may require a much more precise measure if the expected changes are relatively small.

Levels of measurement

There are four distinct levels of measurement; nominal, ordinal, interval, and ratio. The interpretations that can be placed on results and the ways in which they can be manipulated in analyses are dependent on the level of measurement achieved. It is essential, therefore, to choose an instrument which achieves a level of measurement which will permit the sorts of analyses required of it.

Nominal scales represent the lowest level of measurement. They consist of systematic identification and labelling of classes of objects or events. At one extreme, the classification male/female is a nominal scale for sex, at the other, the *International classification of diseases* (ICD) is a nominal scale for classifying all diagnoses and presenting problems. The fact that, for practical purposes, numbers may be attached to different values (e.g. 1 male, 2 female) does not imply any ordering or other relationship between values. There is no inherent logic in the ordering of values. Thus it would be equally valid to code females 1 and males 2 or to reverse the numeric codes employed in the ICD. Nominal scales can be used only to determine how often an event or attribute occurs.

Ordinal scales differ from nominal in that their descriptions of classes of objects or events are ordered along a continuum of some sort (e.g. least to most, worst to best). An ordinal scale does not permit the user to determine how far apart are points on the scale, simply to hierarchically rank each point. Perhaps the most common sort of ordinal scale in medicine is severe, moderate, mild as a means of classifying the severity of disease. We know that moderate is worse than mild and severe worst than moderate, but we do not know by how much. Neither do we know how far they are from absolute values at either end of the spectrum. Thus knowing that a person suffers from mild arthritis tells us nothing about how far away that person is from complete health at one end of the spectrum, or death at the other. Another example of an ordinal scale is the rating of patients' satisfaction with a service, from very satisfied to very dissatisfied. Scores on ordinal scales cannot be added or subtracted. It is therefore not appropriate to apply even basic statistics such as means or standard deviations, unless scaling techniques have been used to convert them to higher-order scales. It would be meaningless to rate arthritic patients on a one to three scale (mild to severe) and calculate an average for a group of patients.

Interval scales not only provide a rank ordering, but also specify the distance between points on the scale. They do not, however, provide an absolute zero point. Temperature measured in Fahrenheit or Celcius is a good example of an interval scale. It is possible to add or subtract values and thus calculate basic statistics, such as the average daytime temperature in Manchester, but the absence of an absolute zero means that scores on an interval scale cannot be multiplied or divided. Thus it is incorrect to say that a temperature of 60 degrees is twice as hot as a temperature of 30 degrees. Many measures of health-related variables claim to achieve interval level measurement, but such claims are often open to question.

The highest level of measurement is the *ratio scale* which, in addition to meeting all the criteria for an interval scale, also has an absolute zero point or defined point of origin. This permits values to be multiplied or divided.

Time and distance measures are examples of ratio scales. Not only is it possible to calculate the mean age of a group, it is also legitimate to say that a person of 60 years is twice as old as someone of 30 years.

Recognition of the differences between levels of measurement is important because of their respective limitations. The level of measurement achieved will determine the appropriate level of analysis. It is, unfortunately, all too common to see results obtained using ordinal or even nominal levels of measurement subjected to wholly inappropriate statistical analyses.

Constructing measures and scaling

To understand the strengths and limitations of a measure, including the level of measurement achieved, it helps to know how it was constructed. It is beyond the scope of this book to provide a detailed account of methods of constructing scales, but the potential user should be aware of the basic steps in the development of measures and alternative approaches to scaling. All of the measures included in subsequent chapters consist of a number of questions or items, responses to which are scored and may be aggregated in some way to form either a single index or a number of values representing different dimensions. It is important that the intending user should have at least a basic understanding of the terms commonly used in the development and testing of instruments and the methods of scaling used.

Single-item versus multi-item measures

The simplest measures employ a single item to measure a particular concept. This may be as broad as, 'How would you describe your health at present?', or as narrow as 'How far are you able to walk without assistance?'. However, most of the instruments included in later chapters are multi-item measures. They use a number of questions or statements, and responses are combined in some way to produce a score. Thus, for example, mobility might be covered by five items: walking, running, transfer from bed or chair, climbing stairs, using public transport.

Response categories

Whether a single item is used or a number of items, appropriate response categories will have to be provided. There are only four basic types of response category. Firstly, questions can be phrased to produce simple yes/no responses. Secondly, a number of descriptions can be placed in rank order (e.g. unable to walk, walks less than 50 yards, walks more than 50 yards). Thirdly, responses to statements can be classified as a number of points on a single dimension (e.g. strongly agree, agree, neutral, disagree, strongly disagree). This type of response category used in Likert scaling (see below) is closely related to the fourth method, the visual analogue. Here the respondent is presented with a line anchored at both ends and asked to place a mark anywhere on the line (e.g. very sad———————very happy).

Indices versus profiles

The purpose of multi-item measures is to combine the items in some way in order to create a score or scores. In some cases all items relate to a single dimension and are therefore combined to produce a single score (e.g. depression). Where a number of different dimensions are covered (e.g. mobility, household tasks, pain, emotional state), these can either be presented as separate scores (profile) or combined to produce an aggregated score (index). The index is an attempt to create a truly multidimensional measure. Some indices are constructed so that scores can either be presented as profiles or as an overall score.

Scaling techniques

A wide variety of scaling techniques have been used to construct measures of health status and patient satisfaction. It is impossible here to provide a detailed description and discussion of the various approaches, but it will be helpful for the potential user of measures to have a basic understanding of the commonly used techniques. Table 3.1 provides a brief summary of these. Some, such as rank ordering and category rating, are closely related to each other, and might more properly be considered subdivisions of the same general approach. The choice of scaling technique will depend on various considerations, such as whether the measure is unidimensional or multi-dimensional, the intended uses, the level of measurement required, theoretical considerations, and practical constraints in both development and use of the measure. It should be remembered that the method of scaling used will have been determined by the criteria applied by the original authors, which may not be the same as those of another researcher or practitioner seeking an 'off the peg' instrument.

It will be apparent from the descriptions of the instruments in later chapters that scaling techniques are employed with varying degrees of rigour. In some cases development and testing bear only a passing resemblance to systematic scaling techniques, and in others the researchers have used a more rigorous psychometric approach to scaling.

Item generation

The initial step with all measures based on self-report or descriptions of health states is to generate the questions, statements, or descriptions to be

Table 3.1   Scaling techniques

Rank ordering

One of the simplest techniques for deriving an ordinal scale is to ask a panel of judges to rank items or states in an appropriate order (e.g. severity, importance, desirability, etc.). Thus, for example, five descriptions of different sorts of pain could be ranked 1 to 5 in order of severity. However, such an approach is only possible with a small number of items, and, by forcing judges to rank each item, does not permit ties where two or more items might be considered of equal severity. Also, because the resulting scale is only ordinal, there is no way of establishing the relationship between points on the scale.

Guttman scaling

Guttman-type scales are also rank-ordered ordinal scales, and have been particularly useful in the field of disability. Scale items may be designed by the author or derived from analysis of a larger number of items. The key features of the resulting scale are that it should tap a single dimension and that the items should be cumulative. Thus in the following example of a simple Guttman scale each item builds on the previous item(s): (1) able to walk 10 metres; (2) able to walk 100 metres; (3) able to walk 1 kilometre. One of the standard tests for a Guttman scale is the extent to which responses are consistent. An inconsistent set of responses to the above example would be 1 Yes, 2 No, 3 Yes. In practice Guttman scales are neither as simple nor as consistent as this example. One of the problems faced by the user is how to deal with inconsistent (non-scale) responses, which may account for up to a quarter of all respondents.

Likert scaling

One of the most popular psychometric rating techniques is the Likert scale. All items in the pool are given the same graded responses (e.g. strongly agree to strongly disagree, very important to not important, frequently to never), usually on a five-point scale. They are then administered to a population and the responses analysed for internal consistency. Items which correlate well with total scores (high, low, average, etc.) are retained and those which are inconsistent are discarded. Likert scales are suitable for measuring a single dimension, but there is no provision for differential weighting of items.

Category rating/equal appearing intervals

These are both direct methods of scaling in that panels of judges are asked to rate each of the proposed items. Judges are asked either to sort statements into categories or to place them on a scale of equal-appearing intervals. Thus, for example, judges may be given a series of descriptions of symptoms and asked to sort them into eleven categories according to degree of severity. Items on which there is little agreement are rejected. Remaining items are weighted according to the median category for that item. Thus if twenty judges rated an item as follows: three placed it in category 7, four in category 8, eight in category 9, three in category 10, two in category 11; the median category for weighting that item would be category 9. Items are selected from the remaining pool to represent the full range of categories. The method produces an interval level scale for a single dimension.

Table 3.1 *cont'd.*

Paired comparisons

Each item from a pool is paired with every other item in the pool and judges are asked to decide which of each pair is more severe, more important, preferable, etc. It is rather cumbersome, so that 20 items will produce 190 possible pairs. Item weights are based on the proportions of judges selecting each item in relation to all other items. The method can be used to discard items on which there is little agreement between judges but it is too cumbersome to deal with a large number of items.

Utility estimation

Economic evaluations have employed a variety of methods designed to construct interval scales based on the concept of utility. In this context utility refers to desirability or preference rather than usefulness. Scales constructed in this way have tended to start from descriptions of health states rather than components of health. Judges are asked to make a series of paired comparisons of different states and to express preferences. Three techniques have been used: standard gamble, time tradeoff, and equivalence. In the standard gamble, judges are offered a choice between alternative states of health with different outcomes. Probabilities are attached to the different outcomes and varied until the judge is indifferent between the alternatives. In the time tradeoff method judges choose between a defined health state for a defined period of time followed by death and remaining well for a shorter period of time and then dying. The time period in the second alternative is adjusted until the judge becomes indifferent. Lastly, the equivalence method aims to identify the judge's point of indifference between keeping alive a group of people in perfect health and keeping alive a larger group of less well people. All three methods are complicated and difficult for judges to understand. However, they have a sound theoretical foundation and any health state can be evaluated in this way and weighted relative to all other states.

Magnitude estimation

Attempts to construct a ratio scale of health states have used the technique of magnitude estimation. Judges are asked to directly scale the magnitude of differences between health states. One or both ends of the scale are defined and judges asked to place alternative states relative to this/these points. For example, one day spent in perfect health might be given a value of 1000 and all other states are then rated between 0 and 1000. Although less complicated than utility estimation, this method has less theoretical foundation. It also requires very careful application if the ratings given by judges are to be valid.

---

included in the instrument. Methods of doing this can be broadly divided into those which rely on professional judgements and those which draw directly or indirectly on the experiences of the people for whom the measure is intended, although in many instances there are elements of both. It is surprising how many measures seem, at least in the first instance, to have been constructed solely on the basis of the authors' own experience. Somewhat more sophisticated are those which generate statements from a panel of professional judges or from the professional literature. In some instances this will be the most appropriate method, but where the purpose is to measure subjective experience of needs or outcomes, the most appropriate technique will be to ask intended respondents what problems they have experienced, how they rate these in terms of importance or severity, and what they feel are important criteria of need or outcome. This can be done through semi-structured interviews or group discussions, or, more economically, by reviewing other studies which have reported the perceptions of target populations.

Selection of judges

Many scaling methods require the use of judges both to select items and to allocate weights or values to items or states. Since the judgements of these individuals are fundamental to the validity of the scale, it is essential that they are chosen carefully, and that they are adequately described by the authors. Non-professional judges should be drawn from the population on whom the measure will be used. Other users should note that procedures for standardization and weighting derived from one group of judges may not be applicable in a different context (for example, weights derived from American judges may not apply in Britain). Also it should be noted that more sophisticated measurement procedures impose more complex tasks on the judges. It seems unlikely, for example, that utility estimation techniques such as the standard gamble could be applied in a general population sample.

Item reduction

With scales derived from a large pool of items, generated by potential respondents or from existing literature, it will be necessary to reduce the number of items to manageable proportions. The standard scaling techniques described in Table 3.1 are accompanied by standard techniques for item reduction based on consistency and representativeness. Thus, for example, in the analysis of initial versions of a Likert-type scale, those items which produce inconsistent responses are excluded. Statistical techniques are often employed to achieve item reduction. Procedures designed to measure internal consistency (see section on reliability) can be used to maximize the precision of the instrument to measure a given construct and to reduce the number of items to a minimum. Such procedures are entirely appropriate for a measure designed to discriminate between groups. However, where a measure is required for evaluative purposes the criteria for item reduction may be different. Measures of internal consistency focus on consistency between respondents at a point in time, but the evaluator is interested in consistency within individuals over a period of time. Also, for evaluative research it may be less important to minimize the number of items and more important to ensure that any item which may show a difference is retained.

Weighting

Techniques for attributing weights to individual items in order to construct a total score are provided within each of the scaling methods. The purpose of differentially weighting items is to permit the inclusion of items at different levels of severity without distorting the overall scale score. Weights will be based on the importance attached to items by the judges, whatever the particular method of scaling used. It should be remembered that a different group of judges might produce different weights.

Variability of scores

A good instrument will produce scores which are spread across the full range and which are distributed 'normally' (i.e. a bell-shaped distribution). One of the most common problems in measures of health status is that scores tend to be skewed to one end of the scale. This is because most instruments focus on dysfunction, so that all subjects who do not experience dysfunction will score zero or the maximum, depending on the direction of scoring. Such skewed distributions of scores are problematic for two reasons. Firstly, many statistical techniques are based on the assumption that scores are normally distributed, and are therefore not appropriate. Secondly, they do not permit the measurement of improvement in subjects who have already achieved the scale maximum or minimum.

Even where scores are normally distributed there may still be problems. If the distribution is so heavily concentrated around the mean that the ends of the spectrum are virtually unused, this suggests that many of the scale items are redundant. Lastly, it should be remembered that the distribution of scores will depend on the population of interest. Thus, although measures of activities of daily living might produce normally distributed scores in hospital populations, they may produce highly skewed distributions when applied to people living independently in the community.

Reliability

One of the objectives of any measurement should be to reduce to a minimum both random and non-random error. All measurement includes some degree of random error (i.e. it follows no systematic pattern). The more reliable a measure is, the lower the element of random error. Non-random error or bias is assessed by testing validity, which is dealt with in the following section.

The reliability of a measure is the extent to which it yields the same results in repeated applications on an unchanged population or phenomenon. A speedometer which one day gives a reading of 70 m.p.h., the next day 60 m.p.h. and the third day 80 m.p.h., although on all three occasions the car was travelling at 70 m.p.h., is clearly unreliable, and therefore likely to expose the driver to the risk of a fine for speeding. The reliability of clinical, social, and psychological instruments is less easily established, but equally or even more important. Three types of reliability are generally considered important in the assessment of instruments. Firstly, consistency over time is assessed using repeated applications of the instrument (test–retest reliability). Secondly, consistency between different users of the instrument may need to be established (inter-rater reliability). Thirdly, the internal consistency of items within the instrument can be assessed (i.e. to what extent do all of the items measure the same dimension?)

Test–retest reliability is assessed by applying the measure to the same population at different points in time under the same conditions. The correlation between the two sets of results is used as an estimation of the reliability of the measure. However, there are important difficulties in this approach. Firstly, there may have been real changes in the population between the two test administrations. The importance of this problem depends on the length of time which elapses between test administrations and the stability of the variable being measured. Secondly, there is a danger that subjects either undergo a learning process or remember the responses they gave at the first administration. Thus, for example, if a group of children are given the same spelling test at two-week intervals, correlations between the results on different occasions are likely to be influenced by a learning process. One might expect the results to have improved. It is possible to overcome this problem by using statistical techniques, but this can have the effect of causing one to reject an instrument which shows little between-subject variation but is sensitive to changes within subjects over time.[8] In other words, the changes observed in the assessment of test–retest reliability are real changes which reflect the responsiveness of the measure rather than random errors.

Consistency between different observers or users of an instrument, *inter-rater reliability*, is important for any measure which requires judgements or observations to be made by the person administering the measure. This is ideally measured by different raters interviewing the same respondents with a very short gap between interviews. However, it is usually impractical to fulfil these conditions, so a less satisfactory alternative of using tape-recorded interviews with different raters is commonly adopted. In either case, careful attention should be given to the conditions under which inter-rater reliability is assessed. The fact that high reliability has been achieved using a small number of highly trained interviewers working as part of a team should not be taken to imply that a similar degree of consistency will be achieved by a larger group of untrained interviewers working in isolation. The most appropriate measure of inter-rater reliability is the Kappa coefficient of agreement.[4] Simple correlation analysis makes no allowance for chance agreement. In contrast, Kappa takes chance agreement into consideration and produces a coefficient between -1 and $+1$, negative values indicating levels of agreement worse than chance.

In addition to reliability tests based on repeated administration, there are statistical tests of *internal consistency*, which can be carried out on a single data set. These tests assess the extent to which individual items are correlated with each other and with overall scale scores. They thus provide an estimate of homogeneity. The split-half method divides the items in the schedule randomly into two halves and correlates the results achieved. More sophisticated measures of internal consistency such as Cronbach's alpha and Kuder and Richardson's formulae[3] are based on the average correlation between items included in the instrument. The internal consistency is only relevant to measures containing items related to a single dimension. Multidimensional measures would not be expected to have high internal consistency, although it would be possible to assess the internal consistency of individual dimensions of a health profile.

It is safe to assume that all measurement suffers from some random error, but that measurements in the psychosocial and health fields are more prone to this than measurements in the physical world. The important question is what level of random error we should treat as acceptable. This will depend to a considerable extent on the use of the measure. If we are concerned to take life-threatening decisions with respect to individuals, we might be prepared to accept only a tiny element of random error in an instrument. However, in situations where the concern is to monitor progress or to make comparisons between groups the accepted standard may be much lower. For coefficients ranging between zero and one, the commonly accepted reliability standard is 0.5,[10] since random error will tend to average out in large samples. This should not, however, induce a sense of complacency. In most circumstances samples will not be large and considerably higher levels of reliability are desirable.

Whatever the evidence of reliability presented by the proponents of a particular instrument, the potential user should bear in mind that there can be no universal test of reliability. At best, the conscientious researcher will have demonstrated reliability under a set of specified circumstances. It is unlikely that the potential user's circumstances will match these. It may therefore be necessary to re-establish the reliability of the measure for particular conditions of use.

Validity

The validity of an instrument relates to the effects of non-random or systematic error. Reliability is a necessary but not sufficient condition for a useful measure. A speedometer may be, as near as possible, perfectly reliable if it always shows 70 m.p.h. when the true speed is 80 m.p.h., but, as the driver will find to his or her cost, it is not a valid indicator of the number of miles travelled per hour. An instrument is valid to the extent that it measures what it purports to measure. But like reliability, validity is not determined in the abstract. A measure may be valid for the specific purpose for which it was developed, but it will not necessarily be valid for a related but not equivalent purpose. The potential user of a measure should examine evidence of validity in the context of the practical use to which it is intended to put the measure. There are three basic types of validity: content, criterion, and construct. Table 3.2 offers basic definitions in terms of the questions asked.

Table 3.2 Types of validity

Content validity	Is the choice of, and relative importance given to, each component of the index appropriate for the domains they are supposed to measure?
Criterion validity	Does the measure produce results which correspond with those obtained using a superior measure simultaneously (concurrent) or which forecast a future criterion value (predictive)?
Construct validity	Do the results obtained confirm the expected pattern of relationships or hypotheses derived from the theoretical constructs on which the measure is based?

Content validity

There are no standard procedures appropriate to the demonstration of content validity. It is necessary to specify the domain of content relevant to the measure and the relative importance of each of the components within that domain, and to show that the items cover all components in a representative fashion. Thus, for example, the content validity of spelling tests for 12-year-olds can be demonstrated by reference to the total universe of words they should be able to spell, subdivided according to length of words or type (e.g. adjectives, nouns). However, the demonstration of content validity for measures dealing with health and illness is more difficult. There is unlikely to be universal agreement on the domain of content relevant, and it is impossible to sample content in the same way as for a spelling test. Therefore, the demonstration of content validity tends to rest mainly on an appeal to reason regarding the adequacy with which the domain has been defined and sampled. Content validity may be claimed on the grounds that a large number of representative judges were used to generate and select items, and the resulting measure includes all commonly mentioned items. It may also be demonstrated by reference to existing literature on the subject, showing that the new instrument covers all of the topics which have previously been regarded as important. Content validity is sometimes confused with face validity, which seems to carry little meaning other than that the selection of items should appear sensible to an intelligent audience. This seems to be a less stringent criterion.

Criterion validity

By definition, if a measure is to be validated against a criterion this should be demonstrably superior to the measure, i.e. a 'gold standard'. Thus, for example, one might assess the validity of a speedometer against a stopwatch over a measured distance. If a criterion exists, the only justification for developing a new measure must be that it is more practicable, more economical, or produces a result sooner than would otherwise be possible. Concurrent tests of criterion validity require that the measure under test be administered at the same time as the criterion. Thus, a functional test intended to identify potential for rehabilitation might be tested against a full multi-professional clinical assessment procedure. However, even such a comprehensive assessment might not constitute a true 'gold standard'. For this reason such tests of validity are sometimes referred to as 'criterion related' validity. In other instances the criterion will be a future outcome (e.g. death, development of disease, restoration to independent living). Demonstration of the ability of an instrument to accurately predict such outcomes will constitute the main test of validity for measures designed with the specific purpose of predicting behaviour or events external to the measure itself. In the case of general purpose measures predictive validity will constitute only one element in the process of validation.

Construct validity

Where there is no true or quasi 'gold standard' against which to validate an instrument, the researcher becomes involved in collecting empirical evidence to support the inference that a particular measure has meaning. This may involve comparisons with related measures and/or predictions about the distribution of scores among different groups of respondents. A measure of physical health may be tested against a measure of activities of daily living, with the prediction that there should be a positive correlation, but not a one to one correspondence. If this is demonstrated to be the case it would be evidence of convergent validity. To the extent that it can be demonstrated that the measure does not correlate with variables to which it should not be related, this is evidence of discriminant validity. Thus, for example, a measure of function should not be highly correlated with a measure of depression.

One of the most common approaches to the assessment of construct validity is to apply the instrument to groups known to differ in terms of the concept being measured. Thus patients suffering from a chronic illness might be compared with a general population sample, or young adults compared with elderly people. It should be noted that the choice of groups for comparison is very important. The ability of a measure to distinguish between patients suffering from arthritis at different levels of severity is a far more stringent criterion than its ability to distinguish between patients with arthritis and people with no chronic illness.

Lastly, construct validity is sometimes assessed using a multi-trait, multi-method approach.[2] In this approach, the correlation between alternative methods of measuring the same variable (e.g. self-report and observation) is compared with the correlation between measures using the same method to measure different variables.

The demonstration of validity using any or all of the methods outlined here is not a 'once and for all' exercise. It should be seen as an ongoing exercise similar to the accumulation of evidence to support a scientific theory. No single piece of evidence is sufficient in itself, but is a contribution to a cumulative process. All serious measures should be able to advance some evidence of validity, but the available evidence may not be appropriate to the particular purpose the user has in mind. It may therefore be necessary to consider further tests of validity appropriate to the purpose and context of any particular application.

Response bias

One form of systematic error common in self-report measures is response bias. There are two commonly recognized forms; acquiescent response sets and socially desirable response sets. The tendency of some respondents to agree with any statement regardless of content is known as acquiescent response. It can be reduced by keeping questions or statements short, by using several questions to measure each concept, and by alternating the wording of different items (e.g. I feel tense/I feel relaxed). The second category of response bias concerns the tendency for respondents to be unwilling to report feelings or behaviour which they perceive as socially undesirable. This problem tends to be reduced in self-completion measures as opposed to face to face interviews and can be further minimized by writing questions or statements in such a way as to make it easy to give an 'undesirable' response.

Responsiveness

In a series of papers concerning the usefulness of health status and quality of life measures as evaluative instruments Guyatt and his colleagues[8,9,11] and Deyo[5-7] have drawn attention to the failure of existing measures to identify small but clinically significant changes. They have argued that the criteria for selecting a measure for evaluative purposes should include its sensitivity to change. We have chosen to use the term responsiveness rather than sensitivity to avoid confusion with the more common clinical use of the term sensitivity, where it refers to the ability of a measure to detect a high proportion of true cases. Our concern here is with the ability of a measure to detect small changes. Responsiveness is closely related to validity, and some authors include it under the heading of discriminant validity. However, responsiveness is not essential to validity, rather it is a characteristic of the measure and is thus perhaps better dealt with separately.

Although responsiveness to clinically significant change in individuals over time is likely to be a major consideration in any study concerned to evaluate the impact of treatment, it tends not to be routinely included in the development of measures. Because the development of many measures of health and health-related variables has emphasized validity and reliability rather than responsiveness, there is often inadequate information about how useful such measures would be in evaluative research. Indeed the usually preferred methods of establishing validity and reliability tend to militate against responsiveness. They tend to focus on the ability to discriminate between individuals or groups, correlation with other measures, and internal consistency. Measures which are good at discriminating will tend to have very limited response categories (e.g. yes/no) so as to minimize the problem of respondents placing different interpretations on response categories. They will tend to exclude items that only apply to small numbers of respondents, and they will keep the number of items to a minimum in order to maximize internal consistency. In contrast, a measure which is responsive to small changes over time in the same individuals may require a more refined grading of responses to items and the inclusion of any item which might show change. Such a measure may be poor at discriminating between groups, it may exclude items which are good discriminators but not amenable to change, and it may include others which only affect a few respondents or are treated inconsistently. Nevertheless, it may be perfectly valid as a measure of change in individuals.

In the reviews of instruments which follow in later chapters, we have been forced to remark far too often that there is an absence of evidence concerning responsiveness to change. This partly reflects the purposes for which measures were originally developed and partly a lack of sophistication in our methods for evaluating responsiveness. However, techniques are now being developed and we might expect to see considerably better evidence of responsiveness over the next few years.

Administration and practical issues

Whilst scientific criteria are vitally important in the selection of an appropriate measure, they cannot and should not be applied to the exclusion of more practical considerations. The choice of the best measure for a particular job will often be a compromise between scientific rigour and practical constraints. The user needs to consider the practical problems of administering the measure, both from his or her own point of view, from the point of view of the respondents, and in relation to problems of analysing and using the data once they have been collected.

Perhaps the most important decision in terms of the administration of the measure is whether it is to be self-administered by respondents or administered by an interviewer. Clearly there are considerable time savings in the former if the researcher/practitioner's presence is not required. The measures can be distributed by post or given to respondents in the course of other activities (e.g. consultation, clinic attendance). In contrast, the interviewer administered measure by definition requires a clinician, researcher, or qualified interviewer to be present. For research purposes, the constraints of time and resources will inevitably mean that it is possible to obtain a far smaller number of responses than would be the case with a postal questionnaire. It is likely also that the study would have to be restricted to a small geographical area. For the practitioner, normal service routines including consultations may be disrupted. Against these considerations there are undoubted advantages to using interviewer-administered measures. Firstly, although the total number of respondents will be smaller than if a self-administered measure were used, the response rate (the proportion of those approached who actually respond) will be higher. Secondly, it will be possible to collect more information from each respondent, perhaps using a variety of measures and some open-ended questions. Thirdly, it is possible in a face-to-face interview to deal with more complex sensitive issues which would be difficult or impossible to raise through the impersonal medium of a postal questionnaire. The choice between self-administered or interviewer-administered measures will depend on the particular purposes for which the measure is required and the circumstances in which it is to be administered.

Related to the problem of the type of administration is the issue of proxy responses. If the user is concerned with severely ill or infirm people, there will be instances in which the patient/respondent is unable to complete the measure or unwilling to be interviewed. Rather than treating such cases as non-responses, the user may wish to complete the measures using information from a third party (e.g. spouse, other relative, nurse, residential care worker, etc.). Indeed it is not uncommon, even where the respondent is able to answer the questions, to find that a relative or friend 'helps' with the answers. Some measures are intended to be completed by a third party and thus present no problem, but most are intended to be completed by the respondent. Evidence concerning their reliability and validity will be based on them being applied in this way. Thus, if third-party responses are to be used they should be clearly identified for analysis. If this is likely to be a common problem, it may be worth mounting a study to test the use of the measure in this way.

Whatever the measure chosen and the method of administration, it is essential to calculate carefully the resources required for administration. For research purposes, these will include the time taken to draw a sample, negotiating access with appropriate authorities, printing and stationery costs, postage, travelling time, and costs of following up non-respondents. Even the most experienced researchers tend to underestimate how much time and effort is necessary to the successful administration of a survey questionnaire. It is always advisable to carry out a small pre-test which will enable the user to calculate exactly how much time has to be allocated for each task. In calculating the resources required, the researcher should not forget the demands being made on respondents and others. Respondents will be asked to devote some of their time and energy to helping the researcher, usually free of charge. Is it reasonable to expect them to give up their time, particularly if they are feeling unwell? If the demands made on respondents are unreasonable, it is likely that a substantial proportion will refuse to complete the measure. Thus, for example, asking patients to complete a lengthy schedule immediately after a visit to the doctor is unlikely to generate a high response rate.

For the clinician, the calculation of costs and the impact on normal routine is at least as important as it is for the researcher. There will be little point in using an instrument which disrupts the clinical routine and irritates patients and office staff. However, the costs should not be over emphasized. Many measures take no longer than ten minutes to complete and there is evidence that patients appreciate being given the opportunity to describe their problems in a different way from the normal clinical interview. Nevertheless, the inclusion of an additional step in the consultation process must involve some costs. It is therefore desirable to undertake some sort of pre-test and to examine the perceived usefulness of assessments to both clinicians and patients.

One of the most commonly ignored issues, in both research and clinical applications, is how the data will be processed and analysed. The golden rule should be to avoid collecting data which will not be used, either because of the amount of material collected or the complexity of analysis required. In selecting a measure(s), the user should carefully consider how the information is to be processed and how it will be used. The needs of the researcher and the clinician will clearly differ. The researcher will usually be able to enter data into a computer for statistical analysis, but even very basic data entry can be extremely time consuming for a large-scale study. Although most of the measures reviewed in later chapters provide for relatively straightforward analysis, it is likely that they will form only part of a larger battery of questions and tests. In these circumstances the researcher should have a clear idea at the outset of how the information can be used so that any redundant items can be excluded at this stage.

The clinician's concern will be primarily with the individual patient. If the information collected is to be of value it must be easily and quickly interpreted, so that it can be immediately incorporated into the clinical process. It will also be important to consider how the information should be stored for future use, both in terms of monitoring individual patients and in terms of research or audit of clinical practice.

Selection and presentation of instruments

In the following seven chapters we have reviewed 40 instruments which measure aspects of health status, quality of life and patient satisfaction. In selecting instruments for inclusion we have had in mind the needs of the researcher, practitioner, and manager concerned with the provision of primary health care services. However, it will be apparent to the reader that many of these were not developed specifically for use in primary health care. Indeed, some have never been used in this setting. Nevertheless, we consider that all 40 measures have potential applications in research or clinical practice in primary health care.

It is in the nature of a selective review such as this one, that there are many instruments which we have chosen to leave out that might be felt by others to warrant a place. We have made our judgements on the basis of both methodological criteria and how widely the instruments have been used by other researchers, as well as their applicability to primary health care. We have also tried in each chapter to offer a range of different approaches which will suit different circumstances. Perhaps the most important omissions are instruments which are currently in use but which have not yet been published. The technology of measurement in health services and clinical research is rapidly developing, but we decided that it was essential that our readers should have access to published source material for all of the measures included. We would recommend, however, that before adopting a particular instrument readers should consult recent literature and perhaps contact the designers of the measure so as to take account of more recent developments.

The headings under which we have reviewed each of the measures (Table 3.3) broadly correspond to the issues dealt with in this chapter. The objectives and intended purposes are described, with comments on the extent to which it has been used in ways not envisaged by the original authors. The background and development are described. The method of scoring and scaling is summarized, and available evidence on reliability and validity reviewed. Our appraisal of reliability and validity does not include reporting of

Table 3.3   Standard format for the presentation of measures

Purpose	Brief statement of the purpose and intended uses of the measure.
Background	Description of the conceptual basis and history of development and use.
Description	Description of the content of the instrument, alternative versions, sub-scales and response categories. Includes illustration of whole or part of the instrument, method of scoring individual items, and constructing overall scores.
Administration and acceptability	How the instrument is administered (e.g. self, trained interviewer, doctor). Time taken to complete questions and costs of administration. Is the instrument acceptable to respondents in terms of content, length, and ease of understanding?
Reliability and validity	A brief summary of the extent and nature of testing for reliability and validity. For detailed evidence of reliability and validity, the reader should consult the original paper.
Populations/service settings	Groups for which the scale was originally developed and subsequent use with other client groups (e.g. healthy, sick, specific disease groups, adults, elderly). Use in different service settings (e.g. hospital, general practice, community nursing).
Comments	General comments on the value of the measure as compared with alternatives and its application in primary health care.

coefficients, since we believe that these can be misleading when taken out of context. We also comment on the ease or difficulty of administering the measure, and the populations and service settings for which it is appropriate. Such brief reviews clearly cannot provide sufficient detail on which to make a final decision. Each entry therefore includes a list of key references which can be followed up for more detailed information. We consider it essential that the intending user should do this before making a final decision on a measure.

Conclusions

The intending user of measures of needs or outcomes in the field of health care does not need to become an expert in the various aspects of research methodology discussed in this chapter. However, the user does require a knowledge of the basic principles involved in the design and testing of measures, in order to be able to make an informed choice and in order to use the chosen measure appropriately. None of the measures we have reviewed will perform well against all of the criteria discussed in this chapter. They all have strengths and weaknesses which make them more or less suitable for particular purposes. In making a selection the intending user should be aware of these strengths and weaknesses. This requires at least a basic understanding of the principles of psychometric techniques. What we have presented here is no more than this. For the reader who would like to obtain a better grasp of these there are some excellent general texts which deal with the issues in greater depth.[1,12,13,15] In addition, Anita Stewart in her introductory chapter to the WONCA volume on *Functional status measurement in primary care* provides a more focused discussion.[14] For anyone considering modification of an existing instrument or the development of a new one we consider these or similar texts essential reading.

References

1. Bergner, M. and Rothman, M. L. (1987). Health status measures: an overview and guide for selection. *American Review of Public Health*, **8**, 191–210.
2. Cambell, D. T. and Fiske, D. W. (1959). Convergent and discriminant validation by the multitrait–multimethod matrix. *Psychological Bulletin*, **56**, 81–105.
3. Carmines, E. G. and Zeller, R. A. (1979). *Reliability and validity assessment*. Sage University Paper Series on Quantitative Applications in the Social Sciences, No. 07–017. Sage, Beverley Hills.
4. Cohen, J. (1968). Weighted Kappa: nominal scale agreement with provision for scaled disagreement or partial credit. *Psychological Bulletin*, **70**, 213–58.
5. Deyo, R. A. (1984). Measuring functional outcomes in therapeutic trials for chronic disease. *Controlled Clinical Trials*, **5**, 223–40.
6. Deyo, R. A. and Centor, R. M. (1986). Assessing the responsiveness of functional scales to clinical changes: an analogy to diagnostic test performance. *Journal of Chronic Disease*, **39**, 897–906.
7. Deyo, R. A. and Inu, T. S. (1984). Toward clinical applications of health status measures: sensitivity of scales to clinically important changes. *Health Services Research*, **19**, 787–805.
8. Guyatt, G., Walters, S., and Norman, G. (1985). Measuring change over time: assessing the usefulness of evaluative instruments. *Journal of Chronic Disease*, **40**, 171–8.
9. Guyatt, G., Bombardier, C., and Tugwell, P. (1986). Measuring disease specific

quality of life in clinical trials. *Canadian Medical Association Journal*, **134**, 889–95.

10. Helmstadter, G. C. (1964). *Principles of psychological measurement*. Appleton Century Crofts, New York.

11. Kirshner, B. and Guyatt, G. (1985). A methodological framework for assessing health indices. *Journal of Chronic Disease*, **38**, 27–36.

12. McDowell, T. Y. and Newell, C. (1987). *Measuring health: a guide to rating scales and questionnaires*. Oxford University Press, New York.

13. Nunnally, J. C. (1978). *Psychometric theory*, (2nd edn). McGraw Hill, New York.

14. Stewart, A. L. (1990). Psychometric considerations in functional status instruments. In *Functional status measurement in primary care* p. 3–26 (WONCA Classification Committee). Springer, New York.

15. Streiner, D. L. and Norman, G. R. (1989). *Health measurement scales: a practical guide to their development and use*. Oxford University Press, New York.

4 Measures of functioning

Introduction

The measures included in this chapter all deal with disablement and handicap. They all have common roots in the concept of activities of daily living (ADL) and most have been developed with the purpose of describing the impact of chronic illness on the lives of sufferers. As modern medicine has gradually had to come to grips with the problems presented by chronic disabling illness, emphasis in recording and classifying problems and in evaluating the impact of care has shifted from a predominant concern with impairment and diagnosis to a concern to establish the impact of illness in terms of the restrictions it places on the ability of individuals to lead normal lives. It might be argued that this has always been the legitimate focus of primary health care, but the development of systematic ways of measuring it has had to wait upon the growth of specialist rehabilitation medicine in areas such as geriatric medicine, rheumatology, and cardiology. Since the 1950s there has been a proliferation of instruments designed to summarize the nature and extent of restrictions on ADL. Many such measures have simply evolved out of clinical practice, paying scant attention to conceptual foundations or to the host of measures already in existence. Initially they tended to focus on a range of basic activities of daily living (mobility, dressing, toileting, etc.) reflecting a concern with the sort of severe disablement commonly found among institutionalized patients. During the 1970s, with the increased emphasis on people living in the community and on restoration to normal social roles, a new generation of more broadly based measures began to appear. These measures included instrumental activities of daily living (laundry, housework, managing money, employment, etc.). They thus extended the disability theme of ADL scales to include elements of handicap. In selecting and organizing measures for presentation in this chapter, our concern has been firstly with their relevance to the sorts of problems encountered in primary health care, secondly with the evidence of validity and reliability, and thirdly with the extent to which they have been used. The availability of a large number of measures has meant that we have been more selective than in other sections of this review. The measures represent two distinct categories. Firstly, there are the ADL measures dealing primarily with basic activities of daily living (Katz's Index of ADL, Barthel Index). Secondly, there are the more broadly based measures of limitations on activities (Lambeth Disability Screening Questionnaire, Functional Status Index, Rand Functional Status Indexes).

Before considering the available measures there are three issues which need to be considered in respect of all measures of functional limitation. Firstly, there is the problem of how to define the norms against which performance can be assessed. Secondly, problems can be encountered in attributing causes to the failure of individuals to meet norms. Thirdly, there is the issue of whether to measure actual performance of an activity or the individual's capacity to perform the activity, possibly under hypothetical conditions.

All measures face the problem of defining norms of behaviour against which to assess performance. The further one moves away from basic physiological function the more difficult it becomes to define such norms in any absolute sense. Whilst independence in mobility and basic self-care (washing, dressing, feeding, etc.) might be regarded as universal norms (at least for adults), ability to cook, wash clothes, go shopping, or hold paid employment are potentially more problematic. There will be differences between cultures and even between groups within the same culture. Perhaps the most commonly experienced problem for those involved in using IADL scales is their failure to make any differentiation on the basis of gender. Norms of behaviour with regard to domestic activities such as cooking, cleaning, and washing clothes are clearly different in our society for men and women. The intending user of a measure which includes these items should consider in advance how to classify responses, and where appropriate should separate responses in analyses, so that, for example, results for men and women could be analysed and presented separately.

Related to the problem of culturally defined norms is that of attempting to attribute causes to the failure of individuals to meet those norms. Disability is defined as a restriction or lack of ability to perform an activity resulting from an impairment. In other words we are concerned with the disabling effects of illness. But measures of activity describe functional limitations regardless of cause, so that a physically fit mentally alert man who has never cooked a meal may be described as 'unable to prepare a meal'. One way around this problem is to attempt to determine whether limitations are consequences of health problems. However, this is also fraught with difficulty. How are we to classify a man who has never cooked a meal in his life and is known to have arthritis which limits manual dexterity?

Lastly, and related to each of the previous problems, is the issue of whether to rate actual performance or capacity. This is particularly problematic for people living in institutions where many 'normal' activities (e.g. cooking, laundry, shopping) may be performed for them. But it can also apply to people living in their own home. Thus a person with ground-floor accommodation may never have to climb stairs or a relative may always do the shopping. In such circumstances a performance-based rating would assess the respondent as not performing the task. A capacity-based rating would ask whether she or he could do it. The validity of responses to such a hypothetical question is clearly uncertain.

None of the measures reviewed in this chapter succeeds in satisfactorily resolving all of the problems discussed in a way which would satisfy all intending users. The user must therefore make an informed choice between measures, depending upon the requirements of the particular research.

Index of Independence in Activities of Daily Living (ADL) (Katz and colleagues 1959)

Purpose

The Index of ADL was developed to measure and objectively evaluate the degree of functional incapacity or independence of people suffering from chronic conditions, especially the elderly. It has been used as a predictor of the course of illness, needs for care and functional/'sociobiological' outcomes of chronic diseases. The intention of the authors was also to develop a measure which could be used in both research and clinical practice to evaluate the effectiveness of different treatments.

Background

The original instrument, which has been subject to only minor modifications, was developed by staff of the Benjamin Rose Hospital in Cleveland in 1959.[14] Katz noted that, as a consequence of chronic disease, functional capacities are lost in a particular order, and that this order is then reversed in the reacquisition of abilities as a result of rehabilitation.[9] This concept of an ordered progression is fundamental to the Index of ADL. Katz showed that ability to undertake more complex activities (e.g. bathing, dressing, etc.) was lost first in the onset of chronic illness, and less complex activities (e.g. continence, feeding) later. He compared this pattern to the acquisition of skills in children and in primitive societies, and claimed that the index is based on primary biological and psychosocial function, reflecting the adequacy of organized neurological and locomotor response. However, it should be noted that the achievement of a set of tasks which could be ordered hierarchically was only possible by omitting activities such as walking and climbing stairs, which did not fit the pattern.

The Index of ADL was developed and tested using observations by physicians, nurses, sociologists, and other professionals of a large number of activities performed by patients with a fracture of the hip. Standardized observations were made at various points during the course of treatment. Grades of 'better' and 'worse' were defined for each area of function and the resulting patient profiles were used to identify a set of hierarchical relationships among the variables. The resulting index was subsequently applied to patients suffering from a variety of other chronic conditions, such as cerebral infarction, multiple sclerosis, arthritis, and stroke.[8-11]

Description

Six activities are included in the index; bathing, dressing, toiletting, transfer, continence, and feeding. The individual is rated on a three-point scale of independence for each activity using the form shown in Exhibit 4.1.

Exhibit 4.1   Index of ADL

(Adapted with permission from Katz, S., Downs, T. D., Cash, H. R., and Grotz, R. C. (1970). Progress in development of the Index of ADL. *Gerontologist*, **10**, 24)

Evaluation Form

Name _____   Day of evaluation _____

For each area of functioning listed below, check description that applies. (The word 'assistance' means supervision, direction, or personal assistance.)

Bathing—either sponge bath; tub bath, or shower

Receives no assistance (gets in and out of tub by self if tub is usual means of bathing)	Receives assistance in bathing only one part of the body (such as back or a leg)	Receives assistance in bathing more than one part of the body (or not bathed)

Dressing—gets clothes from closets and drawers—including underclothes, outer garments and using fasteners (including braces if worn)

Gets clothes and gets completely dressed without assistance	Gets clothes and gets dressed without assistance except for assistance in tying shoes	Receives assistance in getting clothes or in getting dressed, or stays partly or completely undressed

Toiletting—going to the 'toilet room' for bowel and urine elimination; cleaning self after elimination, and arranging clothes

Goes to 'toilet room', cleans self and arranges clothes without assistance (may use object for support such as cane, walker, or wheelchair and may manage night bedpan or commode, emptying same in morning)	Receives assistance in going to the 'toilet room' or in cleansing self or in arranging clothes after elimination or in use of night bedpan or commode	Doesn't go to room termed 'toilet' for the elimination process

Transfer

Moves in and out of bed as well as in and out of chair without assistance (may be using object for support such as cane or walker)	Moves in and out of bed or chair with assistance	Doesn't get out of bed

Continence

Controls urination and bowel movement completely by self	Has occasional 'accidents'	Supervision helps keep urine or bowel control; catheter is used, or is incontinent

Exhibit 4.1 (continued)

Feeding

Feeds self without assistance	Feeds self except for getting assistance in cutting meat or buttering bread	Receives assistance in feeding or is fed partly or completely by using tubes or intravenous fluids

Scoring

The Index of Independence in Activities of Daily Living is based on an evaluation of the functional independence or dependence of patients in bathing, dressing, going to toilet, transferring, continence, and feeding. Specific definitions of functional independence and dependence appear below.

A   —Independent in feeding, continence transferring, going to toilet, dressing, and bathing.
B   —Independent in all but one of these functions.
C   —Independent in all but bathing and one additional function.
D   —Independent in all but bathing, dressing, and one additional function.
E   —Independent in all but bathing, dressing, going to toilet, and one additional function.
F   —Independent in all but bathing, dressing, going to toilet, transferring, and one additional function.
G   —Dependent in all six functions.
Other—Dependent in at least two functions, but not classifiable as C, D, E, or F.

The observer records the most dependent degree of performance during a two-week period, using the brief descriptions of behaviour as guides. More comprehensive descriptions of these activities are provided by Katz.[12] Having completed the three-point rating, the information is converted into an Index of ADL grade with the aid of the definitions shown in the second part of Exhibit 4.1. First, the three-point ratings are converted to independent/dependent. For bathing, dressing, and feeding the middle categories are treated as representing independence, but for the other three items they are rated dependent. Second, a grading from A to G is arrived at as illustrated. However, this system leaves some cases unclassified. In a later paper the authors suggest an alternative classification ranging from 0–6, representing simply the number of activities in which the individual is dependent, regardless of the order in which dependencies appear.[8]

Although the development of the Index of ADL was based on the proposition that dependency could be assessed using a Guttman-type scale (i.e. cumulative and unidimensional), the final scale fails to achieve this. Indeed the modified index moves further from this approach by simply scoring the number of areas in which the individual is dependent.

Attempts have been made in recent years to extend the scope of the Index of ADL to include instrumental activities of daily living. Katz and his colleagues have reported work on expanding it to include shopping, transport and housekeeping.[13] They have not yet published this revised version. Two Swedish researchers have, however, published a five-item supplement including shopping, cleaning, transportation, washing and cooking in addition to the original self-care items.[3] Each of these is rated on a three-point scale (independent, partly dependent, and dependent) in exactly the same way as the original index. They have suggested a thirteen-point classification of grades using the combined version.

Administration and acceptability

Unlike most of the measures included in this book, the Index of ADL is designed for completion by an observer. The definitions are easily learned and there should be little difficulty in training observers to make systematic and consistent ratings. Where the observer knows the subject well, assessments can be completed in two or three minutes. For these reasons the instrument is well suited for use in routine professional practice, where the clinician is seeing the patient regularly.

Reliability and validity

For a scale which has been in existence for a long time and has been widely used, it is surprising how little evidence is available on either reliability or validity. Whilst clear and unambiguous scoring instructions should ensure high levels of reliability, it would be desirable to have more direct evidence of reliability. The authors report that, with adequate training, differences between raters occurred only once in twenty evaluations or less frequently.[9] A more recent study carried out in Sweden reported adequate coefficients of scalability in a Guttman analysis of scale items,[5] although another study showed that both the original Katz classification and a new Guttman scale were able to describe only two thirds of cases.[15] This seems a poor result, given that 48 per cent of the sample in this study were dependent in all six categories. Evidence of construct validity is mainly restricted to the work carried out in developing the index, although the claim to measure fundamental biological and psychosocial function has been questioned.[6] The best evidence available of validity relates to the ability of the Index to predict outcomes in chronic illness.[5,7,8,12] However, these studies have mainly looked at gross outcomes such as death, admission to hospital, and discharge. Even with such gross outcomes the Index of ADL may not be a very accurate predictor. In one study, although scores were marginally better predictors of death than physician ratings, neither was very good.[1] The Index of ADL is unlikely to be responsive to small but clinically significant changes in patients' conditions.

Populations/service settings

The Index of ADL was originally developed for use with elderly people suffering from chronic illness, and most applications have been with these groups. It has been used in a wide variety of chronic conditions.[8] It has also been applied in surveys of elderly people, regardless of chronic condition.[4]

The index is best suited for use in an institutional environment, where observation is feasible, and it was originally developed for use in a hospital setting. However, it has been used in community studies and in primary health care.[2] Provided that raters have adequate opportunity to observe behaviour over a time period or to use a reliable informant, it is suitable for use in primary health care settings.

Comments

The Index of ADL is one of the earliest, best known, and most extensively used measures of functioning. It is easily understood and readily applicable in a clinical situation. It has also been extremely influential in the development of subsequent measures of function and multidimensional instruments. It is thus somewhat surprising that more evidence of reliability and validity is not available. Intending users should pay particular attention to reliability and validity, where possible conducting their own tests in the particular research or clinical setting. Despite these reservations the index is worthy of consideration for use in clinical practice concerned with care of patients suffering from chronic illness, particularly in assessing needs for care. For research purposes, other more recent ADL scales or multidimensional measures have better evidence of reliability and validity.

Although work on expanding the Index of ADL to include instrumental activities of daily living such as shopping, transport and housekeeping[13] has begun, further work remains to be done on the validity and reliability of an extended index.

References

1. Asberg, K. H. (1987). Disability as a predictor of outcome for the elderly in a department of internal medicine. A comparison of predictions based on index of ADL and physician predictions. *Scandinavian Journal of Social Medicine,* **15**, 261–5.
2. Akpom, C. A., Katz, S., and Densen, P. M. (1973). Methods of classifying disability and severity of illness in ambulatory care patients. *Medical Care,* **2**, Suppl, 125–31.
3. Asberg, K. H., and Sonn, U. (1989). The cumulative structure of personal and instrumental ADL. A study of elderly people in a health service district. *Scandinavian Journal of Rehabilitative Medicine,* **21**, 171–7.
4. Branch, L. G., Katz, S., Kneipmann, K., and Papsidero, J. A. (1984). A prospec-

tive study of functional status among community elders. *American Journal of Public Health,* **74**, 266–8.

5. Brorsson, B., and Asberg, K. H. (1984). Katz Index of Independence in ADL: Reliability and validity in short term care. *Scandinavian Journal of Rehabilitative Medicine,* **16**, 125–32.

6. Chen, M. K., and Bryant, B. E. (1975). The measurement of health: a critical and selective overview. *International Journal of Epidemiology,* **4**, 257–64.

7. Harrel, J. S., McConnell, E. S., Wildman, D. S., and Samsa, G. P. (1989). Do nursing diagnoses affect functional status? *Journal of Gerontological Nursing,* **15**, 13–19.

8. Katz, S., and Akpom, C. A. (1976). A measure of primary sociobiological functions. *International Journal Health Services,* **6**, 493–507.

9. Katz, S., Ford, A. B., Moskowitz, R. W., Jackson, B. A., and Jaffe, M. W. (1963). Studies of illness in the aged: the Index of ADL: A standardised measure of biological and psychosocial function. *Journal of the American Medical Association,* **185**, 914–19.

10. Katz, S., Ford, A. B., Chinn, A. B., and Newill, V. A. (1966). Prognosis after strokes: II longterm course of 159 patients with stroke. *Medicine,* **45**, 236–46.

11. Katz, S., Vignos, P. J., Moskowitz, R. W., Thompson, H. M., and Svec, K. H. (1968). Comprehensive outpatient care in rheumatoid arthritis: a controlled study. *Journal of the American Medical Association,* **206**, 1249–54.

12. Katz, S., Downs, T. D., Cash, H. R., and Grotz, R. C. (1970). Progress in development of the Index of ADL. *The Gerontologist,* **10**, 20–30.

13. Spector, W. D., Katz, S., Murphy, J. B., and Fulton, J. P. (1987). The hierarchical relationship between activities of daily living and instrumental activities of daily living. *Journal of Chronic Disease,* **40**, 481–9.

14. Staff of the Benjamin Rose Hospital (1959). Multidisciplinary studies of illness in aged persons: II a new classification of functional status activities of daily living. *Journal of Chronic Disease,* **9**, 55–62.

15. Travis, S. S., and McAuley, W. J. (1990). Simple counts of the number of basic ADL dependencies for long-term care research and practice. *Health Services Research,* **25**, 349–60.

The Barthel Index (Mahoney and Barthel 1965, revised by Granger 1979)

Purpose

The Barthel Index was originally developed and used in clinical practice as a means of assessing the degree of independence in patients with neuromuscular or musculoskeletal disorders. It was used to assess patients before admission to hospital and after discharge, but has subsequently been used to identify patients who could benefit from rehabilitation programmes, predict length of stay, estimate prognosis, anticipate outcomes and evaluate services.

Background

Although first published in 1965,[9] the index had been in use since 1955. Its conceptual focus is on patients' dependence on others for actual physical assistance. Its origins in the routine assessment of patients entering hospital are reflected in the fact that the scoring system was developed to reflect the amount of, and time spent on, actual physical assistance for patients in a range of daily activities. The content of the index and its scoring seem to have developed out of clinical practice rather than the more academic approach used in many other measures. For this reason the assessment of reliability and validity in more formal terms was not undertaken until long after the original publication. However, the strength of the measure in terms of its usefulness in practice has led to its use in many studies. The original Barthel Index was modified in the 1970s by Carl Granger who increased the number of items and extended the rating categories.[4] Both modified and original versions have been further amended by subsequent users, often on mainly pragmatic grounds.

Description

The original Barthel Index consists of ten items, each of which is rated in terms of whether the patient is unable to perform the task, requires help, or can manage independently. Detailed definitions of the criteria to be applied in rating each item are provided by the authors.[9] Patients are classified in one of three categories on each item: dependent, performs task with help, independent. Dependent scores zero on all items. Other scores are intended to reflect the amount of, and time taken in providing, help. Thus, for example, independence in bathing scores only 5 because it is relatively infrequent, whilst walking scores 15, and there are three items (total score 30) dealing with incontinence and the ability to use the toilet. There are, however, inconsistencies in the scoring, so that, for example, full independence using a wheelchair scores 5, whilst someone who is able to walk only with help scores 10. Scores are totalled to give an overall score out of 100. Although a score of 100 implies complete independence for this range of activities, it is pointed out that individuals scoring 100 are not necessarily able to live alone, since the index does not cover household tasks.

Exhibit 4.2 shows a slightly modified version of the original index. Collin and colleagues at the Rivermead Rehabilitation Centre in Oxford have retained the original ten items, but have used a simpler scoring system and made minor amendments to the rating instructions.[1] This version gives a total score ranging from 0 (dependent on all items) to 20 (independent).

Granger's modification of the Barthel Index, which he called the Barthel Rating Scale or the Modified Barthel Index, incorporates the fifteen items

Exhibit 4.2   The Barthel ADL Index

Reproduced with permission from Collin, C., Wade, D. T., Davies, S., and Horn, V. (1988). The Barthel ADL Index: A reliability study. *International Disability Studies*, **10**, 61-3.

Bowels
  0 = incontinent (or needs to be given enema)
  1 = occasional accident (once/week)
  2 = continent

Bladder
  0 = incontinent, or catheterized and unable to manage
  1 = occasional accident (max. once per 24 hours)
  2 = continent (for over 7 days)

Grooming
  0 = needs help with personal care
  1 = independent face/hair/teeth/shaving (implements provided)

Toilet use
  0 = dependent
  1 = needs some help, but can do something alone
  2 = independent

Feeding
  0 = unable
  1 = needs help cutting, spreading butter, etc.
  2 = independent (food provided in reach)

Transfer
  0 = unable—no sitting balance
  1 = major help (one or two people), physical, can sit
  2 = minor help (verbal or physical)
  3 = independent

Mobility
  0 = immobile
  1 = wheel-chair independent including corners, etc.
  2 = walks with help of one person (verbal or physical)
  3 = independent (but may use any aid, e.g. stick)

Dressing
  0 = dependent
  1 = needs help, but can do about half unaided
  2 = independent (including buttons, zips, laces)

Stairs
  0 = unable
  1 = needs help (verbal, physical, carrying aid)
  2 = independent up and down

Bathing
  0 = dependent
  1 = independent (or in shower)

TOTAL (0-20)

Exhibit 4.2 (continued)

The Barthel ADL Index guidelines

General

The index should be used as a record of *what a patient does*, NOT as a record of *what a patient could do*.

The main aim is to establish *degree of independence from any help*, physical or verbal, however minor and for whatever reason.

The need for *supervision* renders the patient, NOT *independent*.

A patient's performance should be established *using the best available evidence*. Asking the patient, friends/relatives and nurses will be the usual source, but direct observation and common sense are also important. However, *direct testing is not needed*.

Usually the performance over the *preceding 24–48 hours** is important, but occasionally longer periods will be relevant.

Unconscious patients should score '0' throughout, even if not yet incontinent. Middle categories imply that patient supplies *over 50 per cent of the effort*.

Use *of aids* to be independent is *allowed*.

Bowels (preceding week)	If needs enema from nurse, then 'incontinent'* Occasional* = once a week
Bladder (preceding week)	Occasional = less than once a day A catheterized patient who can completely manage the catheter alone is registered as 'continent'
Grooming (preceding 24–48 hrs)	Refers to personal hygiene: doing teeth, fitting false teeth, doing hair, shaving, washing face. Implements* can be provided by helper.
Toilet use	Should be able to reach toilet/commode, undress sufficiently, clean self, dress and leave. With help = can wipe self, and do some other of above.*
Feeding	Able to eat any normal food (not only soft food*). Food cooked and served by others. But not cut up. Help = food cut up, patient feeds self.*
Transfer	From bed to chair and back. Dependent = NO sitting balance (unable to sit); two people to lift. Major help = one strong/skilled, or two normal people. Can sit up. Minor help = one person easily, OR needs any supervision for safety.
Mobility	Refers to mobility about house or ward, indoors. May use aid. If in wheelchair, must negotiate corners/doors unaided. Help = by one, untrained person, including supervision/moral support.

Exhibit 4.2 (continued)

Dressing	Should be able to select and put on all clothes, which may be adapted.
	Half = help with buttons, zips, etc. (check!), but can put on some garments alone.
Stairs	Must carry any walking aid used to be independent.
Bathing	Usually the most difficult activity.
	Must get in and out unsupervised and wash self.
	Independent in shower = 'independent' if unsupervised/unaided.*

* = items added or modified after study; asterisk at end, whole item added; asterisk in middle, phrase added or clarified.

---

shown in Exhibit 4.3, each of which is rated on a three-point scale. The scoring is based on the same principles as the original and detailed definitions are available from the author. Scores range from −2 to 100. Granger has also incorporated the modified Barthel Index into the Long Range Evaluation System (LRES),[3] where a four-point classification system (with ease, with difficulty, with some help, totally dependent) is used. This is a comprehensive computerized assessment method that measures functional abilities, activities, and environmental support. Granger also reports use of a twelve item version (excluding drinking, putting on brace or artificial limb, and bathing).[6] Lastly, a group of Australian researchers has presented a five-point scoring system which is claimed to increase sensitivity.[10]

Administration and acceptability

The index can be completed by a doctor, nurse, or other health professional on the basis of observation and clinical assessment or from information available from existing records. However, the unreliability of much information contained in records will mean that other sources of information will usually be required. It can also be completed on the basis of self-report in 2–5 minutes, but nobody has yet published a structured questionaire designed to elicit Barthel item scores. One study has reported using the modified index in a telephone interview.[11] Although the Barthel Index requires interview or observation, the fact that it can be completed in a few minutes means that it can be incorporated into a consultation with little or no disruption. All studies report high response rates and no problems in administration.

Exhibit 4.3   Modified Barthel Index

(Reproduced with permission from Granger, C. V., Albrecht, G. L., and Hamilton, B. B. (1979). Outcome of comprehensive medical rehabilitation: measurement by PULSES Profile and Barthel Index. *Archives of Physical Medicine and Rehabilitation*, **60**, 145–54)

The following presents the items or tasks scored in the Barthel Index with the corresponding values for independent performance of the tasks:

	'Can do by myself'	'Can do with help of someone else'	'Cannot do at all'
Self-care subscore			
1. Drinking from a cup	4	0	0
2. Eating	6	0	0
3. Dressing upper body	5	3	0
4. Dressing lower body	7	4	0
5. Putting on brace or artificial limb	0	– 2	0 (not applicable)
6. Grooming	5	0	0
7. Washing or bathing	6	0	0
8. Controlling urination	10	5 (accidents)	0 (incontinent)
9. Controlling bowel movements	10	5 (accidents)	0 (incontinent)
Mobility subscore			
10. getting in and out of chair	15	7	0
11. Getting on and off toilet	6	3	0
12. Getting in and out of tub or shower	1	0	0
13. Walking 50 yards on the level	15	10	0
14. Walking up/down one flight of stairs	10	5	0
15. If not walking: Propelling or pushing wheelchair	5	0	0 (not applicable)

Barthel Total: best score is 100; worst score is 0.
Note: Tasks 1–9, the self-care subscore (including control of bladder and bowel sphincters), have a total possible score of 53.
Tasks 10–15, the mobility subscore, have a total possible score of 47. The two groups of task combined make up the total Barthel Index with a total possible score of 100.

Reliability and validity

Until recently, little attention seemed to have been paid to reliability, despite the fact that the index has been in use for more than thirty years. Recent papers have reported high levels of agreement between raters and between different methods of assessment.[1,11] Granger's modified version has also achieved good inter-rater agreement.[4,8] There has been very little attention paid to internal consistency, but one recent study of stroke patients yielded high levels of internal consistency for the original version and a version wtih modified scoring.[10] Factor analysis of results obtained using the version shown in Exhibit 4.2 confirms that it is measuring a single dimension.[13]

Predictive validity, which is one of the most important criteria for a measure designed for use in clinical practice, has been tested in many studies. The index has been shown to predict survival, length of stay, and progress among stroke patients.[14-16] In stroke patients, there seems to be a predictable progression through the items as recovery occurs.[13] Granger and his colleagues also demonstrated predictive validity for stroke patients, and showed that a score of 60 appeared to be the pivotal point for distinguishing between dependence and assisted independence.[5] The Index has been shown to correlate well with the PULSES profile[4] and the modified version with patients' actual behaviour at home.[2] The same study provides evidence of construct validity in demonstrating associations with age, psychological problems, and role performance. In a review of evidence concerning validity, Wade and Collin cite extensive evidence of concurrent predictive and construct validity.[12]

Despite the evidence that the Barthel Index is able to detect changes in the process of rehabilitation following a stroke, there is insufficient evidence of its responsiveness to change. Substantial change can occur within the broad categories without altering Index scores. Although revised scoring systems may improve responsiveness, the gain is relatively small.[10]

Populations/service settings

Like most of the measures of function and activities of daily living, the Barthel Index is most suited to patients suffering moderate to severe disability. It has been used with people suffering from a wide range of chronic illnesses which result in substantial disability and with infirm elderly people, but its main application has been with patients suffering from strokes. Although developed originally for use in a hospital setting it has also been used in home care programmes. However, it is not self-administered and requires that the rater has considerable knowledge of the individual's abilities and circumstances. In the setting of community health services it would usually be completed by a professional in the patient's own home.

Comments

The original Barthel Index is one of the oldest measures included in this volume and is very limited in the scope of activities covered. However, it has been widely used in both clinical practice and research, and has become one of the most widely known ADL measures. Partly because of its widespread use, it has spawned a bewildering array of variants. In a review of its applications, Wade and Collin recommended choosing a very simple version with simple scoring methods.[12]

Within its limitations of scope the Barthel Index is one of the best brief assessments of basic ADL currently available. Its validity as a measure of needs for care, potential for rehabilitation and likely outcomes is well established. For these reasons it should be considered where a measure is required which focuses on the degree of dependence in basic activities of daily living in a relatively disabled population. A joint working part of the Royal College of Physicians and the Royal College of General Practitioners has recently recommended its use for screening elderly people in general medical practice. However, for less disabled populations and where assessment of a broader range of function is required, other instruments are likely to be more appropriate. Where outcomes of treatment are of concern, the crude categories employed in the Barthel Index may be insufficient to detect important changes.

References

1. Colin, C., Wade, D. T., Davies, S., and Horne, V. (1988). The Barthel ADL Index: a reliability study. *International Disability Studies,* **10**, 61-3.
2. Fortinsky, R. H., Granger, C. V., and Seltzer, G. B. (1981). The use of functional assessment in understanding home care needs. *Medical Care,* **19**, 489-97.
3. Granger, C. V., and McNamara, M. A. (1984). Functional assessment utilisation: The Long Range Evaluation System (LRES). In *Functional assessment in rehabilitation medicine*, p. 99-121 (ed. C. V. Granger and G. E. Gresham), Williams & Williams, Baltimore.
4. Granger, C. V., Albrecht, G. L., and Hamilton, B. B. (1979). Outcome of comprehensive medical rehabilitation: Measurement by PULSES Profile and the Barthel Index. *Archives of Physical Medicine and Rehabilitation,* **60**, 145-54.
5. Granger, C. V., Dewis, L. S., Peters, N. C., Sherwood, C. C., and Barrett, J. E. (1979). Stroke rehabilitation: Analysis of repeated Barthel Index measures. *Archives of Physical Medicine and Rehabilitation,* **60**, 14-17.
6. Granger, C. V., Hamilton, B. B., Gresham, G. E., and Kramer, A. A. (1989). The stroke rehabilitation outcome study: Part II. Relative merits of the total Barthel Index score and a four-item subscore in predicting patient outcomes. *Archives of Physical Medicine and Rehabilitation,* **70**, 100-3.
7. Kane, R. A., and Kane, R. L. (1981). *Assessing the elderly: a practical guide to measurement*. Lexington Books, Lexington.
8. Loewen, S. C., and Anderson, B. A. (1988). Reliability of the Modified Motor Assessment Scale and the Barthel Index. *Physical Therapy,* **68**, 1077-81.
9. Mahoney, F. I., and Barthel, D. W. (1965). Functional evaluation: The Barthel Index. *Maryland State Medical Journal,* **14**, 61-5.

10. Shah, S., Vanclay, F., and Cooper, B. (1989). Improving the sensitivity of the Barthel Index for stroke rehabilitation. *Journal of Clinical Epidemiology,* **42**, 703–9.
11. Shinar, D., Gross, C.R., Bronstein, K.S., Licata-Gehr, E.E., Eden, D.T., Cabrera, A.R., Fishman, I.G., Roth, A.A., Barwick, J.A., and Kunitz, S.C. (1987). Reliability of the activities of daily living scale and its use in telephone interview. *Archives of Physical Medical Rehabilitation,* **68**, 723–8.
12. Wade, D.T., and Collin, C. (1988) The Barthel ADL Index: a standard measure of physical disability? *International Disability Studies,* **10**, 64–7.
13. Wade, D.T., and Langton Hewer, R. (1987). Functional abilities after stroke: measurement, natural history and prognosis. *Journal of Neurology, Neurosurgery and Psychiatry,* **50**, 177–82.
14. Wylie, C.M. (1967). Gauging the response of stroke patients to rehabilitation. *Journal of the American Geriatrics Society,* **15**, 797–805.
15. Wylie, C.M. (1967). Measuring end results of rehabilitation of patients with stroke. *Public Health Report,* **82**, 893–8.
16. Wylie, C.M., and White, B.K. (1964). A measure of disability. *Archives of Environmental Health,* **8**, 834–9.

The Functional Status Index (FSI) (Jette 1978, 1980)

Purpose

The FSI is designed to measure the degree of dependence, pain, and difficulty experienced by people suffering from arthritis living in the community. It is intended to be used as both an adjunct to clinical practice and as an evaluative tool in research.

Background

Jette and his colleagues in the Pilot Geriatric Arthritis Program in Michigan required an evaluative measure which matched the goals of the programme, which were to prevent disability, restore activity, reduce pain, and encourage social and emotional adjustment.[1] They were critical of existing measures of function, which emphasized dependence and independence at the expense of other important dimensions. It was argued that, in clinical practice, it was sometimes desirable to provide assistance (i.e. increase dependence) in order to alleviate pain and reduce difficulty. Existing measures, by treating increased dependence as loss of health, ignored the importance of pain and difficulty in performing tasks. Jette also criticized existing instruments for their use of broad categories of activity, such as dressing, which incorporated a number of complex activities each involving different joints and muscles.[4]

The FSI was based on a number of existing instruments (Katz Index of ADL, Barthel, PULSES) but the number of activities and their specificity were increased to make them more sensitive to modest changes in function. The original version contained 44 items (later 45) each dealing with a specific aspect of function in daily living.[7] Each item was rated in terms of level of dependence, difficulty and pain, giving a total of 132 questions (45 item version 135 questions) which took between one and one and a half hours to administer. Factor analysis of responses to this full version was used to reduce the total number of items and group them under five headings.[4,5]

Description

The 18-item FSI groups activities under the five headings shown in Exhibit 4.4. Respondents are asked to use a time frame of the previous seven days and to base their response on their experience on average during that period. For each item they are asked first the degree to which they used help with that activity. Responses are rated 1 to 5 as shown in Exhibit 4.4. If they did not undertake the activity for reasons other than health, the item is not scored. Second, they are asked, for each item they undertook, how much pain they experienced, and third how difficult it was to perform the activity. These sections can either be scored on four point scales as shown in Exhibit 4.4, or they can use a seven-point ladder scale.[5]

An overall score for all dimensions and all activities is not recommended. In the users' instructions, Jette recommends either fifteen summated rating scales or three overall function scores.[3] One rating score is calculated for each dimension (dependence, difficulty, pain) for each group of activities. Thus, for example, dependence in personal care is calculated by adding dependency scores for each of the four activities under this heading and dividing by the number of activities. Overall function scores are calculated by adding all scores in each dimension (dependence, difficulty, pain) and dividing by the number of activities. In both cases any activity that is not undertaken out of preference or for other non-health reasons is not counted.

Administration and acceptability

It is designed to be administered by a health professional or trained interviewer in 20–30 minutes. The questionnaire on which FSI ratings are based has not been published, although interviewer instructions and questionnaires are available from Alan Jette. Although a self administered version has been used, it is recommended that the FSI be completed by an interviewer who presents respondents with 'show cards' to determine the appropriate rating. The interviewer is expected to probe as necessary, particularly to establish why an activity is not performed, and whether it could be performed if necessary. This relatively open ended style of interviewing has the advantage of making the assessment more conversational, but the disadvantage of introducing more potential sources of error if inter-

Exhibit 4.4   Functional Status Index

(Adapted with permission from Jette, A. M. (1980). Functional Status Index: reliability of a chronic disease evaluation instrument. *Archives of Physical Medicine and Rehabilitation*, **61**, 395–401)

Tasks

Gross mobility
  walking inside
  stair climbing
  chair transfers

Hand activities
  opening containers
  writing
  dialling a phone

Interpersonal activities
  driving a car
  visiting family or friends
  attending meetings
  performing your job

Personal care
  washing all parts of the body
  putting on pants
  putting on a shirt
  buttoning a shirt
Home chores
  doing laundry
  reaching into low cupboards
  doing yard-work
  vacuuming a rug

Response categories

Assistance: 1 = Independent
                 2 = Uses devices
                 3 = Uses human assistance
                 4 = Uses devices and human assistance
                 5 = Unable or unsafe to do activity

Pain: 1 = No pain
                 2 = Mild pain
                 3 = Moderate pain
                 4 = Severe pain

Difficulty: 1 = No difficulty
                 2 = Mild difficulty
                 3 = Moderate difficulty
                 4 = Severe difficulty

viewers use different approaches. The detailed instructions to interviewers are designed to overcome this problem. There do not seem to be any difficulties arising from understanding or acceptability to respondents.

Despite the claim that the FSI is useful in clinical practice, it is unlikely that many primary health care professionals will be able to spare 20–30 minutes to complete an assessment. For this reason, unless a self-administered version is used, the FSI is likely to be more useful in research applications.

Reliability and validity

The 18-item version was tested for internal consistency, inter-observer, and test–retest reliability on 149 adults suffering from rheumatoid arthritis.[2,5] The results were satisfactory in each case, although internal consistency of dependency in hand activities was poor. The level of inter-observer reliability was generally higher than test–retest reliability (time interval 1–3 days). Whilst reliability coefficients were generally satisfactory, there appears to be room for improvement in the reliability of the FSI.

Content validity is perhaps better than other measures of function because of the sound conceptual foundations of this measure. However, comparisons between FSI scores, patient self-ratings, and staff ratings produced extremely varied results.[1] It seems likely that the questions put to patients and staff were assessing different dimensions from those covered in the FSI. Moderate positive correlations have been reported between FSI scores, the American Rheumatism Association Functional Classification, and professional global assessments.[6,10] Concurrent validity of nine dependency items was tested on inpatients suffering from hip fracture, by comparing them to the results of direct performance tests.[2] All correlations were above 0.7 and disagreements most commonly arose from under reporting of functional ability on the FSI. Factor analysis of the 18-item version provided support for the grouping of items into the five categories shown in Exhibit 4.4.[5] Although more evidence on validity would be desirable, it is worth pointing out that FSI scores might be expected to differ from those achieved using other measures because of its broader definition of function. There is relatively little evidence of the responsiveness of the FSI to changes resulting from treatment interventions. In one study of patients following hip fracture, FSI scores were able to plot the pattern of recovery of function.[8] However, in a comparison of five health status instruments for orthopaedic evaluation, Liang reported that the FSI was less responsive than other measures to changes in mobility and global function.[9]

Populations/service settings

The FSI has been used with elderly people suffering from arthritis living in the community, but is intended to be applicable to any adult suffering from arthritis. It has also been used in hip fracture patients and patients who have had hip or knee replacements. Whilst it may be applicable to other patient groups, it would need to be tested on these groups. It is suitable for use in a primary health care setting or in hospital out-patient care.

Comments

The FSI is unique among measures of function in attempting to operationalize a concept which is more broadly based than dependence/

independence. For this reason alone it is worthy of serious consideration. It is, however, unfortunate that more has not been done to develop and further test the FSI. The available evidence on reliability and validity is limited and inconclusive.

References

1. Denniston, O. L., and Jette, A. M. (1980). A functional status assessment instrument: Validation in an elderly population. *Health Services Research,* **15**, 21–34.
2. Harris, B. A., Jette, A. M., Campion, E. W., and Cleary P. D. (1986). Validity of self report measures of functional disability. *Topics in Geriatric Rehabilitation,* **1**, 31–41.
3. Jette, A. M. (undated). *Users' Instructions: Functional Status Index*, Available from the author.
4. Jette, A. M. (1980). Functional capacity evaluation: An empirical approach. *Archives of Physical Medical Rehabilitation,* **61**, 85–9.
5. Jette, A. M. (1980). The Functional Status Index: reliability of a chronic disease evaluation instrument. *Archives of Physical Medicine and Rehabilitation,* **61**, 395–401.
6. Jette, A. M. (1987). The Functional Status Index: reliability and validity of a self-report functional disability measure. *Journal Of Rheumatology,* **14**, Suppl, 15–21.
7. Jette, A. M., and Denniston, L. O (1978). Inter-observer reliability of a functional status assessment instrument. *Journal of Chronic Disease,* **31**, 575–80.
8. Jette, A. M., Harris, B. A., Cleary P. D., and Campion, E. W. (1987). Functional recovery after hip fracture. *Archives of Physical Medical Rehabilitation,* **68**, 735–40.
9. Liang, M. H., Fossel, A. H., and Larson, M. G. (1990). Comparisons of five health status instruments for orthopedic evaluation. *Medical Care,* **28**, 632–42.
10. Shope, J., Barnwell, B., and Jette, A. M. (1983). Functional status outcome after treatment of RA. *Rheumatology in Practice,* **1**, 243–8.

Lambeth Disability Screening Questionnaire (Patrick and others 1980, 1983)

Purpose

The screening questionnaire is intended to identify adults living in the community who have some degree of disability. Although originally designed for use in planning health and social services, it could be used to estimate needs for care at a more localized level. It could also be used to identify individuals who require more comprehensive assessment.

Background

For the purposes of conducting a population survey of the prevalence of disability in Lambeth, the authors devised a postal screening questionnaire, which was tested in a populaton of patients registered with general practitioners.[6] The purpose of the questionnaire was to identify disabled people who were subsequently interviewed using the Functional Limitations Profile (FLP) (see p. 133). Items used fell into four broad categories: ambulation and mobility, body care and movement, sensory and motor activity, and social activity.[4] This version of the questionnaire was completed by one member of each household who was asked to identify any household members who experienced difficulty in each area of activity. A subsequent shorter version was developed for completion by individuals.[4]

Description

The household disability screening questionnaire shown in Exhibit 4.5 contains 25 items. Respondents are asked to identify any member of the

---

Exhibit 4.5   Lambeth Disability Screening Questionnaire (households)

(Adapted with permission from Patrick, D. L. and Peach, H (1989) (ed.). *Disablement in the community*. Oxford University Press, Oxford)

---

1. *WHO has difficulty with any of the following?*	The first names and ages of everyone having this difficulty are:	No-one
a. Walking without help		
b. Getting outside the house without help		
c. Crossing the road without help		
d. Travelling on a bus or train without help		

(Sections 2, 3, and 4—adopt same format as for 1 above)

Exhibit 4.5 (continued)

2. *WHO has difficulty with any of the following?*
a. Getting in and out of bed or chair without help
b. Dressing or undressing without help
c. Kneeling or bending over without help
d. Going up or down stairs without help
e. Having a bath or all-over wash without help
f. Holding or gripping (for example a comb or a pen) without help
g. Getting to and using the toilet without help

3. *WHO has difficulty with any of the following?*
a. Difficulty with spells of giddiness
b. Frequent falls
c. Weakness or paralysis of arms
d. A stroke
e. Difficulty seeing newspaper print even with glasses
f. Difficulty recognizing people across the road even with glasses
g. Hearing difficulties
h. Loss of whole or significant part of an arm, hand, leg, or foot
i. Controlling bowels or bladder

4. *WHO is limited in doing any of the following BECAUSE OF ILLNESS OR DISABILITY?*
a. Working at all
b. Doing the job of their choice
c. Doing housework
d. Visiting family or friends

5. If you have written ANY names in Questions 1–4, *please tell us what their major illness or disability is.*

First names and ages of anyone mentioned in Questions 1–4.	Please describe their major illness or disability below.

6. *Does* anyone else *in your household have any illness or disability which affects their activities in any way?*

First names and ages of anyone with illness/disability	What is the major illness or disability?	Please describe activity (e.g. playing sports, sewing, going to the pub)

household who has difficulty with a range of activities. Questions also cover
a range of specific medical problems and any major illnesses. Since there is
no attempt to classify severity of problems, difficulty can range from mild
discomfort to being completely unable to perform an activity. Questions are
oriented towards performance (Do you do?) rather than capacity (Could you
do?)

The version shown in Exhibit 4.6 is designed for completion by individuals

---

Exhibit 4.6   Lambeth Disability Questionnaire (individuals)

(Reproduced with permission, from Charlton, J. R. H., Patrick, D. L., and Peach, H. (1983). Use of multivariate measures of disability in health surveys. *Journal of Epidemiology and Community Health*, **37**, 304)

Because of illness, accident or anything related to your health, do you have difficulty
with any of the following? (**Read out individually and code.**)

  a. Walking without help
  b. Getting outside the house without help
  c. Crossing the road without help
  d. Travelling on a bus or train without help
  e. Getting in and out of bed or chair without help
  f. Dressing or undressing without help
  g. Kneeling or bending without help
  h. Going up or down stairs without help
  i. Having a bath or all over wash without help
  j. Holding or gripping (e.g. a comb or pen) without help
  k. Getting to and using the toilet without help
  l. Eating or drinking without help

Because of your health, do you have . . .
  m. Difficulty seeing newspaper print even with glasses
  n. Difficulty recognizing people across the road even with glasses
  o. Difficulty in hearing a conversation even with a hearing aid
  p. Difficulty speaking

Because of your health, do you have difficulty . . .
  q. Preparing or cooking a hot meal without help
  r. Doing housework without help
  s. Visiting family or friends without help
  t. Doing any of your hobbies or spare time activities
  u. Doing paid work of any kind (if under 65)
  v. Doing paid work of your choice (if under 65)

and attempts to identify only health related difficulties. This version can be scored using item weights derived from regression analysis of responses with scores on the FLP.[1]

Administration and acceptability

The household version is designed for postal administration and achieved very high response rates in the Lambeth survey.[4] Nevertheless, non-response does present problems in prevalence surveys and the authors have discussed methods of reducing bias from this source.[6]

The 22-item version is designed for interviewer administration. However, there seems to be no reason why it should not be adapted for use as a postal screening questionnaire or for self-completion in other settings, since this was the method used in earlier versions. No information is provided on the time taken to complete either questionnaire, but we would expect the household screening version to take 10–15 minutes and the individual version no more than 5 minutes. A recent postal survey carried out by the present authors using the 22-item questionnaire produced a response rate of more than 80 per cent.

Reliability and validity

Little evidence of reliability is available for either instrument. Test–retest reliability of the household version was assessed by comparison with results of personal interviews after three to six months.[6]

Comparisons of self-ratings with ratings by general practitioners showed low levels of agreement.[5,6] However, this is more likely to suggest ignorance on the part of the doctors than lack of validity in the questionnaire. Comparisons between disabled people identified by the household screening questionnaire and a control group of non-disabled in terms of FLP scores obtained at personal interview showed the screening questionnaire to have good sensitivity and specificity in identifying disablement.[3] Scores obtained using the individual version were strongly correlated with FLP physical dimension scores but less well correlated with psychosocial scores, as might be expected.[1]

Populations/service settings

The Lambeth questionnaires were originally developed for epidemiological purposes and are therefore intended as population screening tools. They are not suitable for the assessment of individuals or for the evaluation of specific treatments, unless quite large changes in performance are predicted. Their main use in primary health care is likely to be in identifying needs for treatment/care at the level of populations or the desirability of more comprehensive assessment for individuals.

Comments

The Lambeth Disability Screening Questionnaires provide an economical method of estimating levels of disability in a population and thus estimating needs for services. The fact that they are suitable for self-completion and for use in postal surveys makes them particularly attractive for situations in which resources are severely limited. The evidence available on reliability and validity is encouraging.

References

1. Charlton, J.R.H., Patrick, D.L., and Peach, H. (1983). Use of multivariate measures of disability in health surveys. *Journal of Epidemiology and Community Health,* **37**, 296–304.
2. Locker, D., Wiggins, R., Sittampalam, Y., and Patrick, D.L. (1981). Estimating the prevalence of disability in the community: the influence of sample design and response bias. *Journal of Epidemiology and Community Health,* **35**, 208–12.
3. Patrick, D.L., and Peach, H. (1989). *Disablement in the community*, Oxford University Press, Oxford.
4. Patrick, D.L., Darby, S.C., Green, S., Horton, G., Locker, D., and Wiggins, R.D. (1981). Screening for disability in the inner city. *Journal of Epidemiology and Community Health,* **35**, 65–70.
5. Patrick, D.L., Peach, H., and Gregg, I. (1982). Disablement and care: a comparison of patient views and general practitioner knowledge. *Journal of the Royal College of General Practitioners,* **32**, 429–34.
6. Peach, H., Green, S., Locker, D., Darby, S., and Patrick, D.L. (1980). Evaluation of a postal screening questionnaire to identify the physically disabled. *International Rehabilitation Medicine,* **2**, 189–93.

Rand Functional Status Indexes (Stewart, Ware and Brook 1978)

Purpose

These indexes are designed to measure physical health in terms of functioning in general populations. Functioning is assessed in three broad areas: personal limitations, role limitations, and physical capacities. The questionnaires and indexes derived from them are primarily research instruments suitable for both epidemiological surveys and evaluation of service programmes.

Background

Among measures of functional status, those produced by the research team at the Rand Corporation in California are perhaps the most carefully developed and tested. They were developed for use in the Health Insurance

Experiment conducted in six sites across the USA. Stewart and her colleagues identified five categories of activities commonly included under functional status: (1) self-care activities, (2) mobility, (3) physical activities, (4) role activities, (5) leisure activities.[7] A review of existing measures of function suggested that although scales for all five categories of function existed, evidence of reliability and validity was limited and sometimes non-existent. Where evidence of reliability and validity was available for measures dealing with particular areas of physical function, there appeared to be scope for reduction in the number of measures that must be scored and interpreted separately to define functional status.[8] Also, to the extent that measures had been used to successfully detect differences in function related to use of services this research focused on disabled or chronically ill populations. The Rand Corporation researchers therefore developed a set of measures which would be suitable for use with a general population and which could be used to construct aggregate indices.

Following an extensive review of both the methodological and empirical literature on functional status, the researchers established clear criteria for the selection of measures.[7] Two questionnaire batteries were developed: the Functional Limitations Battery based on work by Bush and his colleagues[4] and the National Center for Health Statistics;[2] and the Physical Abilities Battery based on the work of Hulka and Cassel.[1] Additional questions on disability days (e.g. work-loss days, school-loss days) were included, but are not dealt with here. A number of versions of these questionnaires was used in the Health Insurance Experiment sites on nearly 6000 adults between the ages of 14 and 66 years. Data from these studies were used to develop aggregate functional status indexes.

Description

The two batteries of questions shown in Exhibit 4.7 deal with similar areas of function, but differ in a number of respects: item structure and response choices; time frame of the questions; whether the items describe favourable or unfavourable health states; emphasis on performance of activity or capacity to perform.

The Functional Limitations Battery consists of 13 items covering mobility, physical activities, role activities, and self-care. In the original version each item carried two questions, the first established the existence of any limitation (yes/no) and the second for how long it had existed. However, the authors recommend using a single question for each item with the response categories shown in Exhibit 4.7.[9]

The Physical Capacities Battery consists of 12 items concentrated on physical activity, but also including items on self-care and household activities. Endorsement of these items indicates ability to perform the activity, but an intermediate response category (yes, but only slowly) is also provided. In

Exhibit 4.7 Rand functional status questions

(Adapted from Stewart, A., Ware, J. E., Brook, R. H., and Davies-Avery, A. (1978). *Conceptualization and measurement of health for adults in the Health Insurance Study: Vol. II Physical health in terms of functioning.* Rand Pub. No. 1987/2-HEW, Santa Monica)

Functional Limitations Battery

8. Are you able to drive a car?
9. When you travel around your community, does someone have to assist you because of your health?
10. Do you have to stay indoors most or all of the day, because of your health?
11. Are you in bed or a chair for most or all of the day because of your health?
12. Does your health limit the kind of vigorous activities you can do, such as running, lifting heavy objects, or participating in strenuous sports?
13. Do you have any trouble either walking several blocks or climbing a few flights of stairs, because of your health?
14. Do you have trouble bending, lifting, or stooping because of your health?
15. Do you have any trouble either walking *one* block or climbing *one* flight of stairs because of your health?
16. Are you unable to walk unless you are assisted by another person or by a cane, crutches, artificial limbs, or braces?
17. Are you unable to do certain kinds or amounts of work, housework, or schoolwork because of your health?
18. Does your health keep you from working at a job, doing work around the house, or going to school?
19. Do you need help with eating, dressing, bathing, or using the toilet because of your health?
20. Does your health limit you in any way from doing anything you want to do?

Response categories:
All items except item 8: (1) No, not limited; (2) Yes, for 3 months; (3) Yes, for more than 3 months.
Item 8: (1) No, because of my health; (2) No, for some other reason; (3) Yes, able to drive car.

Physical Capacities Battery

Questions about physical limitations
These next questions are about any physical limitations you might have and what causes them. For these activities, please circle a number for the statement which best describes you.

227. Can you do hard activities at home, heavy work like scrubbing floors, or lifting or moving heavy furniture?
228. If you wanted to, could you participate in active sports such as swimming, tennis, basketball, volleyball, or rowing a boat?
229. Could you do moderate work at home like moving a chair or table, or pushing a vacuum cleaner?

Exhibit 4.7 (continued)

230. Can you do light work around the house like dusting or washing dishes?
231. If you wanted to, could you run a short distance?
232. Can you walk uphill or up stairs?
233. Can you walk a block or more?
234. Can you walk around inside the house?
235. Can you walk to a table for meals?
236. Can you dress yourself?
237. Can you eat without help?
238. Can you use the bathroom without help?

Response categories
(1) Yes,
(2) Yes, but only slowly
(3) No, I can't do this

the original version, respondents were also asked why they were unable to perform the activity and given a list of 21 possible health reasons. Inability to peform an activity for reasons other than health was not counted as a limitation of function.

Results from the two batteries can be presented in simple descriptive terms, but Stewart and her colleagues have developed aggregate functional status measures.[8-10] These are summarized in Exhibit 4.8. All are ordinal scales developed using Guttman scalogram analysis of results from the Health Insurance Experiment. The Personal Limitations Index is a six-level scale based on nine of the items from the Functional Limitations Battery and aggregates data on self-care, mobility, and physical activities. Where a number of items are combined, endorsement of any one of them counts as limitation in that area. Scale levels are determined by the response patterns shown. Where responses do not follow the predicted pattern, levels can be assigned on a case by case basis (see Stewart *et al*,[10] for detailed description). The Role Limitations Index is constructed in the same way using three items from the Functional Limitations Battery and has four levels. The Physical Capacities Index uses all 12 items from the Physical Capacities Battery, although all except one are combined and treated in the same way as combined items on the Personal Limitations Index. This produces one index with seven levels.

Further experimentation with aggregating these indexes showed that personal limitations cannot be combined with role limitations to form a cumulative unidimensional scale. However, it was possible to produce an index which combined Personal Limitations and Physical Capacities.[8,9] This combined index is called a Personal Functioning Index and has the advantage of identifying those slightly disabled individuals who score as

Exhibit 4.8   Aggregate indexes of functional health

(Adapted from Stewart, A., Ware, J. E., Brook, R. H., and Davies-Avery, A. (1978). Conceptualization and measurement of health for adults in the Health Insurance Study: Vol. II Physical health in terms of functioning. Rand Pub. No. 1978/2-HEW, Santa Monica)

Personal limitations index

Item	19	8–11	15	13	12 or 14
Scale level	Limited in self-care	Limited in mobility	Trouble walking one block or climbing one flight of stairs	Trouble walking several blocks or climbing a few flights of stairs	Limited in vigorous activities or in bending lifting, or stooping
5	yes	yes	yes	yes	yes
4	no	yes	yes	yes	yes
3	no	no	yes	yes	yes
2	no	no	no	yes	yes
1	no	no	no	no	yes
0	no	no	no	no	no

Role limitations index

Item	18	17	20
Scale level	Unable to work	Limited in work	Limited in any way
3	yes	yes	yes
2	no	yes	yes
1	no	no	yes
0	no	no	no
– 1	missing		

Physical capacities index

Item	236, 237, 238	234, 235	230	229, 233	231, 232	227, 228
Scale level	Limited in self-care activities	Limited in walking around inside house	Limited in light housework	Limited in moderate housework or in walking a block or more	Limited in running a short distance or walking uphill or up stairs	Limited in hard activities at home or in active sports
1	yes	yes	yes	yes	yes	yes
2	no	yes	yes	yes	yes	yes
3	no	no	yes	yes	yes	yes
4	no	no	no	yes	yes	yes
5	no	no	no	no	yes	yes
6	no	no	no	no	no	yes
7	no	no	no	no	no	no

limited on one of the indices but not on both. In addition to these aggregate indexes, a number of scales measuring more specific aspects of functioning are available. These were developed and tested using an earlier version of the instruments.[7] Where global indexes do not provide sufficient detail, scales dealing separately with mobility, self-care, strenuous activity, etc., may be more appropriate.

Administration and acceptability

The Functional Limitations Battery and Physical Capacities Battery are designed for self-completion and should be completed in approximately ten minutes by most people. No problems in terms of acceptability to respondents are reported by the authors, and a study of patients attending primary care physicians achieved a response rate of more than 90 per cent.[3]

Reliability and validity

The measures developed for the Rand Health Insurance Experiment have been more thoroughly tested for reliability and validity than most measures of functional status. The original versions of the Functional Limitations Battery and Physical Capacities Battery were assessed in terms of test–retest reliability and internal consistency.[7] All of the aggregated indexes recommended for use exceed the standard requirements for Guttman scales in terms of reproducibility.[8]

Content validity of the Rand measures was studied by assessing their representativeness in terms of the universe of content of physical health measures identified in the literature. Construct validity was examined in terms of associations between measures of functioning, associations between measures of functioning and socio-demographic variables, and associations between measures of functioning and other health-related variables.[7] The validity of the aggregated indexes is demonstrated in terms of the reproducibility and scalability criteria appropriate to a Guttman scale.[8] They constitute valid and reliable ordinal scales. The Rand instruments were not designed for the purpose of assessing the outcomes of particular patterns of care for specific diseases, and there is no evidence concerning their responsiveness to clinically significant change. There is, however, evidence that they are capable of detecting differences associated with five years of age in group comparisons.[5]

One of the strengths of the research conducted by the researchers at the Rand Corporation is the recognition of the limitations of their measures as well as their strengths. Measurement at the interval level is not claimed for the aggregate indexes, so that the distance between scale points is likely to vary. Also the authors point out that although the scales are reliable and valid for general populations, they may not be appropriate to older populations or to populations of disabled people.[8] Further research in these areas is necessary.

Populations/service settings

These measures were developed specifically for use in surveys of the general adult population. They are suitable for group comparisons, but are not intended as individual assessments. They were intended primarily for research purposes with people registered with different types of health insurance schemes. They appear to be suitable for use in a primary health care setting where the research is concerned with the adult (non-elderly) population, and have been used successfully in a study of patients attending primary care physicians in the USA.[3]

Comments

The Rand Health Insurance Experiment has made a major contribution to the measurement of health status in terms of functioning. Within the constraints indicated by the researchers (ordinal measurement of function in adult populations) the indexes are well validated and reliable measures of physical function and roles. For elderly people and populations suffering high levels of disability, other measures may be more appropriate.

The Rand functional status measures have become something of a benchmark and reference point for health status measurement in the USA. Many other researchers have used them in whole or in part, and a number of other instruments have drawn heavily on the Rand measures. It is unfortunate that the actual questionnaires have not been published in journals which would have made them more accessible to a wider range of potential users.

The original instruments referred to in this entry have been revised and extensively tested in the Medical Outcomes Study (see p. 153). The revised schedules and comprehensive information on their reliability and validity have recently been published and the reader should refer to this latest work when considering the suitability of the Rand functional status measures.[6]

References

1. Hulka, B.S., and Cassel, J.C. (1973). The AAFP-UNC study of the organisation, utilisation and assessment of primary medical care. *American Journal of Public Health,* **63**, 494–501.
2. National Center for Health Statistics (1974). *Limitation of activity and mobility due to chronic conditions: United States 1972.* National Center for Health Statistics, DHEW Publication No (HRA), 75–1523, Rockville, Maryland.

3. Nelson, E., Conger, B., Douglass, R., Gephort, D., Kirk, J., Page, R., Clark, A., Johnson, K., Stone, K., Wasson, J., and Zubkoff, M. (1983). Functional health status levels of primary care patients. *Journal of the American Medical Association,* **249**, 3331–8.

4. Patrick, D. L., Bush, J. W., and Chen, M. M. (1973). Toward an operational definition of health. *Journal of Health and Social Behaviour,* **14**, 6–23.

5. Rogers, W. H., Williams, K. N., and Brook, R. H. (1979). *Conceptualization and measurement of health for adults in the health insurance study: Vol. 7 power analysis of health status measures.* Rand: Publication No R-1987/7-HEW, Santa Monica.

6. Stewart, A. L., and Ware, J. E. (ed.) (1992). *Measuring functioning and wellbeing: the Medical Outcomes Study approach,* Duke University Press, Durham, North Carolina, and London.

7. Stewart, A., Ware, J. E., Brook, R. H., and Davies-Avery, A. (1978). *Conceptualization and measurement of health for adults in the health insurance study: Vol. II physical health in terms of functioning,* Rand: Publication No 1987/2-HEW, Santa Monica.

8. Stewart, A. L., Ware, J. E., and Brook, R. H. (1981). Advances in the measurement of functional status: construction of aggregate indices. *Medical Care,* **19**, 473–88.

9. Stewart, A. L., Ware, J. E., and Brook, R. H. (1981). *Construction and scoring of aggregate functional status indexes: Vol. I,* Rand: Publication No 2-2551-HHS, Santa Monica.

10. Stewart, A. L., Ware, J. E., and Brook, R. H. (1982). *Construction and scoring of aggregate functional status measures: Vol. II appendices,* Rand: Publication No N-1706-1-HHS, Santa Monica.

Conclusions

Instruments for assessing physical functioning played a pioneering role in the history of the development of measures of health status. During the 1950s and 1960s many instruments were produced to evaluate clinical care in the emerging specialties of geriatric medicine, rheumatology, and rehabilitation medicine. The proliferation of these measures stemmed from the need to evaluate patient care in areas of medicine where the traditional criteria of mortality and morbidity were inappropriate. Because they grew out of clinical practice, many of these early measures were in use long before they were formally reported and they often lacked formal conceptualization and testing. Nevertheless, measures of ADL drawn from clinical practice have been extremely influential in the development of many more comprehensive measures reviewed in later chapters. Of the measures reviewed in this chapter Katz's Index of ADL and the Barthel Index clearly belong to this earlier generation of instruments. Jette's Functional Status Index lies somewhere in between the older clinically derived measures and more recent development of research-based measures.

Instruments such as the Lambeth screening questionnaires and the Rand Functional Status indexes clearly belong in the research camp in terms of their origins. They tend to be conceptually more sophisticated and to be designed according to more formal criteria, although Katz's Index of ADL also has a conceptually sophisticated foundation. Although measures such as those developed by the Rand Corporation have been far more thoroughly evaluated than many earlier instruments, some of these older measures remain in use. This is not simply a reflection of conservatism on the part of clinicians. It stems from their established value in clinical practice which many newer instruments have yet to achieve. However, there is a need to improve on older instruments. As mentioned above, these instruments played an important part in the development of sophisticated multidimensional measures. There may now be scope for this process to be reversed. Some of the multidimensional measures reviewed in Chapter 7 contain excellent measures of activities of daily living, and readers looking for measures in this area should consider whether sections of such instruments might be a better choice than some of the older measures of physical and role function described in this chapter.

5 Measures of mental illness and mental health

Introduction

The selection of measures appropriate for inclusion in this chapter proved more difficult than for most others because of the large number of well researched measures available. In contrast to physical functioning and activities of daily living, the development of measures of mental illness and mental health has been founded on explicit conceptual analysis and careful validation of instruments. This emphasis on systematic measurement stems in large part from the needs of professionals (psychiatrists and psychologists) to describe and categorize the problems with which they are dealing in clinical practice. The result is a wealth of concepts dealing with the spectrum from psychotic illness to psychological well-being. The corresponding range of measures designed to tap these concepts draws upon an equally wide range of measurement techniques, from the in-depth clinical interview to the self-completed pencil and paper test.

A review of even the most commonly used measures in the whole field is not only beyond the scope of this book, but also beyond the abilities of the authors. Our selection of seven measures for inclusion was based on considerations of their relevance to primary health care, their reliability and validity, and their practicality.

Needs for and outcomes of care at the primary level in the field of mental health are predominantly defined in terms of the presence and severity of illness, rather than in terms of psychological well-being. The most useful measures for the general practitioner will be those which assist in the identification of needs for treatment and which are capable of measuring the benefits of treatment. This means primarily measures designed to assess the presence and severity of depression and anxiety. Whilst psychotic disorders are seen in general practice, the numbers are small and many will be referred to specialists. In contrast, as many as 30 per cent of patients consulting will be suffering from depression and/or anxiety and the vast majority of these will be treated without resort to specialists. There is a need for measures capable of identifying those individuals who might benefit from treatment and capable of assessing responses to treatment. For these reasons five out of the seven measures we have included are designed specifically to detect the presence or absence of neurotic disorders defined in clinical terms. Of these five, four are concerned specifically with depression and anxiety, and the fifth (the General Health Questionnaire) with the identification of 'cases' of mental disorder regardless of diagnostic category. The remaining two measures adopt a broader perspective on mental health and do not focus exclusively on illness. The Mental Health Inventory encompasses mental distress in terms easily recognizable to the clinician, but also incorporates a measure of positive well-being in an attempt to focus on positive health as well as illness. Lastly, the Life Satisfaction Index, which has been widely used in studies of elderly people, completely abandons the notion of mental illness, although some of the items would be clearly recognizable to the clinician in terms of illness. However, we believe it is important to extend measurement into the areas of morale and life satisfaction in ways which do not label problems in terms of illness.

In selecting measures for inclusion, we have avoided those designed for use with hospital in-patients or those which require administration by a psychiatrist or psychologist. Despite their sophistication, and their ability to detect a wider range of disorders and to assess severity, we do not consider such measures suitable for use in either research or clinical practice in primary health care.

Zung Self-rating Depression Scale (SDS) (Zung 1965)

Purpose

The SDS is designed to provide a simple quantitative measurement of the subjective experience of depression as characterized by affective, cognitive, behavioural, and psychological symptoms. It was not intended to be either a substitute for, nor equivalent to, a clinical diagnosis. It has been widely used in monitoring changes during treatment, differentiating depressed patients from other diagnostic groups and measuring depressive symptomatology in the general population. It has also been extensively used in cross-cultural studies of patients with diagnoses of depressive disorder.

Background

Zung developed the SDS in the 1960s because existing measures were too long or relied too much on interpretation by the interviewer. A measure was required for patients whose primary diagnosis was depressive disorder which would be: inclusive with respect to symptoms of the illness, short and simple, quantitative, self-administered, and indicate the patient's own response at the time it was administered.[8] The content of the SDS was based on an analysis of verbatim reports of patient interviews. Using a set of factors characteristic in depressive disorders, those statements most representative of a particular symptom were selected for inclusion. They covered pervasive affect, physiological equivalents, and psychological equivalents.

Description

The 20 items included in the SDS are evenly divided between positive and negative phrasing (Exhibit 5.1). This is intended to avoid respondents being able to detect a trend in their responses. Each item has four response categories in order to avoid the tendency to tick the centre column. Respondents are asked to rate each item according to how it applied to them during the past week,[11] although the instrument itself does not specify a time-scale.

Exhibit 5.1   The Zung Self-rating Depression Scale

Name_____ Age___ Sex___ Date_____	None or a little of the time	Some of the time	Good part of the time	Most or all of the time
1. I feel down-hearted, blue and sad	1	2	3	4
2. Morning is when I feel the best	4	3	2	1
3. I have crying spells or feel like it	1	2	3	4
4. I have trouble sleeping through the night	1	2	3	4
5. I eat as much as I used to	4	3	2	1
6. I enjoy looking at, talking to and being with attractive women/men	4	3	2	1
7. I notice that I am losing weight	1	2	3	4
8. I have trouble with constipation	1	2	3	4
9. My heart beats faster than usual	1	2	3	4
10. I get tired for no reason	1	2	3	4
11. My mind is as clear as it used to be	4	3	2	1
12. I find it easy to do the things I used to	4	3	2	1
13. I am restless and can't keep still	1	2	3	4
14. I feel hopeful about the future	4	3	2	1

Exhibit 5.1 (continued)

15. I am more irritable than usual	1	2	3	4
16. I find it easy to make decisions	4	3	2	1
17. I feel that I am useful and needed	4	3	2	1
18. My life is pretty full	4	3	2	1
19. I feel that others would be better off if I were dead	1	2	3	4
20. I still enjoy the things I used to do	4	3	2	1

SDS index	Equivalent clinical global impression
Below 50	Within normal range, no psychopathology
50–59	Presence of minimal to mild depression
60–69	Presence of moderate to marked depression
70 & over	Presence of severe to most extreme depression

$$\text{SDS Index} = \frac{\text{raw score total}}{\text{maximum score of 80}} \times 100$$

Items are scored 1–4 and the scoring is reversed for positive phrasing. Raw scores are calculated by summing item scores, with no weighting of items. Raw scores, which range between 20 and 80, are converted to an index with a range from 25 to 100 by dividing by 80 and multiplying by 100. High scores indicate severe depression. Zung suggests that scores below 50 are within normal range, 50–59 reflect presence of minimal to mild depression, 60–69 moderate to marked depression and 70 plus severe to extremely depressed.[10] There seems to be no clearly agreed cut off point to define psychiatric caseness, and scores of 50, 55 and 60 have been used in different studies.

Administration and acceptability

The instrument is self administered, although it is usually introduced and explained by a doctor or researcher. It is not therefore designed for use in a postal survey, although there seems no obvious reason why it could not be adapted for postal administration. It can be completed in around three minutes and does not seem to generate any resistance from respondents. However, low response rates have been reported among elderly people.[7] Where it has been used in general practice it has usually been administered by a researcher (psychologist) prior to the patient's appointment with the clinician.[4,13]

Reliability and validity

For a scale which has been so widely used (Zung in 1986 reported over 300 publications using SDS2) there is surprisingly little evidence of reliability. Tests of internal consistency produced satisfactory results,[9,2] but more evidence would be desirable. Test–retest reliability has not been adequately demonstrated. Although there are problems in distinguishing between real change and error in test–retest correlations, evidence of consistency over different time periods would be useful, particularly in the light of known problems with retest reliability in other self completed psychiatric instruments such as the General Health Questionnaire.

In contrast to reliability, there are many published studies of validity. Content validity is claimed by virtue of the method of generating scale items, but others have argued that the SDS is inadequate in its coverage of depressive symptomatology[1] and includes items which do not necessarily indicate the presence of a mental illness.[6] Construct validity has been tested in comparisons with the Hamilton Rating Scale for Depression, the Beck Depression Inventory, and the Minnesota Multiphasic Personality Inventory.[3] Some studies report quite good correlations between the SDS and interviewer administered assessments of depression, but other investigators have failed to corroborate these findings.[3] With elderly patients the SDS has been shown to have a lower correlation with physicians' judgements than a rater administered interview.[7] SDS factor profiles have been used to discriminate between groups of patients, but some researchers have found the SDS a poor predictor of response to treatment. Disagreements also remain over whether the SDS is responsive to treatment induced change. Summing up these findings in their review of reliability and validity, Hedlund and Vieweg suggest that the evidence on validity supports the use of SDS as a screening instrument and as an adjunctive clinical tool, but not as an independent measure of depression.[3] In support of this recommendation, one study of the use of the SDS in primary care showed a significant increase in recognition of depression and change to treatment as a result of feedback to clinicians.[5]

Populations/service settings

Although originally devised for use in a mental illness service with depressed patients, the SDS has subsequently been widely used in non-hospital settings on 'normal' populations. It has been recommended for use as a screening tool in general practice.[12-14] However, despite its widespread use with many different patient groups, in different service settings, and in different countries, there remain doubts as to its general applicability. In particular there is some doubt as to its value with non-patient groups where the same dimensions can convey different meanings to different segments of the population.[1]

Comment

The Zung SDS is one of the most widely used self-evaluation measures of depression. However, there remain some serious questions concerning its validity in situations where something more than a screening instrument is required. To some extent these are common to all self-rating assessments of depression, and concern the issue of whether a self-assessment can be comparable with an observer (i.e. clinical) assessment. In addition to this, there remain questions about the validity of SDS even as a self-evaluation measure. Various researchers have questioned the content of the instrument, and results in both treatment evaluation and population studies are equivocal. Used as a screening tool and adjunct to clinical practice, the SDS is easily administered and helpful, but there are other equally suitable instruments. For more systematic assessments of need for care and outcome of care, we recommend that the researcher should compare the SDS with other measures of depression, taking into consideration the results of validation studies.

References

1. Blumenthal, M. (1975). Measuring depressive symptomatology in a general population. *Archives of General Psychiatry*, **32**, 971–78.
2. Giambra, L. (1977). Independent dimensions of depression: A factor analysis of three self report depression measures. *Journal of Clinical Psychology*, **33**, 928–35.
3. Hedlund, J. L. and Vieweg, B. W. (1979). The Zung self rating depression scale: A comprehensive review. *Journal of Operational Psychiatry*, **10**, 51–64.
4. Magill, M. K. and Zung, W. W. K. (1982). Clinical decisions about diagnosis and treatment for depression identified by screening. *Journal of Family Practice*, **14**, 1144–9.
5. Magruder-Habib, K., Zung, W. W., Feussner J. R. (1990). Improving physicians' recognition and treatment of depression in general medical care. Results from a randomized clinical trial. *Medical Care*, **28**, 239–50.
6. Snaith, R. P. (1987). The concept of mild depression. *British Journal of Psychiatry*, **150**, 387–93.
7. Toner, J., Gurland, B., Teresi, J. (1988). Comparison of self-administered and rater-administered methods of assessing levels of severity of depression in elderly patients. *Journal of Gerontology*, **43**, 136–40.
8. Zung, W. W. K. (1965). A self rating depression scale. *Archives of General Psychiatry*, **12**, 63–70.
9. Zung, W. W. K. (1972). The depression status inventory: an adjunct to the self rating depression scale. *Journal of Clinical Psychology*, **28**, 539–43.
10. Zung, W. W. K. (1974). The measurement of affects: Depression and anxiety. In *Psychological measurement in psychopharmacology. Modern problems of pharmacopsychiatry, Vol. 7*, p. 170–88 (ed. P. Pichot). Karger, Basel.
11. Zung, W. W. K. (1986). Self Rating Depression Scale and Depression Status Inventory. In *Assessment of Depression*, p. 221–31 (ed. N. Sartorius and T. A. Ban). Springer, Heidelberg.

12. Zung, W.W. (1990). The role of rating scales in the identification and management of the depressed patient in the primary care setting. *Journal of Clinical Psychiatry*, **51** Suppl, 72–6.
13. Zung, W.W.K. and King, R.E. (1983). Identification and treatment of masked depression in a general medical practice. *Journal of Clinical Psychiatry*, **44**, 365–8.
14. Zung, W.W.K. and Zung, E.M. (1986). Use of the Zung self rating depression scale in the elderly. *Clinical Gerontologist*, **5**, 137–48.

Beck Depression Inventory (BDI) (Beck 1961)

Purpose

The BDI is intended to assess the existence and severity of depression for clinical and research purposes. It also highlights any affective, cognitive, motivational, or physiological symptoms which may need immediate attention. It can be used as a screening instrument to detect undiagnosed depression in normal populations, to assess the severity of depression in established cases, and to monitor the effectiveness over time of therapeutic interventions.

Background

The first version of the BDI was published in 1961[4] in an attempt to provide a standard self-rating instrument of depression in patients. Existing measures were felt to be inadequate for a variety of reasons (require professional administration, too narrow or too heterogeneous, unsuitable for psychiatric patients, etc.). Minor amendments have been made since 1961, but the content and structure of the BDI has remained broadly the same as the original version. The form of the BDI is based on the observation that the number of symptoms increases with the severity of depression; the frequency of depressive symptoms progresses in a step-like manner from non-depressed to severely depressed; the more depressed an individual is the more intense a particular symptom is likely to be. The inventory was designed 'to include all symptoms integral to the depressive constellation, and at the same time to provide for grading the intensity of each'.[1] Items for inclusion were derived from clinical observation of the characteristic attitudes and symptoms of depressed patients. Those which appeared specific to depression and consistent with descriptions in the literature were selected. Neither the original paper nor subsequent reviews provide any further information on exactly how items were generated and selected for inclusion.

Description

The BDI consists of 21 items which stress the cognitive rather than affective or somatic symptoms of depression. Each item describes a particular manifestation of depression in the areas particularly of self-esteem, general life satisfaction, mood, relationships with others, appetite and sleep. Items consist of four self-evaluative statements which are scored 0 to 3 to indicate the degree of severity. Total scores are obtained by simply adding the scores on each of the 21 items, without applying any weighting. Where a respondent circles more than one statement, only the highest score is counted for that item. Exhibit 5.2 illustrates six items from the Inventory which cannot be reproduced in its entirety due to copyright restrictions.

Total scores range from 0 to 63. There is no universally applicable cut-off point to represent psychiatric caseness. The authors recommend that cutting points should be varied to suit the particular purposes of a study. Thus lower

---

Exhibit 5.2   Sample Items from The Beck Depession Inventory

(Copyright on The Beck Depression Inventory is held by the Psychological Corporation, 555 Academic Court, San Antonio, Texas 78204-2498, to whom all enquiries relating to reproduction and use should be directed.)

Beck Inventory

Name _____   Date _____

On this questionnaire are groups of statements. Please read each group of statements carefully. Then pick out the one statement in each group which best describes the way you have been feeling the PAST WEEK, INCLUDING TODAY! Circle the number beside the statement you picked. If several statements in the group seem to apply equally well, circle each one. *Be sure to read all the statements in each group before making your choice.*

0 I do not feel like a failure.
1 I feel I have failed more than the average person.
2 As I look back on my life, all I can see is a lot of failures.
3 I feel I am a complete failure as a person.

0 I have not lost interest in other people.
1 I am less interested in other people than I used to be.
2 I have lost most of my interest in other people.
3 I have lost all of my interest in other people.

0 I get as much satisfaction out of things as I used to.
1 I don't enjoy things the way I used to.
2 I don't get real satisfaction out of anything anymore.
3 I am dissatisfied or bored with everything.

0 I don't feel I look any worse than I used to.
1 I am worried that I am looking old and unattractive.
2 I feel that there are permanent changes in my appearance that make me look unattractive.
3 I believe that I look ugly.

0 I am no more irritated now than I ever am.
1 I get annoyed or irritated more easily than I used to.
2 I feel irritated all the time now.
3 I don't get irritated at all by the things that used to irritate me.

0 I can sleep as well as usual.
1 I don't sleep as well as I used to.
2 I wake up 1-2 hours earlier than usual and find it hard to get back to sleep.
3 I wake up several hours earlier than I used to and cannot get back to sleep.

cutting points might be used for a 'normal' population than for a population of psychiatric patients. As a screening device to detect depression among psychiatric patients a cutting point of 13 is recommended,[1] but for screening depression among medical patients a score of 10 has been suggested.[13] For purposes of assessing severity, scores below 14 have been classed as mild, 14 to 20 moderate, and 21 and above severe.[15] However, for general practice studies, Salkind recommends the following classification: no depression 0–10; mild depression 11–17; moderate depression 18–23; severe depression 23 and above.[11]

A 13-item short version of the BDI has been developed, specifically for screening non-psychiatric populations in a family practice setting.[2] This was designed to have a high correlation with scores on the full version and with clinicians' ratings of depression[6] and was used in some studies.[12,16] However, it is not currently available. A revised version has also been published.[3,5] In this section, attention has been restricted to the standard 21-item version.

Administration and acceptability

The original version was intended to be administered by an interviewer to respondents, but most users now seem to treat it as a straightforward self-completion instrument which does not require supervision. It is relatively economical, taking ten minutes to complete (short version five minutes) and producing data which can be easily interpreted and analysed. Most respondents can complete the BDI without difficulty. Studies of therapeutic interventions have reported that the BDI can be repeated at one-week intervals without inducing boredom or resentment,[10] although in these circumstances it would be necessary to control for the effects of repeat testing.

Reliability and validity

Both the reliability and the validity of the BDI have been extensively tested in a wide variety of circumstances.[1] A review published in 1986[15] reports over 500 published studies which have used the measure, many of which have contributed to information on reliability and/or validity. Indeed there has been a trend for the BDI to be included in other psychological test batteries as a touchstone against which to compare assessments derived from other measures.

Test–retest reliability results are good, although the time period used might be expected to affect this. Thus, if respondents are asked how they feel today, it is likely that stability on retest will be much lower than if they are asked how they have been feeling during the past week. Tests of internal consistency using a split half method and item consistency have produced excellent results.[15]

Validation studies have been carried out on in-patients, out-patients and 'normal' populations. BDI scores correlate well with independent clinical judgements of depression and other psychometric instruments. It is also claimed to be predictive of outcome, able to discriminate between different levels of severity of depression, and appears to be sensitive to change associated with pharmacological trials and other psychotherapeutic techniques.[15] However, a recent study in patients with rheumatoid arthritis showed that the BDI had poor discriminant validity.[7] The authors suggested that the BDI is a measure of general distress, but is unable to distinguish among degrees of anxiety and depression.

The factor structure of the BDI has been examined in a number of studies, typically reporting four or more factors. However, a recent examination of the factor structure in a large predominantly male sample suggested that it is not factorially complex.[8] Rather, it measures depressive severity in a nearly unidimensional manner, relying heavily on cognitive symptoms. The authors suggest that it may be relatively weak as a measure of the vegetative symptoms of depression.

Some authors have criticized the validity of the BDI for its lack of items dealing with somatic components of depression.[16] They have suggested modifications to items dealing with sleep, appetite, and weight as well as the inclusion of additional items. However, Beck has not accepted these changes.[14] It has been argued that the relative weakness on somatic components is a positive advantage for use in non-psychiatric populations, where somatic symptoms may be attributable to physical illness.

Populations/service-settings

Although originally developed for use with adult psychiatric patients, the BDI has been used extensively with normal and physically ill populations (for a review of applications see Steer *et al.* 1986[15]). It has been specifically recommended for use in general practice.[11,9] Apart from ease of administration, the relatively small contribution of somatic symptoms to total scores seems to make it particularly suitable for clinical or research purposes in which patients might be expected to be also suffering from physical illness. There is, however, a need for more evidence concerning population norms, appropriate cut-off points, and applications in various groups within the population. Large between-study variations in family practice studies using the BDI indicate a need to collect normative data for the population to be studied.[18] There is some evidence that BDI factor structures may vary for men and women.[17]

Comments

The BDI is one of the most widely used assessments of the existence and severity of depression. Although it has some critics, it is so well established as to require serious consideration for any study requiring a self-evaluation measure of depression. It seems particularly well suited to the needs of general practice, both because of its brevity and because it has been extensively used in non-hospital populations. However, more evidence is needed concerning population norms, and applicability to different groups.

References

1. Beck, A. T. and Beamesderfer, A. (1974). Assessment of depression: The depression inventory. In *Psychological measurements in psychopharmacology. Modern problems in pharmacopsychiatry*, Vol. 7. (ed. Pichot, P.). Karger, Basel.
2. Beck, A. T. and Beck, R. W. (1972). Screening depressed patients in family practice. *Postgraduate Medicine*, **Dec**, 81-5.
3. Beck, A., and Steer, R. (1984). Internal consistencies of the original and revised Beck Depression Inventory. *Journal of Clinical Psychology*, **40**, 1365-7.
4. Beck, A. T., Ward, C. H., Mendelson, M., Mock, J., and Erbaugh, J. (1961). An inventory for measuring depression. *Archives of General Psychiatry*, **4**, 561-71.
5. Beck, A., Rush, J., Shaw, B., and Emery, G. (1979). *Cognitive therapy of depression*. Guilford Press, New York.
6. Beck, A. T., Rial, W. Y. and Rickels, K. (1974). Short form of depression inventory: Cross validation. *Psychological Reports*, **34**, 1184-6.
7. Hagglund, K. J., Roth, D. L., Haley, W. E., and Alarcon G. S. (1989). Discriminant and convergent validity of self-report measures of affective distress in patients with rheumatoid arthritis. *Journal of Rheumatology*, **16**, 1428-32.
8. Louks, J., Hayne, C., and Smith, J. (1989). Replicated factor structure of the Beck Depression Inventory. *Journal of Nervous Mental Disease,* **177**, 473-9.
9. Rawnsley, K. (1968). The early diagnosis of depression. *Early Diagnosis, Paper 4*. Office of Health Economics, London.
10. Rush, A. J., Beck, A. T., Kovacs, M., and Hollon, S. (1977). Comparative efficacy of cognitive therapy and pharmacotherapy in the treatment of depressed outpatients. *Cognitive Therapy and Research*, **1**, 117-37.
11. Salkind, M. R. (1969). Beck Depression Inventory in general practice. *Journal of the Royal College of General Practitioners*, **18**, 267-71.
12. Scogin, R., Beutler, L., Corbishley, A., and Hamblin, D. (1988). Reliability and validity of the short form Beck Depression Inventory with older adults. *Journal of Clinical Psychology*, **44**, 853-7.
13. Scwab, J. J., Bialow, M., Brown, J. M. and Holzer, C. E. (1967). Diagnosing depression in medical inpatients. *Annals of Internal Medicine*, **67**, 695-707.
14. Steer, R. A. and Beck, A. T. (1985). Modifying the Beck depression inventory: Reply to Vredenburg, Krames and Flett. *Psychological Reports*, **57**, 625-6.
15. Steer, R. A., Beck, A. T. and Garrison, B. (1986). Applications of the Beck depression inventory. In *Assessment of depression*, p. 123-42 (ed. N. Sartorius and T. Ban). Springer, Heidelberg.

16. Vredenburg, K., Krames, L., and Flett, G. L. (1985). Re-examining the Beck Depression Inventory: The long and short of it. *Psychological Reports*, **56**, 767–78.
17. Williamson, M. T. (1987). Sex differences in depression symptoms among adult family medicine patients. *Journal of Family Practice* **25**, 591–4.
18. Williamson, H. A. Jr., and Williamson, M. T. (1989). The Beck Depression Inventory: normative data problems with generalizability. *Family Medicine*, **21**, 58–60.

Montgomery–Asberg Depression Rating Scale (MADRS) (Montgomery and Asberg 1979)

Purpose

The MADRS is designed to evaluate quickly and with precision the severity of depression and changes in severity with treatment. It is not intended as a screening or diagnostic instrument, but for purposes of assessing severity in individuals where the diagnosis of depression is already established. It is thus particularly useful as a means of evaluating treatment outcomes.

Background

The MADRS was developed from the authors' earlier 65-item Comprehensive Psychopathological Rating Scale,[1] by selecting those items which proved most sensitive to change.[4] The objective was to produce a measure which would be both more sensitive to change and relatively economical to administer. This was achieved by selecting those items which occur most frequently in depression, and from these selecting the items which were most sensitive to change, rather than attempting to be comprehensive.

Description

The scale consists of ten items, each rated between 0 and 6 (Exhibit 5.3). Descriptions are provided for only four of the possible ratings on each item, the remaining scores (1,3, and 5) being used for unspecified intermediate points. Ratings are based not only on responses from the patient, but also on any other available information (e.g. observations, nursing staff, relatives, etc.). The items do not include somatic symptoms which might result from physical illness. The time period covered in making an assessment is not specified, and will therefore depend on the requirements of the particular study.

Total scores are constructed by simply adding the scores on each item, giving a range between 0 and 60. A recent study has offered the following grouping of scores: 0–6 recovered; 7–9 mild; 20–34 moderate; 35–60

Exhibit 5.3   Montgomery and Asberg Depression Rating Scale

(Adapted, with permission, from Montgomery, S. A. and Asberg, M. (1979). A new depression scale designed to be sensitive to change. *British Journal of Psychiatry*, **134**, 382–9)

1. Apparent sadness

Representing despondency, gloom, and despair, (more than just ordinary transient low spirits) reflected in speech, facial expression, and posture. Rate by depth and ability to brighten up.

- 0 No sadness.
- 2 Looks dispirited but brightens up occasionally.
- 4 Appears sad and unhappy all of the time.
- 6 Extreme and continuous gloom and despondency.

2. Reported sadness

Representing subjectively experienced mood, regardless of whether it is reflected in appearance or not. Includes depressed mood, low spirits, despondency, and the feeling of being beyond help and without hope. Rate according to intensity, duration and the extent to which the mood is influenced by events. Elated mood is scored zero on this item.

- 0 Occasional sadness may occur in the circumstances.
- 2 Predominant feelings of sadnes, but brighter moments occur.
- 4 Pervasive feelings of sadness or gloominess. The mood is still influenced by external circumstances.
- 6 Continuous experience of misery or extreme despondency.

3. Inner tension

Representing feeling of ill-defined discomfort, edginess, inner turmoil, mental tension mounting to panic, dread, and anguish. Rate according to intensity, frequency duration, and the extent of reassurance called for.

- 0 Placid. Only fleeting inner tension.
- 2 Occasional feelings of edginess and ill-defined discomfort.
- 4 Continuous feelings of inner tension, or intermittent panic which the patient can only master with some difficulty.
- 6 Unrelenting dread or anguish. Overwhelming panic.

4. Reduced sleep

Representing a subjective experience of reduced duration or depth of sleep compared to the subject's own normal pattern when well.

- 0 Sleeps as usual.
- 2 Slight difficulty dropping off to sleep or slightly reduced, light, or fitful sleep.
- 4 Sleep reduced or broken by at least two hours.
- 6 Less than two or three hours sleep.

5. Reduced appetite

Representing the feeling of a loss of appetite compared with when well.

- 0 Normal or increased appetite.
- 2 Slightly reduced appetite.
- 4 No appetite. Food is tasteless. Need to force oneself to eat.
- 6 Must be forced to eat. Food refusal.

Exhibit 5.3 (continued)

6. Concentration difficulties
Representing difficulties in collecting one's thoughts mounting to incapacitating lack of concentration. Rate according to intensity, frequency, and degree of incapacity produced.

    0   No difficulties in concentrating.
    2   Occasional difficulties in collecting one's thoughts.
    4   Difficulties in concentrating and sustaining thought which interferes with reading or conversation.
    6   Incapacitating lack of concentration.

7. Lassitude
Representing difficulty in getting started or slowness in initiating and performing everyday activites.

    0   Hardly any difficulty in getting started. No sluggishness.
    2   Difficulties in starting activities.
    4   Difficulties in starting simple routine activities which are carried out only with effort.
    6   Complete inertia. Unable to start activity without help.

8. Inability to feel
Representing the subjective experience of reduced interest in the surrounding, or activities that normally give pleasure. The ability to react with adequate emotion to circumstances or people is reduced. Distinguish from lassitude.

    0   Normal interest in the surroundings and in other people.
    2   Reduced ability to enjoy usual interests. Reduced ability to feel anger.
    4   Loss of interest in the surroundings. Loss of feelings for friends and acquaintances.
    6   The experience of being emotionally paralysed, inability to feel anger or grief, and a complete or even painful failure to feel for close relatives and friends.

9. Pessimistic thoughts
Representing thoughts of guilt, inferiority, self-reproach, sinfulness, remorse, and ruin.

    0   No pessimistic thoughts.
    2   Fluctuating ideas of failure, self-reproach, or self-depreciation.
    4   Persistent self-accusations, or definite but still rational ideas of guilt or sin. Increasingly pessimistic about the future.
    6   Delusions of ruin, remorse, and unredeemable sin. Absurd self accusations.

10. Suicidal thoughts
Representing the feeling that life is not worth living, that a natural death would be welcome, suicidal thoughts, and preparations for suicide. Suicidal attempts should not in themselves influence the rating.

    0   Enjoys life or takes it as it comes.
    2   Weary of life. Only fleeting suicidal thoughts.
    4   Much better off dead. Suicidal thoughts are common, and suicide is considered as a possible solution, but without specific plans or intention.

Exhibit 5.3 (continued)

---

    6   Explicit plans for suicide when there is an opportunity. Active preparations for suicide.

Each item can also be scored 1,3,5, when assessment is respectively between 0 and 2, 2 and 4, and 4 and 6.

The rating should be based on a clinical interview moving from broadly phrased questions about symptoms to more detailed ones which allow a precise rating of severity. The rater must decide whether the rating lies on the defined scale steps (0,2,4,6) or between them (1,3,5).

It is important to remember that it is only on rare occasions that a depressed patient is encountered who cannot be rated on the items in the scale. If definite answers cannot be elicited from the patient all relevant clues as well as information from other sources should be used as a basis for the rating in line with customary clinical practice.

The scale may be used for any time interval between ratings, be it weekly or otherwise but this must be recorded.

---

severe,[7] but the most widely used cut-off points appear to be 12 for mild depression, 24 for moderate, and 35 for severe.[5]

Administration and acceptability

Ratings should be made on the basis of a clinical interview, but this can be undertaken by a nurse or general practitioner as well as by a psychiatrist. Training in the use of the scale is, however, desirable. Interviews take between 20 and 60 minutes depending on the patient's condition and the ability of the rater. In comparison with some psychiatric rating scales the instrument is brief and easily administered with clear instructions about the allocation of scores. Nevertheless, in terms of professional time, it is expensive to administer and would be difficult to incorporate into routine clinical practice. It is, therefore, more likely to find applications as a research instrument.

Reliability and validity

Evidence of both reliability and validity from a number of studies is good. Inter-rater reliability is particularly important with a measure such as the MADRS, which calls upon raters to form judgements based upon a loosely structured interview. The authors report very high levels of inter-rater reliability,[4] and although a subsequent study showed lower levels of agreement, they remained satisfactory.[3] No evidence of test–retest reliability has been produced, but there is good evidence of internal consistency. However, Davidson and colleagues suggest that the items dealing with appetite, sleep, and suicidal thoughts do not correlate well with the rest of the scale.[3]

Validation studies have been carried out on both hospital in-patients and out-patients. Several studies have compared the MADRS with the Hamilton Rating Scale for Depression.[2-4] These have demonstrated both concurrent validity and greater sensitivity to change in the MADRS. Davidson has also shown that the scale is able to discriminate between endogenous and non-endogenous depression.[3] Lastly, Snaith and Taylor in a study of concurrent validity, suggested the removal of the two items dealing with psychic anxiety and insomnia in order to improve its ability to distinguish depression from anxiety without impairing its validity as a depression scale.[6]

Populations/service settings

The MADRS is not a population screening tool. Its main application will be in therapeutic trials with patients having an established depressive illness. Although it has been used mainly in a hospital setting, the fact that it has been used with both in-patients and out-patients suggests that it would also be applicable in primary health care.

Comments

The MADRS is unlikely to be widely used in primary health care because of the time taken to administer it and the training requirement. However, it may be of value for research into the treatment of depression in general practice. Reliability and validity seem to be well established and, most importantly, it is responsive to change as a result of treatment. There is a need for further research into its reliability and validity when used by non-psychiatrists out-side hospital with patients suffering varying degrees of severity of depression.

References

1. Asberg, M., Montgomery, S., Perris, C., Schalling, D., and Sedval, G. (1978). A comprehensive psychopathological rating scale. *Acta Psychiatrica Scandinavica*, **271**, Suppl, 5–27.
2. Davidson, J.R.T. and Turnbull, C.D. (1984). The importance of dose in isocarboxazid therapy. *Journal of Clinical Psychiatry*, **45**, 49–52.
3. Davidson, J., Turnbull, C.D., Strickland, R., Miller, R., and Graves, K. (1986). The Montgomery–Asberg depression scale: reliability and validity. *Acta Psychiatrica Scandinavica*, **73**, 544–8.
4. Montgomery, S.A. and Asberg, M. (1979). A new depression scale designed to be sensitive to change. *British Journal of Psychiatry*, **134**, 382–9.
5. Montgomery, S.A., Montgomery, D., Baldwin, D., and Green, M. (1989). Intermittent 3-day depressions and suicidal behaviour. *Neuropsychobiology*, **22**, 128–34.
6. Snaith, R.P. and Taylor, C.M. (1985). Rating scales for depression and anxiety: A current perspective. *British Journal of Clinical Pharmacology*, **19**, 175–205.
7. Snaith, R.P., Harrop, F.M., Newby, D.A. and Teale, C. (1986). Grade scores

of the Montgomery–Asberg depression and the clinical anxiety scales. *British Journal of Psychiatry*, **148**, 599–601.

Hospital Anxiety and Depression (HAD) Scale (Zigmond and Snaith)

Purpose

The HAD Scale is designed to detect the presence and severity of relatively mild degrees of mood disorder likely to be found in non-psychiatric hospital out-patients. It is intended both as a screening device and to chart progress over time.

Background

Because many measures of mood disorder include somatic symptoms and provide insufficient distinction between one mood disorder and another, the authors felt that there was a need for a new self-completion rating scale which could be used in non-psychiatric settings. The HAD Scale specifically excludes reference to symptoms such as dizziness and headaches which might be attributable to physical illness. Items for the depression sub-scale concentrate on the concept of anhedonia (loss of pleasure response) since 'this is probably the central psychopathological feature of that form of depression which responds well to anti-depressant drug treatment'.[7] Items for the anxiety sub-scale were chosen from a study of the appropriate section of the Present State Examination[6] and the authors' own research into the psychic manifestations of anxiety neurosis.

Description

The scale consists of fourteen items, seven of which relate to depression and seven to anxiety (Exhibit 5.4). Each item provides four response categories ordered in terms of frequency or severity. The wording of questions and response categories is positive (i.e. 0–3) for six items and negative (i.e. 3–0) for the remaining eight. Responses relate to feelings during the past week and respondents are encouraged to give their immediate reaction, rather than a carefully considered answer. Item scores for each sub-scale are summed and indicate non-cases (7 or less) doubtful cases (8 to 10), and definite cases (11 plus).[7] Although a threshold score of 8 was suggested as a means of including all possible cases, a more recent study carried out in general practice advocated using a score of 11 because of the large proportion (51 per cent) of cases identified using the lower threshold score.[3] However, this study summed the two subscales, contrary to the original authors' recommendations.

Exhibit 5.4   Hospital Anxiety and Depression Scale

Items labelled 'D' are summed to produce the depression score and those labelled 'A' are summed to produce the anxiety score. Scores and labels are not printed on the self-administered questionnaire. (Reproduced, with permission, from Zigmond, A. S. and Snaith, R. P. (1983). The Hospital Anxiety and Depression Scale. Acta Psychiatra Scandinavica, **67**, 361–70.)

Name: _____   Date _____

Doctors are aware that emotions play an important part in most illnesses. If your doctor knows about these feelings he will be able to help you more.

This questionnaire is designed to help your doctor to know how you feel. Read each item and place a firm tick in the box opposite the reply which comes closest to how you have been feeling in the past week.

Don't take too long over your replies: your immediate reaction to each item will probably be more accurate than a long thought-out response.

Tick only one box in each section.

I feel tense or 'wound up':   **A**
Most of the time	3
A lot of the time	2
Time to time/occasionally	1
Not at all	0

I feel as if I am slowed down: **D**
Nearly all the time	3
Very often	2
Sometimes	1
Not at all	0

I still enjoy the things I used to enjoy: **D**
Definitely as much	0
Not quite so much	1
Only a little	2
Hardly at all	3

I get a sort of frightened feeling like 'butterflies' in the stomach: **A**
Not at all	0
Occasionally	1
Quite often	2
Very often	3

I get a sort of frightened feeling as if something awful is about to happen: **A**
Very definitely and quite badly	3
Yes but not too badly	2
A little but it doesn't worry me	1
Not at all	0

I have lost interest in my appearance   **D**
Definitely	3
I don't take so much care as I should	2
I may not take quite as much care	1
I take just as much care as ever	0

I can laugh and see the funny side of things: **D**
As much as I always could	0
Not quite so much now	1
Definitely not so much now	2
Not at all	3

I feel restless as if I have to be on the move: **A**
Very much indeed	3
Quite a lot	2
Not very much	1
Not at all	0

Exhibit 5.4 (continued)

Worrying thoughts go through my mind:		A
A great deal of the time		3
A lot of the time		2
From time to time but not too often		1
Only occasionally		0

I look forward with enjoyment to things:		D
As much as ever I did		0
Rather less than I used to		1
Definitely less than I used to		2
Hardly at all		3

I feel cheerful:	D	
Not at all	3	
Not often	2	
Sometimes	1	
Most of the time	0	

I get sudden feelings of panic:		A
Very often indeed		3
Quite often		2
Not very often		1
Not at all		0

I can sit at ease and feel relaxed:		A
Definitely		0
Usually		1
Not often		2
Not at all		3

I can enjoy a good book or radio or TV programme:		D
Often		0
Sometimes		1
Not often		2
Very seldom		3

(Copies available from Dr R. P. Snaith, Department of Psychiatry, Clinical Services Building, St James University Hospital, Leeds LS9 7TF.)

Administration and acceptability

The scale is self-administered and can be completed in approximately two minutes. It is therefore ideal for use in a waiting room and can be easily incorporated into clinical practice. Response rates are very high and efforts have been made to ensure that the questions do not imply that patients are suffering from psychiatric disorders.

Reliability and validity

There is less evidence of the reliability of the HAD Scale than of its validity. The authors report satisfactory internal consistency,[7] but do not appear to have assessed test–retest reliability. The scale was initially validated against a 20-minute psychiatric assessment. Against this standard, the depression sub-scale yielded only 1 per cent false positives and 1 per cent false negatives. Figures for the anxiety scale were 5 per cent and 1 per cent. Using the same data, the scales were also shown to be satisfactory measures of severity and to differentiate between anxiety and depression. Subsequent evidence has confirmed the validity of the HAD Scale when tested against other measures of anxiety and depression.[2,4,5] In a comparison of the HAD Scale and the General Health Questionaire (GHQ) (see next section), Wilkinson and Barczak showed that the HAD Scale performed better than the GHQ in identifying cases against the criterion of a research psychiatric interview.[5] There seems to be no evidence concerning the responsiveness of the scale to treatment effects, although the authors do recommend its use as a means of monitoring progress over time in clinical practice.

Populations/service settings

The HAD Scale was originally developed for use in non-psychiatric hospital out-patient settings and has been used in general medical out-patient clinics[7] and in a clinic for inflammatory bowel disease.[1] The authors, however, see no reason why it should not be used in the community or primary health care. A survey of recently published papers shows that the HAD Scale has been used in a wide variety of patients suffering from chronic conditions (e.g. rheumatoid arthritis, respiratory problems, inflammatory bowel disease, cancer, myocardial infarction, and early dementia). In one study, the HAD Scale was compared with the GHQ in general practice and was preferred to the GHQ as a means of identifying cases.[5] However, a further general practice study suggested that the scale might identify more cases than could be reasonably followed up.[3] It is recommended for use with adults between the ages of 16 and 65 years. Further research is required before it could be recommended for use with elderly patients.

Comments

Amid the plethora of well established measures of anxiety and depression, it might seem that there is little reason to produce another. However, the relatively recent HAD Scale does seem to be a very useful addition to those already available, particularly for primary health care. Its brevity, the fact that it is self-administered, and the absence of reference to somatic symptoms which might be attributable to physical illness make it well suited to the demands of primary health care. Its focus is relatively narrow, but anxiety and depression are by far the most common problems seen in primary health care. It is therefore well worth consideration, both as an adjunct to clinical practice and as a research instrument. As with all relatively new instruments there is a need for further testing of reliability and validity, although results so far published seem very encouraging.

References

1. Andrews, H., Barczak, P., and Allan, R. (1987). Psychiatric illness in patients with inflammatory bowel disease. *Gut*, **12**, 1600-4.

2. Aylard, P. R. *et al.* (1987). A validation study of three anxiety and depression self assessment scales. *Journal of Psychosomatic Research*, **31**, 261–8.
3. Dowell, A.C., and Biran, L.A. (1990). Problems in using the hospital anxiety and depression scale for screening patients in general practice. *British Journal of General Practice*, **40**, 27–8.
4. Snaith, R.P., and Taylor, C.M. (1985). Rating scales for depression and anxiety: A current perspective. *British Journal of Clinical Pharmacology*, **19**, Suppl 175–203.
5. Wilkinson, M.J.B., and Barczak, P. (1988). Psychiatric screening in general practice: comparison of the general health questionnaire and the hospital anxiety depression scale. *Journal of the Royal College of General Practitioners*, **38**, 311–13.
6. Wing, J.K., Cooper, J.E., and Sartorious, N. (1974). *The measurement and classification of psychiatric symptoms*. Cambridge University Press, London.
7. Zigmond, A.S. and Snaith, R.P. (1983). The hospital anxiety and depression scale. *Acta Psychiatrica Scandinavica*, **67**, 361–70.

General Health Questionnaire (GHQ) (Goldberg 1972)

Purpose

The GHQ is designed to detect non-psychotic psychiatric illness/affective disorder in a community setting. It is thus not intended to pick up functional psychoses, such as schizophrenia or psychotic depression, although experience has suggested that these conditions can be detected by the instrument. Neither is it intended to provide a firm diagnosis or an assessment of severity. The GHQ identifies potential cases who should then be examined using a more conventional psychiatric interview. However, despite these caveats, the GHQ has been widely used to estimate prevalence of affective disorder and to assess severity. Although originally designed for use in population surveys of psychiatric morbidity, it has been extensively used as a screening instrument in clinical practice, as an aid to clinical teaching, and for the assessment of unmet needs.

Background

The instrument was developed during the 1960s and first published in 1972.[1] It focuses on breaks in normal functioning, rather than lifelong traits, and concerns itself with inability to carry out normal 'healthy' functions and the appearance of new phenomena of a distressing nature.[4] It is based on the principle that psychological distress depends on a critical number of key symptoms, rather than any particular symptom. The emphasis on conditions appropriate to general medical care resulted in a focus on 'just clinically significant psychiatric illness'.[1]

The initial pool of statements from which items for the GHQ were selected was derived from existing instruments and clinical experience. Statements were selected to represent four main areas; depression, anxiety, objectively observable behaviour (including social impairment), and hypochondriasis. Criteria for initial selection included ability to reflect changing psychological functioning and universality (i.e. all items must be applicable to the entire population). The selection yielded 140 items which were then applied in a calibration exercise involving severely ill, mildly ill, and 'normal' people. Factor analysis of the results showed one general factor (labelled 'severity of illness') which accounted for 46 per cent of the variance in scores. On the basis of this work 60-items were selected for inclusion in the final version.[2] Although the final 60-item version remains intact, a number of variants have been developed over the years. Some of these are shorter than the original, others have introduced modifications to the wording, response categories, and scoring.

Description

Although Goldberg has recommended using the full 60-item version of the GHQ because of its superior validity, shorter versions have commonly been used in both research and clinical practice. Twelve- and thirty-item versions were designed to exclude those items which tended to be endorsed by physically ill respondents. A 28-item version with four sub-scales (somatic symptoms, anxiety and insomnia, social dysfunction, severe depression) was developed using factor analysis.[4] The choice of which version to use for a particular application will depend on a variety of factors. The excellent *User's Guide to the General Health Questionnaire*[5] provides a detailed account of the different versions and advice on which to choose.

Exhibit 5.5 shows sample items from the 28-item version. All items have four response categories of the general form: the same, worse than usual, much worse than usual. An even number of categories was chosen in order to avoid a tendency to tick the middle category. The time period covered is the past few weeks and the emphasis throughout is on departures from usual state. A recent paper reported the development of a 'worst ever' version of the GHQ which changed the wording to elicit information about previous episodes of illness.[10]

Although four response categories are provided in the standard versions, these are reduced to a simple distinction between present and absent for the purposes of scoring. Better or same as usual both score 0 and worse or much worse score 1. Goldberg compared this simple method of scoring with a more conventional method (i.e. 0, 1, 2, 3) and with weights applied to individual items, but showed no advantage in the more sophisticated approaches in terms of their ability to discriminate between cases and non-cases.[4] Scores can be interpreted as indicating the severity of psychological disturbance

Exhibit 5.5   Sample items from the 28-item version of the General Health Questionnaire

Please read this carefully:
We should like to know if you have had any medical complaints, and how your health has been in general, *over the past few weeks*. Please answer ALL the questions on the following page simply by underlining the answer which you think most nearly applies to you. Remember that we want to know about present and recent complaints, not those that you had in the past.

It is important that you try to answer ALL the questions.

Thank you very much for your cooperation.

Have you recently:
  been feeling run-down and out of sorts?
  felt that you are playing a useful part in things?
  thought of the possibility that you might make away with yourself?
  been getting edgy and bad-tempered?

Response categories:	All items have four response categories of the same general form but with slightly different wording. See *User's Guide*[4] for details.
Sub-scales:	somatic symptoms; anxiety and insomnia; social dysfunction; severe depression.

on a continuum. More commonly, they are used to screen cases by applying cut-offs. For the 28-item version the recommended cut off is 4/5. This version also permits scoring of four sub-scales; somatic symptoms, anxiety and insomnia, social dysfunction, and severe depression (see Exhibit 5.5).

There are no universally accepted cut-off points for defining psychiatric 'caseness'. Apart from the particular version chosen, the cut-off point will depend on the purpose for which it is required and the population in which it is being used. The user will have to make decisions about the relative importance of sensitivity (the probability that a 'true case' will be identified) and specificity (the probability that a 'true normal' will be correctly identified) in determining the appropriate cut-off point.

An alternative method of scoring, known as the CGHQ, has been developed and shown to produce a less skewed distribution of scores.[6] This method adopts different scoring for positive and negative items and is claimed to make it more likely to detect chronic disorders. The relative advantages of alternative methods of scoring are discussed in the *User's Guide*.[5]

Administration and acceptability

All versions of the GHQ are self-administered and take from two minutes for the 12-item version to ten-minutes for the 60-item version to complete. It seems to be well accepted by patients, achieving very high response rates, despite the fact that some of the areas covered might appear sensitive. It is easily administered by receptionists to patients awaiting a consultation, although care should be taken to ensure confidentiality.

Reliability and validity

Less attention has been devoted to reliability than to validity, but small-scale studies of the reliability of the 60-item version have been carefully conducted. Internal consistency was demonstrated by using the split-half technique, which showed a high correlation between the two halves. Subsequent investigations of internal consistency have yielded high alpha coefficients for the 12-, 30-, and 60-item versions.[5] Test–retest reliability is more problematic for a measure which focuses on problems which may well be transient. Goldberg overcame this problem by comparing only those cases where an independent assessment showed no change in condition between the two administrations of the GHQ. Under these conditions test–retest reliability appeared to be very good.[2] However, evidence from general population surveys suggests that there may be a significant retest effect resulting in lower scores on repeat administration.[7] A more recent study has demonstrated a similar retest effect in clinical settings.[9]

Many investigators have explored the factor structure of different versions of the GHQ.[5] The number of factors responsible for variance in scores reflects the number of items, so that studies of the 60-item version have identified up to 19 factors whilst studies of the 12 item version have identified only two or three. The 28-item version was developed on the basis of the results of principal components analysis and contains four sub-scales.

The validity of the GHQ has been well researched in a wide variety of settings and cultures. More than 300 references to the GHQ are reviewed in a recently published *Users' Guide*,[5] which is essential reading for anyone interested in using the GHQ. The original validation was carried out on patients of an urban general practice and out-patients at a London teaching hospital.[1] Subsequently more than 70 studies have reported on validity and 40 of these have been carried out in primary health care. The GHQ has most commonly been compared with standard psychiatric interviews to provide a measure of criterion validity. With few exceptions tests of validity have yielded high correlations between GHQ scores and psychiatric diagnoses. Predictive validity has been established in terms of subsequent general practitioner consultations, post-operative distress, and death following myocardial infarction, despite the fact that it was never intended to have predictive validity. Goldberg reports that sensitivity and specificity are high, resulting in an overall misclassification rate of only 10 per cent for the 60-item version and 14 per cent for the 28-item version.[1,4] Where misclassification occurs, false positives will usually be people suffering transient disorders likely to remit spontaneously, and false negatives will be a combination of those suffering from longstanding complaints and those unwilling to report symptoms. Despite the generally very positive results of research on the sensitivity of the GHQ, Tarnopolovsky and colleagues[14] suggested that sensitivity may be lower than that reported by Goldberg and others. This is supported in a recent comparison of the GHQ and the Mental Health Inventory,[15] in which the MHI is shown to be more sensitive in detecting mental disorders in general and anxiety in particular.

One of the most common criticisms of the validity of the GHQ as a means of detecting psychiatric illness is that it fails to detect instances of chronic conditions because of its emphasis on recent change. The CGHQ scoring system was designed to overcome this problem. Although subsequent investigations have produced some evidence that the CGHQ may be more sensitive it is by no means clear that it has a substantial advantage over the original system.[8,13]

It should be noted that the GHQ was never intended to be used as a measure of severity or as a means of measuring treatment effects. This has not, however, prevented its being used in this way, despite the absence of evidence that it is responsive to clinically significant change. Indeed the evidence that there may be a substantial retest effect should indicate a need for extreme caution in interpreting changes over time.[9]

Populations/client groups/service settings

The GHQ is intended primarily for use in community settings and is particularly well suited for use with patients consulting general practitioners or other primary health care professionals. It has also been used extensively by epidemiologists and social psychiatrists in survey work. It is suitable for use with all adults, although there seem to have been few studies on populations of elderly people. It has been used successfully in many different countries and seems to be applicable to different cultural groups.

For any particular application the potential user should consider evidence on reliability and validity relevant to the particular context, and which version might be most appropriate. The shorter versions are likely to be favoured for use among patients consulting in primary health care, because they exclude those items dealing with somatic symptoms which may be attributable to physical illness. It has been suggested that the use of the GHQ in clinical general practice could substantially increase the sensitivity of general practitioners to minor psychiatric disorder.[3,17] However, a recently published comparison of the GHQ with the HAD Scale (see p. 90) recommends the latter for use in general practice.[16] Another study showed that use of the GHQ in a primary care setting led to only marginal effects on overall detection and had no impact on management.[11]

Comments

The GHQ is highly recommended as a reliable and valid method of identifying potential cases of affective disorder. It can also be used to provide some indication of the severity of problems, and the 28-item version can be used to identify in which area problems are concentrated. However, the instrument is somewhat limited in its objectives. In particular, it is intended as a means of identifying problems of recent onset. It will therefore tend to miss people suffering from chronic conditions. Where a measure is required to assess absolute severity of symptoms or to differentiate between conditions, other instruments may be more suitable. But within its design limitations the GHQ is one of the best instruments available as a means of screening for affective disorders. Nevertheless, it should be noted that the value of screening for affective disorder in general practice remains open to question. Indeed, one author has suggested that the routine use of the GHQ and other screening measures runs a real risk of causing distress to patients.[12]

References

1. Goldberg, D.P. (1972). *The detection of psychiatric illness by questionnaire, Maudsley Monograph No. 21.* Oxford University Press, London.
2. Goldberg, D.P. (1978). *Manual of the General Health Questionnaire.* NFER, Windsor .
3. Goldberg, D.P. and Bridges, K. (1987). Screening for psychiatric illness in general practice: the general practitioner versus the screening questionnaire. *Journal of the Royal College of General Practitioners*, **37**, 15–18.
4. Goldberg, D.P. and Hillier, V.F. (1979). A scaled version of the General Health Questionnaire. *Psychological Medicine*, **9**, 139–45.
5. Goldberg, D.P. and Williams, P. (1988). *Users' Guide to the General Health Questionnaire.* NFER-Nelson, Windsor.
6. Goodchild, M.E. and Duncan-Jones, P. (1985). Chronicity and the General Health Questionnaire. *British Journal of Psychiatry*, **146**, 56–61.

7. Henderson, S. H., Byrne, D. G. and Duncan-Jones, P. (1981). *Neurosis and the Social Environment*. Academic Press, Sydney.
8. Huppert, F. A., Gore, M., and Elliott, B. J. (1988). The value of an improved scoring system (CGHQ) for the General Health Questionnaire in a representative community sample. *Psychological Medicine*, **18**, 1001–6.
9. Ormel, J., Koeter, M. W., and Van den Brink, W. (1989). Measuring change with the General Health Questionnaire (GHQ). The problem of retest effects. *Social Psychiatry Psychiatric Epidemiology*, **24**, 227–32.
10. Power, M. J. (1988) The 'worst ever' version of the General Health Questionnaire. *Journal of Clinical Psychology*, **44**(2), 215–16.
11. Shapiro, S., German, P. S., Skinner, E. A., Von Korff, M., Turner, R. W., Klein, L. E., *et al.* (1987). An experiment to change detection and management of mental morbidity in primary care. *Medical Care*, **25**, 327–39.
12. Stoate, H. G. (1989). Can health screening damage your health? *Journal of the Royal College of General Practitioners*, **39**, 193–5.
13. Surtees, P. G. (1987). Psychiatric disorder in the community and the General Health Questionnaire. *British Journal of Psychiatry*, **150**, 828–35.
14. Tarnopolovsky, A., Hand, D. J., McLean, E. K., Roberts, H., and Wiggins, R. D. (1979). Validity and uses of a screening questionnaire (GHQ) in the community. *British Journal of Psychiatry*, **134**, 508–15.
15. Weinstein, M. C., Berwick, D. M., Goldman, P. A., Murphy, J. M., and Barsky, A. J. (1989). A comparison of three psychiatric screening tests using receiver operating characteristic (ROC) analysis. *Medical Care*, **27**, 593–607.
16. Wilkinson, M. J. B., and Barczak, P. (1988). Psychiatric screening in general practice: comparison of the general health questionnaire and the hospital anxiety depression scale. *Journal of the Royal College of General Practitioners*, **38**, 311–13.
17. Wright, A. F. and Perini A. F. (1987). Hidden psychiatric illness: use of the General Health Questionnaire in general practice. *Journal of the Royal College of General Practitioners*, **37**, 164–7.

The Mental Health Inventory (MHI) (Ware and colleagues 1979)

Purpose

The MHI is a measurement of psychological distress and well-being, rather than mental illness defined in clinical terms. It was developed for use in population surveys, to identify unmet needs for care, predict the use of mental and general health care services, and assess the psychological health of populations. It was not intended to be used for the assessment of individuals or the measurement of the effects of specific treatments over time.

Background

The MHI was developed as part of the battery of measures to be used in the Rand Health Insurance Study (HIS) funded by the United States Department of Health Education and Welfare.[7] The HIS was designed to determine the effects of different health care funding systems on demand for services, health status, and patient satisfaction. Because the battery of measures included instruments to measure physical and social health, the MHI does not extend to the somatic and social components of psychological distress which appear in other instruments. The authors of the MHI regarded the inclusion of physical symptoms and rarely occurring manifestations of psychological distress as a weakness of existing measures. They therefore excluded physical symptoms and extended the definition of mental health to include psychological well-being. To reflect the multidimensional nature of psychological well-being, they included five factors; anxiety, depression, loss of behavioural/emotional control, general positive affect, and emotional ties.[5] The inclusion of positive feelings was intended to improve the precision of the measure by distinguishing among the substantial proportion of people who receive 'perfect' scores on negative distress measures.

Items for inclusion in the MHI were selected from a variety of existing measures. Fifteen were drawn from Dupuy's General Wellbeing Schedule (see McDowell and Newell[3] for a description), after evaluation of the 22-item version. Those items which showed good discriminant validity were retained and those dealing with general health and vitality discarded. To these were added a further 20 items of proven reliability and validity drawn from other scales, including the Beck Depression Inventory (see p. 80) and Costello and Comrey's Anxiety and Depression Scales.[1] Only three items dealing with emotional ties were written specifically for the MHI. The resulting measure was tested on over 5000 respondents at six test sites throughout the USA.[5,6]

Description

The MHI consists of 38 items divided between the five factors; anxiety (10), depression (5), loss of behavioural/emotional control (9), general positive well-being (11), emotional ties (3). All are phrased as questions relating to the past month, so that the measure is not concerned with short-term fluctuations in mood. Sixteen of the items are positively worded and 22 negatively. Two items provide five response categories and all of the remainder provide six. Nineteen are rated on time ('all of the time' to 'none of the time') and a further ten on frequency ('always' to 'never'). Examples of items and response categories are provided in Exhibit 5.6. The full 38-item questionnaire is published in the original Rand Corporation report[6] and reproduced in full by McDowell and Newell.[3]

Each of the sub-scales can be scored and interpreted separately or they can be combined into an overall measure known as the Mental Health Index.[5] This overall measure, however, results in a significant loss of information and accords more weight to distress, because of the imbalance between

---

Exhibit 5.6   Examples of items from the Mental Health Inventory

(From: Ware, J. E., Johnston, S. A., Davies-Avery, A., and Brook, R. H. (1979). *Conceptualization and measurement of health for adults in the Health Insurance Study: Vol. III, Mental health*, Rand Publication No. R-1987/6-HEW. Rand Corporation, Santa Monica)

	Response type
Anxiety	
How much of the time, during the past month, were you able to relax without difficulty?	T
How often during the past month did you find yourself having difficulty trying to calm down?	AN
Depression	
During the past month, how much of the time have you been moody or brooded about things?	T
During the past month, how much of the time have you been in low or very low spirits?	T
Loss of behavioural/emotional control	
During the past month, how often did you feel that you had nothing to look forward to?	AN
How often have you felt like crying, during the past month?	AN
General positive well-being	
During the past month, how much of the time have you generally enjoyed the things you do?	T
When you got up in the morning, this past month, about how often did you expect to have an interesting day?	AN
Emotional ties	
How much of the time have you felt lonely during the past month?	T
During the past month, how much of the time have you felt loved and wanted?	T

Response categories
 T   1. All of the time; 2. Most of the time; 3. A good bit of the time; 4. Some of the time; 5. A little of the time; 6. None of the time
 AN 1. Always; 2. Very often; 3. Fairly often; 4. Sometimes; 5. Almost Never; 6. Never

---

positive and negative items. A better method of constructing combined scores is to calculate separate scores for psychological distress (anxiety, depression, loss of control) and psychological well-being (general positive well-being, emotional ties). Reference standards for each section of the MHI are provided by Veit and Ware.[5]

Weinstein and colleagues refer to an 18 item version of the MHI containing the same five sub-scales: anxiety, depression, loss of behavioural/emotional control, positive affect, and interpersonal ties.[10] This shorter version does not, however, appear to have been published yet. A modified version of the MHI has also been developed for the Medical Outcomes Study (see p. 153).

Administration and acceptability

The MHI is a self-administered questionnaire which can be completed in about ten minutes. It is suitable for use in postal surveys, although it could equally well be administered by an interviewer or used in a waiting room or similar situation. Use of an interviewer would clearly increase costs, as would the practice of paying respondents which was done in the Rand studies. High response rates have been achieved, but it is impossible to know how much response was affected by the payments offered.

Reliability and validity

As with other measures produced for the Rand HIS, an extensive programme of testing and evaluation has been undertaken. The fact that the MHI draws on existing instruments, selecting only items with established reliability and validity gives it added strength. Test–retest reliability has been established over a one-year period and tests of internal consistency have produced good results.[5] However, it is difficult to know quite what interpretation to place on test–retest correlations over such a long period of time. Substantial variations in scores might be expected if the MHI is measuring transient changes in distress and well-being. Evidence of test–retest reliability over a much shorter period would be desirable.

The absence of items dealing with somatic components of psychological distress might be seen as a deficiency, but with this exception there seems good evidence of the content validity of the MHI. Exploration of the factorial structure of the instrument seems to confirm the hypothesized five factors and the higher order positive and negative factors.[5] Evidence of predictive validity is derived from studies of the relationship between MHI scores and use of services. In particular there was a strong association between scores and use of ambulatory mental health services.[9] The relationships between MHI scores and criterion variables such as life satisfaction and severe emotional problems provide some evidence of criterion validity.[8] Despite the fact that the MHI was not designed as a psychiatric screening instrument, a comparison of the MHI with the GHQ (see previous section) showed the 18 item version of the MHI to be significantly better than the 30 item GHQ in detecting mental disorders generally and anxiety disorders in particular.[10] There is as yet no evidence of the responsiveness of the MHI to specific treatments or service provision, although it was not intended that it should be a measure of specific treatment outcomes.

Populations/service settings

The MHI was designed specifically for use in population surveys, and is likely therefore to be most useful for research applications. Its original use as an outcome measure in the Health Insurance Experiment has been followed up by its use in the Medical Outcomes Study. Although not intended for clinical application as a screening tool, the results achieved by Weinstein and colleagues in a primary care population suggest that it may well have applications in this area.[10] Other recent studies have reported its use with post-operative lobectomy patients and patients undergoing dialysis.[2,4] However, the fact that it was designed for use in community surveys suggests that it is likely to be useful in primary care settings.

Comments

The MHI is an attempt to combine the best features of a range of existing instruments in a form which has a sound theoretical basis. The Rand researchers have taken great care to elaborate the conceptual basis for their instruments and to build on existing work rather than reinventing the wheel. As a combined measure of distress and well-being it goes beyond the more medically oriented measures, but has been shown to be a useful predictor of service use. We recommend its use in surveys of needs for services, and as a measure to supplement assessments of physical health where these are the principal focus of interest. Its usefulness as a measure of outcome has not yet been adequately established, and it would be desirable to see further studies of the reliability of the MHI and its responsiveness to clinically significant change.

References

1. Costello, C. G., and Comrey, A. L. (1967). Scales for measuring depression and anxiety. *Journal of Psychiatry*, **66**, 303–13.
2. Hermann, B. P., Wyler, A. R., Ackerman, B., and Rosenthal, T. (1989). Short-term psychological outcome of anterior temporal lobectomy. *Journal of Neurosurgery*, **71**, 327–34.
3. McDowell, I., and Newell, C. (1987). *Measuring health: a guide to rating scales and questionnaires*. Oxford University Press, New York.

4. Petrie, K. (1989). Psychological well-being and psychiatric disturbance in dialysis and renal transplant patients. *British Journal of Medical Psychology*, **62**, 91–6.
5. Veit, C.T. and Ware, J.E. (1983). The structure of psychological distress and wellbeing in general populations. *Journal of Consulting and Clinical Psychology*, **51**, 730–42.
6. Ware, J.E., Johnston, S.A., Davies-Avery, A., and Brook, R.H. (1979). *Conceptualization and measurement of health for adults in the health insurance study: Vol III, mental health.* Rand: Publication No R-1987/3-HEW, Santa Monica.
7. Ware, J.E., Brook, R.H., Davies-Avery, A., Williams, K.N., Stewart, A., Rogers, W.H., Donald, C.A., and Johnston, S.A. (1980). *Conceptualization and measurement of health for adults in the health insurance study: Vol 1, model of health and methodology.* Rand: Publication No R1987/1-HEW, Santa Monica.
8. Ware, J.E., Davies-Avery, A., and Brook, R.H. (1980). *Conceptualization and measurement of health for adults in the health insurance study: Vol IV, analysis of relationships among health status measures.* Rand: Publication No R-1987/6-HEW, Santa Monica.
9. Ware, J.E., Manning, W.G., Duan, N., Wells, K.B., and Newhouse, J.P. (1984). Health status and the use of ambulatory mental health services. *American Psychologist*, **39**, 1090–100.
10. Weinstein, M.C., Berwick, D.M., Goldman, P.A., Murphy, J.M., and Barsky, A.J. (1989). A comparison of three psychiatric screening tests using receiver operating characteristic (ROC) analysis. *Medical Care*, **27**, 593–607.

The Life Satisfaction Index (LSI) (Neugarten and Havighurst 1961)

Purpose

The LSI was designed to measure the psychological well-being of older people with the goal of identifying 'successful ageing'. It was intended to provide a short and easily administered instrument that could be used in studies of older people.

Background

The LSI was developed as part of a larger study of psychological and social factors in ageing carried out in Kansas City.[12] Neugarten and Havighurst criticised single-dimensional approaches to measuring morale, and sought to develop a multidimensional measure that would use the individual's own evaluations as the point of reference, and that would be relatively independent of level of activity or social participation.

The study population was 177 adults aged between 50 and 90 years. Using existing measures of adjustment and morale, the authors developed operational definitions of five components: zest (versus apathy); resolution and fortitude; congruence between desired and achieved goals; positive self concept and mood tone. An individual was regarded as being at the positive end of the continuum of psychological well-being to the extent that she or he: takes pleasure from everyday life; regards life as meaningful; feels she or he has succeeded in achieving major goals; holds a positive self image and maintains a happy and optimistic mood. Each of these components was rated on a five-point scale known as the Life Satisfaction Rating using information derived from open-ended interviews.

Detailed definitions of ratings are provided by Neugarten.[12] Two forms of the LSI (LSIA and LSIB) were then developed by selecting statements derived from the interviews which best discriminated between high and low scorers. These were then further tested, and redundant items discarded. In addition to LSIA and B, subsequent studies have produced the LSIZ[15] and a shorter version of the LSIA.[1]

Description

The original LSIA consists of 20 items of which 12 are positive and 8 negative (Exhibit 5.7). Items cover all of the five components of morale or life satisfaction employed in the Life Satisfaction Rating. Respondents are asked simply to indicate whether they agree or disagree with each statement. Adams' modification proposed deleting items 11 and 14, because the former incorporates two questions (i.e. whether you feel old and whether you are bothered about it) and the latter showed poor ability to discriminate.[1] Wood's LSIZ deleted the seven items asterisked in Exhibit 5.7.[15] In the original version of LSIA, a two-point score rated items 0 for responses indicating dissatisfaction and 1 for satisfaction. However, this system made no allowance for 'undecided' responses, so subsequent studies have tended to use the three-point scoring system shown in Exhibit 5.7. A five-point Likert scale ranging from strongly disagree to strongly agree has also been used.[7]

Liang has devised a model which integrates Bradburn's Affect Balance Scale and the LSIA.[9] This incorporates items from both scales to construct a measure which taps four dimensions of subjective well-being: congruence, happiness, negative affect, and positive affect.

Administration and acceptability

All versions of the LSI are designed to be self-administered. Response rates appear to be acceptable in studies where it has been used as a postal questionnaire. It takes about ten minutes to complete and seems to be acceptable to most respondents. However, it should be remembered that elderly respondents with poor eyesight will have difficulty completing the schedule.

Reliability and validity

A number of studies of different versions of the LSI have produced evidence regarding internal consistency.[1,4,5,13,15] All showed satisfactory

Exhibit 5.7   Life Satisfaction Index A

(Reproduced, with permission, from Neugarten, B. L., Havighurst, R. J. and Tobin, S. S. (1961). The measurement of life satisfaction. Journal of Gerontology, **16**, 141. Scoring system based on Wood, V., Wylie, M. L. and Sheafor, B. (1969). An analysis of a short self-report measure of life satisfaction: correlation with rater judgements. *Journal of Gerontology*, **24**, 467)

Here are some statements about life in general that people feel differently about. Would you read each statement in the list, and if you agree with it, put a check mark in the space under 'Agree'. If you do not agree with a statement, put a check mark in the space under 'Disagree'. If you are not sure one way or the other, put a check mark in the space under '?'.

Please be sure to answer every question on the list.

	Agree	Disagree	?
1. As I grow older, things seem better than I thought they would be.	-2-	-0-	-1-
2. I have gotten more of the breaks in life than most of the people I know.	-2-	-0-	-1-
3. This is the dreariest time of my life.	-0-	-2-	-1-
4. I am just as happy as when I was younger.	-2-	-0-	-1-
*5. My life could be happier than it is now.	-0-	-2-	-1-
6. These are the best years of my life.	-2-	-0-	-1-
7. Most of the things I do are boring and monotonous.	-0-	-2-	-1-
*8. I expect some interesting and pleasant things to happen to me in the future.	-2-	-0-	-1-
9. The things I do are as interesting to me as they ever were.	-2-	-0-	-1-
*10. I feel old and somewhat tired.	-0-	-2-	-1-
*11. I feel my age, but it does not bother me.	-2-	-0-	-1-
12. As I look back on my life, I am fairly well satisfied.	-2-	-0-	-1-
*13. I would not change my past life even if I could.	-2-	-0-	-1-
*14. Compared to other people my age, I've made a lot of foolish decisions in my life.	-0-	-2-	-1-
*15. Compared to other people my age, I make a good appearance.	-2-	-0-	-1-
16. I have made plans for things I'll be doing a month or a year from now.	-2-	-0-	-1-
17. When I think back over my life, I didn't get most of the important things I wanted.	-0-	-2-	-1-
18. Compared to other people, I get down in the dumps too often.	-0-	-2-	-1-
19. I've gotten pretty much what I expected out of life.	-2-	-0-	-1-
20. In spite of what people say, the lot of the average man is getting worse, not better.	-0-	-2-	-1-

* Items deleted from LSIZ.

levels of internal consistency, but levels were highest for the subset of items which loaded on factor analysis. The validity of the LSI has been examined in a variety of studies over the past 30 years. In their original work, the authors reported that scores did not correlate with objective indicators such as sex, age, or socio-economic status, thus confirming the subjective nature of the instrument.[12] However, other studies have not replicated this finding and have shown significant correlations between LSI scores and socio-economic status,[3] income, employment and education,[6] perceived health status and social participation,[5] self-rated health, income and education.[11] Neugarten and her colleagues showed moderate correlations between the LSIA and the longer Life Satisfaction Rating.[12] Other researchers have shown correlations between LSI scores and a variety of other measures of morale and life satisfaction.[10,13] Studies which have looked at the factor structure of the LSI have suggested that three factors, representing congruence, mood tone and optimism, provide the best solution.[1,8] Their empirical findings suggest that although the LSI is a multidimensional measure, the original conceptual formulation was inadequate. However, Thomas and Chambers have argued that it is not simply the conceptual formulation which is inadequate.[14] Comparing LSIA scores with qualitative analysis of life satisfaction, they suggest that the quantitative approaches fail to measure life satisfaction because they lack the ability to place responses in context.

Populations/service settings

The LSI has been used largely with older people, and the authors suggest that it is more successful for people over 65 years of age.[12] Although it has been used with people across a wider age range,[2] the majority of applications have been with people aged 65 years or older. It has been used with many different patient groups and in a variety of service settings, from hospitals to community service. Although we are not aware of it having been used among patients consulting primary health care, there seems no reason why it should not be used.

Comments

The LSI has been in use for nearly thirty years and has been used in many studies of older people. Evidence of reliability and validity from many different studies is good, and studies of the factor structure have produced remarkably consistent results. Nevertheless, it has been criticized, particularly on the grounds that it does not reflect the original conceptual model of life satisfaction proposed by its designers. Precisely what it does measure remains the subject of discussion, and further work is necessary in this area. However, this is more a reflection of the difficulty of developing measures which adequately tap the subtle conceptual distinctions in the field of morale, life satisfaction, happiness, etc., than a failing peculiar to the LSI. Of the available measures of morale or life satisfaction in older people, the LSI is one of the strongest currently available. To the extent that researchers working in primary health care require measures of well-being in elderly people which go beyond mental illness, instruments such as the LSI are worth considering.

References

1. Adams, D. L. (1969). Analysis of a life satisfaction index. *Journal of Gerontology*, **24**, 470-4.
2. Burkhardt, C. S. (1985). The impact of arthritis on quality of life. *Nursing Research*, **34**, 11-16.
3. Cutler, S. J. (1973). Voluntary association, participation and life satisfaction: a cautionary research note. *Journal of Gerontology*, **28**, 479-502.
4. Dobson, C., Powers, E. A., Keith, P. M., and Goudy, W. J. (1979). Anomie self esteem and life satisfaction: interrelationships among three scales of wellbeing. *Journal of Gerontology*, **34**, 569-72.
5. Edwards, J. N. and Klemmack, D. L. (1973). Correlates of life satisfaction: a re-examination. *Journal of Gerontology*, **28**, 479-502.
6. Harris, L. (1975). *The myth and reality of aging in America*. National Council on Aging, Washington D.C.
7. Himmelfarb, S. and Murrell, S. A. (1983). Reliability and validity of five mental health scales in older persons. *Journal of Gerontology*, **38**, 333-9.
8. Hoyt, D. R. and Creech, J. C. (1983). The life satisfaction index: a methodological and theoretical critique. *Journal of Gerontology*, **38**, 111-16.
9. Liang, J. (1985). A structural integration of the Affect Balance Scale and the Life Satisfaction Index A. *Journal of Gerontology*, **40**, 552-61.
10. Lohmann, N. (1977). Correlations of life satisfaction, morale and adjustment measures. *Journal of Gerontology*, **32**, 73-5.
11. Markides, K. S. and Martin, H. W. (1979). A causal model of life satisfaction among the elderly. *Journal of Gerontology*, **34**, 86-93.
12. Neugarten, B. L., Havighurst, R. J., and Tobin, S. S. (1961). The measurement of life satisfaction. *Journal of Gerontology*, **16**, 134-43.
13. Stock, W. A. and Okun, M. A. (1982). The construct validity of life satisfaction among the elderly. *Journal of Gerontology*, **37**, 625-7.
14. Thomas, E. L. and Chambers, K. O. (1989). Phenomenology of life satisfaction among elderly men: quantitative and qualitative views. *Psychology and Aging*, **4**, 284-9.
15. Wood, V., Wylie, M. L., and Sheafor, B. (1969). An analysis of a short self-report measure of life satisfaction: correlation with rater judgements. *Journal of Gerontology*, **24**, 465-9.

Conclusions

The seven measures reviewed in this chapter are some of the most widely used and well validated non-specialist measures available in the field of mental health. The more recent instruments, in particular, reflect careful consideration of the conceptual and methodological problems in this area. Nevertheless, there remains scope for further development, particularly in instruments capable of measuring the outcomes of treatment without the need for a specialist clinical interview. Existing measures have established their ability to identify cases of depression and anxiety, but there is less evidence of their responsiveness to changes perceived to be significant by patients and doctors. It should, however, be noted that even the use of instruments to screen for psychiatric problems in primary health care remains controversial. Despite the numerous references to the value of various instruments used in this way, a recent review of studies using the BDI, SDS, GHQ, MHI, and HADS was critical of those studies which purport to demonstrate the benefits of screening.[1] The authors concluded that 'further research and development is required before the widespread use of even the best test can be recommended as part of the periodic health examination'.[11]

The measures presented here are a very small selection from the large number available. Clearly they will not suit all purposes. In particular we have not included more sophisticated measures of depression or measures designed to tap the concept of psychological well-being. For the former we recommend readers to consult *Assessment of depression* by Sartorius and Ban[3] and for the latter McDowell and Newell's *Measuring health*.[2]

References

1. Feightner, J. W. and Worrall, G. (1990). Early detection of depression by primary care physicians. *Canadian Medical Association Journal*, **142**, 1215–20.
2. McDowell, I. and Newell, C. (1987). Measuring Health: A Guide to Rating Scales and Questionnaires. Oxford University Press, New York.
3. Sartorius, N. and Ban, T. (1986). *Assessment of depression*. Springer, Heidelberg.

6 Measures of social support

Introduction

In our planning for this book, we began with the intention of including a chapter which dealt with measures of social health. In the terms of the WHO definition of health as physical, mental, and social well-being it seemed appropriate to include measures of social health in a volume concerned with measures of need and outcome suitable for primary health care. However, we have, like others in this field,[3] come to regard social well-being as separate from individual health. Social well-being can be seen in terms of social adjustment and social support, in so far as it is related to health and health care. In this chapter we concentrate only on measures of social support.

Although there are a number of measures of social adjustment, we have not included them for two reasons. Firstly, the degree to which the individual is adjusted to his or her social environment does not constitute a measure of need for primary health care, except in so far as failure to adjust arises from other health-related causes. Similarly, success or failure in adjustment cannot be seen as an outcome of primary health care provision. Secondly, to the extent that social adjustment is a legitimate focus of health care, this is primarily in the field of psychiatry and psychology, rather than primary health care. It is not surprising, therefore, that many of the measures of social adjustment have been developed in psychiatry, and are of particular relevance to psychotic patients, especially those moving from the hospital to the community (for reviews of measures of social adjustment see McDowell and Newell[5]).

In contrast to social adjustment, social support can be seen as fundamental to the lives of everyone and highly relevant to both the definition of needs for primary health care and success in achieving desired outcomes. The number and quality of social supports available to individuals is both a determinant of health status and dependent on health. Social support thus constitutes an essential component of the health care system. The relationships between social supports, life stress, and health have been extensively researched and there are a number of excellent reviews of the field.[1,2,4] Unfortunately, there are relatively few simple measures of social support suitable for use in a health care setting which tap both quantitative and qualitative dimensions of support.

We have selected only four measures for inclusion in this chapter on criteria of their appropriateness to a primary health care setting and their reliability and validity. Our first consideration was to select only measures which could be completed in a short time, since social support is unlikely to be the main focus of research into needs and outcomes in the field of primary health care. The four measures selected are the Social Activities Questionnaire developed for the Rand Health Insurance Experiment, the Social Relationships Scale, the Duke–UNC Functional Social Support Questiònnaire, and the Norbeck Social Support Questionnaire.

References

1. Broadhead, W.E., Kaplan, B.H., James, S.A., Wagner, E.H., Schoenbach, V.J., Grimson, R., *et al.* (1983). The epidemiologic evidence for a relationship between social support and health. *American Journal of Epidemiology*, **117**, 521–37.
2. Cohen, S. and Syme, S.L. (1985). *Social support and health.* Academic Press, London.
3. Donald, C.A. and Ware, J.E. (1984). The measurement of social support. *Research in Community and Mental Health* 4, 325–70.
4. Kasl, S. (1983). Social and psychological factors affecting the course of disease: an epidemiological perspective. In *Handbook of health, health care and the health professions*, (ed. D. Mechanic), pp. 683–708. Free Press, New York.
5. McDowell, I. and Newell, C. (1987). *Measuring health: a guide to rating scales and questionnaires.* Oxford University Press, New York.

Rand Social Activities Questionnaire (Donald and others 1978)

Purpose

The Social Activities Questionnaire was developed to measure social well-being in the Rand Health Insurance Experiment (HIE). Firstly, it was designed to examine the effects of health care on social contacts and resources in surveys of adults registered with different types of insurance system. Secondly, it was designed to examine the relationships between social support, medical care consumption, and physical and mental health status. It was thus intended to be a survey research instrument suitable for comparing populations.

Background

The questionnaire was developed following an extensive and critical review of the literature on the concept and measurement of social health.[5] Although Donald and her colleagues originally conceptualized social well-being as a dimension of personal health status, they subsequently conceptualized it as external to health, although related to it. They argued, along with others in this field, that the concept of social well-being has two distinct dimensions, quantitative and qualitative. The quantitative is concerned with the number of contacts and the amount of activity, and is thus more objective. The qualitative dimension is concerned with personal evaluations of the adequacy of interpersonal relations, and is thus by definition subjective. In developing the questionnaire and measures derived from it, the Rand researchers have concentrated on objective measures of contacts and activities rather than on subjective evaluations of these. This was in part because subjective evaluations were dealt with in their separate assessment of psychological well-being using the Mental Health Inventory (see p. 100).

The questionnaire drew upon a number of existing instruments by adapting items from these.[2,6,7] The measures were selected to meet a range of specified criteria including conceptual relevance, variability in score distributions, freedom from error, replicability of scaling decisions, independence from other health status components, and sensitivity to the effects of medical care.[3,5]

The authors were critical of the approach taken to scaling of items and the construction of aggregate indices of social support in many existing instruments. Careful attention was therefore devoted to these issues in the analysis of data derived from the questionnaire. Item scaling was accomplished by examining the relationships between responses to each item and three criterion variables: emotional ties, psychological well-being, and current health. Graphs were prepared for each item showing the relationships between response categories and criterion scores, and these were used as a basis for empirically determining the scaling of responses for each item.[3,4] In this way it was possible to ensure that response categories were collapsed only where the pattern of criterion variable scores suggested that this would not result in any loss of information. The generation of multi-item scales was similarly empirically based, using factor analysis to identify those items which could legitimately be combined.

Description

There are 11 items in the Social Activities Questionnaire covering social contacts, group participation, social activities, and subjective evaluation of the quality of relationships (Exhibit 6.1). Pre-coded response categories are converted into scale scores for each item using the scoring rules shown in Exhibit 6.2. Item 7 (letter writing) is excluded from this list because it showed no relationship with the criterion variables. It is also excluded from the development of multi-item scales, and might therefore be considered redundant in future use of the questionnaire.

Three multi-item measures can be generated from the questionnaire and have been used in the HIE analyses (Exhibit 6.3). Social contacts and group participation are relatively homogeneous and can be interpreted straightforwardly. Although an overall summary index of social support is calculated using nine items, the authors suggest that its interpretation is problematic

Exhibit 6.1   Rand Social Activities Questionnaire

(Adapted with permission from Donald, C. A., Ware, J. E., Brook, R. H., and Davies-Avery, A. (1978). *Conceptualization and measurement of health for adults in the Health Insurance Study: Vol. IV Social Health*, Rand Publication No. R-1987/4/HEW. Rand Corporation Santa Monica)

1. About how many families in your neighbourhood are you well enough acquainted with, that you visit each other in your homes?
   _____ families

2. About how many *close* friends do you have—people you feel at ease with and can talk with about what is on your mind? (you may include relatives)
   _____ close friends

3. Over a year's time, about how often do you get together with friends or relatives, like going out together or visiting in each other's homes?
   Every day... 1
   Several days a week................................. 2
   About once a week.................................. 3
   2 or 3 times a month.............................. 4
   About once a month.............................. 5
   5 to 10 times a year.............................. 6
   Less than 5 times a year........................... 7

4. During the *past month*, about how often have you had friends over to your home? (Do *not* count relatives)

5. About how often have you visited with friends at *their* homes during the *past month*? (Do *not* count relatives)

6. About how often were you on the telephone with close friends or relatives during the *past month*?

7. About how often did you write a letter to a friend or relative during the *past month*?

8. In general, how well are you getting along with other people these days—would you say better than usual (1), about the same (2), or not as well as usual (3)?

9. How often have you attended a religious service during the *past month*?

Response categories items 4,5,6,7,9:
   1. Everyday
   2. Several days a week
   3. About once a week
   4. 2 or 3 times in past month
   5. Once in past month
   6. Not at all in past month

10. About how many voluntary groups or organizations do you belong to—like church groups, clubs or lodges, parent groups, etc. ('Voluntary' means because you want to)
   _____ groups or organisations   (Write in number. If none, enter '0')

Exhibit 6.1 (continued)

11. How active are you in the affairs of these groups or clubs you belong to? (If you belong to a great many just count those you feel closest to. If you don't belong to any, circle 4.)

Very active, attend most meetings................	1
Fairly active, attend fairly often...................	2
Not active, belong but hardly ever go............	3
Do not belong to any groups or clubs............	4

Exhibit 6.2 Recoding instructions for individual items

(From Donald, C. A., Ware, J. E., Brook, R. H., and Davies-Avery, A. (1978) *Conceptualization and Measurement of Health for Adults in the Health Insurance Study: Vol. IV, Social Health*, Rand Publication No. R-1987/4 HEW, Rand Corporation Santa Monica, with permission.)

Item	Recoding (original = revised)
Neighbourhood family acquaintances	(0 = 0)(1 = 1)(2 = 2)(3 = 3)(4 = 4) (5 thru 10 = 5)(11 or higher = 6)
Close friends and relatives	(0 = 0)(1 = 1)(2 = 2)(3 = 3)(4 = 4) (5 thru 9 = 5)(10 thru 20 = 6) (21 thru 25 = 7)(26 thru 35 = 8)(36 or higher = 9)
Visits with friends/relatives	(1 thru 3 = 4)(4 = 3)(5'6 = 2)(7 = 1)
Home visits by friends	(1 thru 4 = 3)(5 = 2)(6 = 1)
Visits to homes of friends	(1 thru 3 = 3)(4,5 = 2)(6 = 1)
Telephone contacts	(1 = 5)(2 = 4)(3,4 = 3)(5 = 2)(6 = 1)
Getting along	(1 = 3)(2 = 2)(3 = 1)
Attendance at religious services	(1,2 = 5)(3 = 4)(4 = 3)(5 = 2)(6 = 1)
Voluntary group membership	(0 = 0)(1 = 1)(2 = 2)(3 = 3)(4 = 4) (5 or higher = 5)
Level of group activity	(1 = 4)(2 = 3)(3 = 2)(4 = 1)

---

because of the heterogeneity of item content and weak inter-item correlations. In order to calculate scores for multi-item measures it is necessary to standardize item scores because of substantially differing variances between items.[3,4]

Administration and acceptability

The questionnaire is a straightforward self-completed instrument which can be completed in a few minutes. The content is unlikely to arouse any resis-

Exhibit 6.3   Summary of Rand social support measures

(From Donald, C. A., Ware, J. E., Brook, R. H., and Davies-Avery, A. (1978). *Conceptualization and measurement of health for adults in the Health Insurance Study: Vol. IV social health*, Rand Publication No. R-1987/4 HEW. Rand Corporation, Santa Monica, with permission.

Social support item	Construct-specific measure	Overall index
Visits with friends/relatives Home visits by friends Visits to homes of friends	} Social contacts	
Voluntary group membership Level of group activity	} Group participation	Social Support index
Number of neighbourhood acquaintances* Number of close friends/relatives* Telephone contacts* Attendance at religious services*		
Getting along with others*		

* These items were also retained as single-item social support measures for use in HIE analyses.

tance in respondents, so that good response rates can be expected. The brevity of this measure would make it feasible to include in studies requiring a measure of social activities to supplement measures of physical and mental health.

Reliability and validity

Evidence of reliability and validity is derived from the HIE studies on more than 4000 adults in different sites in the USA. Test–retest reliability of single-item measures of social well-being over short time periods was not possible. However, over one-year intervals all items except 'getting along with others' were sufficiently stable for studies of large differences in group level analyses.[4] The item 'getting along with others' was not stable, but there is no way of knowing whether this is because the measure is unreliable or it is a reliable measure of an unstable construct. There is thus a need for further testing of the reliability of single items. All three of the multi-item measures were tested for internal consistency, the homogeneity of items included and stability over a one-year period.[4] The results showed moderate levels of internal consistency and homogeneity, except for the overall social support index which was least homogeneous because of the diversity of social constructs represented.

Content validity is claimed both in terms of an assessment of the relationship between explicit item content and the labels assigned to measures, and in terms of comparisons with existing literature on social well-being. The construct validity of individual items is supported by their relationships to the criterion variables employed in the scaling procedure. Tests of the discriminant validity of items used to measure social contacts and group participation showed that the items were more sensitive to the constructs they were intended to measure than to other constructs. Construct validity was supported in associations between measures and predictions of mental health.[3,8] Whilst the evidence of validity to date is encouraging, further evidence of predictive validity in terms of health outcomes and comparisons with alternative measures of social support and well-being would be desirable. Finally, there is as yet no evidence concerning the ability of the measures to detect changes in social well-being.

Populations/client groups

The Social Activities Questionnaire was designed for use in large-scale surveys of the adult population in the USA. It has not been used with elderly people, and there are strong grounds for supposing that the relationships between social support and health are different for older people than for adults of working age. The measures are suitable for group comparisons but would not be appropriate for individual assessment and should be used with care in small-scale studies where comparison groups are small. The questionnaire has been used in a variety of other research studies, at least one of which was carried out with patients consulting physicians in primary health care.[1]

Comments

Like other measures used in the HIE, the measures of social well-being are an attempt to build upon available instruments to develop a new 'state of the art' measure. The researchers have carefully documented the development and testing of the questionnaire and measures derived from it, and have adopted a more systematic approach to the problems of scaling than is evident in most measures in this field. Our main criticism of the questionnaire is that it overemphasises the quantitative dimension of social well-being, thus giving insufficient weight to subjective evaluations of the adequacy of social support. For this reason it would be desirable to supplement the questionnaire with a measure such as the DUFSS, or to develop and test additional items which tap this dimension.

References

1. Broadhead, W.E., Gehlbach, S.H., De Gruy, F.V., and Kaplan, B.H. (1989). Functional versus structural social support and health care utilization in a family medicine outpatient practice. *Medical Care*, **27**, 221–3.
2. Dohrenwend, B.S., Dohrenwend, B.P., and Cook, D. (1973). Ability and disability in role functioning in psychiatric patient and non-patient groups. In *Roots of evaluation* (ed. J.D. Wing and H. Hofner), pp. 337–60. Oxford University Press, London.
3. Donald, C.A. and Ware J.E. (1982). *The quantification of social contacts and resources.* Rand: Publication No. R2937-HHS. Rand Corporation, Santa Monica.
4. Donald, C.A. and Ware, J.E. (1984). The measurement of social support. *Research in Community and Mental Health*, **4**, 325–70.
5. Donald, C.A., Ware, J.E., Brook, R.H., and Davies-Avery, A. (1978). *Conceptualization and measurement of health for adults in the health insurance study: Vol. IV social health.* Rand: Publication No. R-1987/4-HEW. Rand Corporation, Santa Monica.
6. Myers, J.K., Lindenthal, J.J., Pepper, M.P., and Ostrander D.R. (1972). Life events and mental status: a longitudinal study. *Journal of Health and Social Behaviour*, **13**, 398–406.
7. Myers, J.K., Lindenthal, J.J., and Pepper, M.P. (1975). Life events, social integration and psychiatric symptomatology. *Journal of Health and Social Behaviour*, **16**, 421–7.
8. Williams, A.W., Ware, J.E., and Donald, C.A. (1981). A model of mental health, life events and social support applicable to general populations. *Journal of Health and Social Behaviour*, **22**, 324–36.

The Social Relationship Scale (SRS)
(McFarlane and colleagues 1981)

Purpose

The SRS was developed to measure the role of social support in cushioning the effects of life stressors on health. It measures both the extent of support and its perceived helpfulness to the individual and was intended primarily as a research instrument.

Background

The authors developed the SRS as part of a two-year prospective study of social support as a cushion or buffer against the effects of life stressors on health. One of the ways in which social networks are thought to function in this task is to provide information as well as encouragement, so that physiological resources can be mobilized to deal with the problem at hand.[2] McFarlane and his colleagues set out to develop a questionnaire which would cover all categories of life stress and the number, type, and quality of relationships available for discussion of problems in each of these categories. They were concerned primarily with relationships as manifested in verbal support. The questionnaire was also designed to provide information about the total number of relationships available and the extent of reciprocity in these. No further information is provided about how the questionnaire was designed and tested, apart from the fact that it originally formed one section in a larger questionnaire concerned with the impact of life changes on emotional well-being.

Description

Respondents are asked to identify all individuals who provide support in each of six separate areas of potential life stress: work, money, finances, home and family, personal and social, and issues that relate to society in general. Exhibit 6.4 shows the questionnaire format applied to the area of home and family. Exactly the same format is used for each of the six areas. Respondents are asked to write down the initials and relationship to the respondent (e.g. spouse, family, friend, neighbour, etc.) of anyone with whom they generally discuss issues of this nature. They are then asked to rate the helpfulness of this particular individual on a seven-point scale (scored −3 to +3) and whether this is a reciprocal relationship (i.e. would the individual discuss his or her problems with the respondent).[1]

The results can be used to present a descriptive account of levels of the quantity and quality of relationships in each of the areas, including the sources of support. They can also be presented in terms of three scores. The quality of relationships is measured by taking an average of the seven-point helpfulness ratings, and the extent of the network is estimated by counting the total number of individuals mentioned.[2] The degree of reciprocity can be measured by expressing the number of people the respondent thinks would come to him or her to discuss problems as a percentage of the total number of individuals mentioned.

Administration and acceptability

The questionnaire was designed as part of a more extensive interview. It is intended to be self-completed, but an interviewer is expected to be present to answer queries and prompt respondents to ensure that they have included everybody. Unfortunately, the authors do not indicate how long it takes to complete or how easy or difficult respondents found the exercise. However, a response rate of 83 per cent in a study of people drawn from the registers of family physicians suggests that there are likely to be few problems.

Exhibit 6.4   Example of the Social
Relationship Scale

(Reproduced from McFarlane, A. H., Neale, K. A., Norman, G. R., Roy, R. J., and Streiner, D. L. (1981). Methodological issues in developing a scale to measure social support. *Schizophrenia Bulletin*, 7, 90–100)

Example 1: Home and family

Please list the people with whom you generally discuss home and family, using the first name or initials only. After each name or set of initials fill in a one- or two-word description of the relation each person has to you.

Then go on to check the circle which indicates the degree of helpfulness or unhelpfulness of your discussions with each person, and lastly, check off yes or no if you feel this person would come to you to discuss home and family.

Don't feel you have to fill up all the spaces provided. If you find you need more spaces, please inform the interviewer.

I discuss my home and family with:

Reliability and validity

The only evidence of reliability and validity is presented in the original report on the SRS.[1] Test–retest reliability of both the extent and helpfulness of relationships was tested on 73 college students over a one-week interval. Correlations were generally high, but lower for more distant relatives and for helpfulness ratings with regard to money and health.

Content validity is claimed for the SRS by virtue of having submitted the questionnaire to a panel of four psychiatrists for review.[1] Although these clinicians concluded that the scale provided useful information about the number and type of relationships in the supportive network, a more thorough appraisal of content validity would be desirable. The SRS seems to tap only limited areas of social relationships, ignoring others which might be equally or more important (e.g. affective component of relationships, assistance with tasks, frequency of contact). The only other evidence of validity is derived from a comparison of parent therapists and parents who had been referred to therapists. The hypothesis that the latter group would rate their spouses as less helpful than the former was supported. This finding is cited as evidence of the discriminant validity of the measure.[3]

In McFarlane's main survey the SRS was administered to a sample of 518 adults drawn from the general population. Although the authors present some of the results from this exercise they have not exploited the data as possible evidence of construct validity. The comparisons between men and women and according to marital status do, however, seem to provide some evidence of construct validity, in that the results show differences in the areas that might be expected. Thus, for example, women reported more relationships with family members than men, and single people reported more friends than those who were married.[3] Also the finding that most support was provided by respondents' families is in accordance with other studies which show that real support is derived from attachment relationships.

Populations/service settings

The SRS was developed for the purposes of research with adults drawn from the registers of family physicians. We are not aware of its having been used in a service setting or with particular categories of people (e.g. patients, disabled people, elderly people). There seems no reason that it should not be applicable to any adults living in the community, but the need for an interviewer to be present would make it difficult to use in a service setting.

Comments

The SRS is a relatively short measure of the number of social relationships and their supportive quality. It is somewhat limited in scope, and provides no information about the nature of any support provided. More evidence of reliability and validity is required before we could recommend the SRS, but the method seems promising. It is unlikely to be the sort of measure which could be incorporated into routine clinical practice, but might be worth considering as a research instrument where detailed information about social networks is required.

References

1. McFarlane, A. H., Neale, K. A., Norman, G. R., Roy, R. G., and Streiner, D. L. (1981). Methodological issues in developing a scale to measure social support. *Schizophrenia Bulletin*, **7**, 90–9.
2. McFarlane, A. H., Norman, G. R., Streiner, D. L., and Roy, R. G. (1983). The process of social stress: stable, reciprocal and mediating relationships. *Journal of Health and Social Behaviour*, **24**, 160–73.
3. McFarlane, A. H., Norman, G. R., Streiner, D. L., and Roy, R. G. (1984). Characteristics and correlates of effective and ineffective social supports. *Journal of Psychosomatic Research*, **28**, 501–10.

The Duke–UNC Functional Social Support Questionnaire (DUFSS) (Broadhead and colleagues 1988)

Purpose

The DUFSS measures qualitative or functional aspects of supportive relationships rather than the number of relationships or the size of the social network. It was designed to be easy to administer in a family practice setting and intended to be of use in studies to detect high-risk psychosocial settings, to examine the effects of social support on health, and to examine the interaction of social support with other determinants of health.

Background

The authors felt that many existing measures of social support ignored the differences between different dimensions of the concept of support. In some cases the quality of support and frequency of social interaction were combined in a summary measure; in others, measures of the amount of support are contaminated with a variety of independent constructs; and in others, measures of tangible support are combined with measures of other types of support. They argued that there was a need for psychometrically sound measures which focused on the qualitative aspects of relationships which are known to be stronger predictors of health outcome than the number of relationships.

The resulting measure was developed with a family practice population to ensure generalisability. Initially 14 items were derived from a longer questionnaire based on a review of the literature concerning the relationship between social support and health.[1] Items were selected for content validity, ease of administration, consistency of response between similar variables, and good variability of response within variables. The content areas defined a priori were: amount of support, confidant support, affective support, and instrumental support. This measure was tested on 401 adult patients consulting at a family medical centre. Three items were removed because they did not satisfy test-retest reliability criteria. Factor analysis of the remaining 11 items showed that three constituted single-item factors and these are not recommended for use without further research.

Description

The eight-item DUFSS measures two dimensions of social support: confidant support (five items) and affective support (three items). Exhibit 6.5 shows the items and response categories. Each item is scored 1 to 5 using a Likert-type response. Separate scores are constructed for confidant and affective support.

Administration and acceptability

A major advantage of the DUFSS over other available measures is the fact that it is a very brief self-completed questionnaire, and can therefore be completed by patients whilst waiting for a consultation. Whilst there are no obvious reasons why there should be any problems of acceptability to patients, the response rate of only 66 per cent achieved in the development study is worrying. Evidence presented by the authors showed that older people, men, and black people were less likely to respond, thus introducing a systematic bias into responses.

Reliability and validity

Evidence of reliability and validity available to date derives from a single study of 401 respondents in family practice.[1] It should be noted that the respondents were predominantly young (18–44 years), white, well educated women of relatively high socio-economic status. The authors are thus rightly cautious about the applicability of the DUFSS with groups which were under-represented in this study.

Test–retest reliability was assessed on only 22 respondents over time periods varying from 6 to 30 days. Three items which showed very poor correlations were deleted following this exercise. Factor analysis and internal consistency analysis of the remaining eleven items provided evidence for five

---

Exhibit 6.5   Duke–UNC Functional Social Support Questionnaire

(Adapted with permission from Broadhead, W. E., Gehlbach, S. H., De Gruy, F. V., and Kaplan, B. H. (1988). The Duke–UNC Functional Social Support Questionnaire: measurement of social support in family medicine patients. *Medical Care*, **26**, 709–23)

Here is a list of some things that other people do for us or give us that may be helpful or supportive. Please read each statement carefully and place a check (✓) in the blank that is closest to your situation.

Here is an example:
I get...

	As much as I would like	Much less than I would like
enough vacation time...	✓	

If you put a check where we have, it means that you get **almost** as much vacation time as you would like, but **not quite** as much as you would like.

Answer each item as best you can. There are NO right or wrong answers.

I get...	As much as I would like			Much less than I would like
1. invitations to go out and do things with other people...				
2. love and affection...				
3. chances to talk to someone about problems at work or with my housework...				
4. chances to talk to someone I trust about my personal and family problems...				
5. chances to talk about money matters...				
6. people who care what happens to me				
7. useful advice about important things in life...				
8. help when I'm sick in bed...				

Scoring: Each item is scored on a five point scale (1 = As much as I would like, 5 = Much less than I would like). Item scores are summed for confidant support (Items 1,3,4,5,7) and affective support (Items 2,6,8) independent types of support, but three of these (visits, praise, and instrumental support) were represented by single items. These cannot be expected to be as reliable as multi-item scales and are therefore not recommended for further use at this stage. The items used to measure confidant and affective support showed acceptable levels of internal consistency.

Validity of the two factors and individual items was assessed by relationships with socio-demographic variables expected to be associated with social support, with health status as measured by the DUHP (Duke–UNC Health Profile; see p. 170), and with alternative measures of social support. Relationships with socio-demographic variables were consistent with the existing literature. Individual items were positively correlated with the health status measures. Correlations between scores for affective and confidant support, the Rand Social Activities support factors (see p. 112), and the social function subscale of the DUHP provide further evidence of validity. However, in all cases the correlations are low, suggesting that the DUFSS is measuring a related but different construct.

Using data from the same study of patients attending family practice, the authors have shown that both confidant and affective support are related to utilization of primary health care.[2] Numbers of contacts, length of consultations, and total expenditure on health care were all higher for respondents with low social support. This potential to predict service use requires further exploration.

Overall, the evidence of reliability and validity is encouraging as far as it goes, but further studies on more representative populations are essential. In addition, there is no information at present on the responsiveness of the measure to changes in circumstances or on the distribution of scores.

Populations/service settings

The DUFSS is designed for use with adults and has been tested on patients attending a family medical centre. As indicated above, caution should be exercised in using it with groups not represented in the original study. In particular there is no evidence of its validity or reliability when used with elderly people, ethnic minorities, or people in lower socio-economic groups. On-going studies are using the DUFSS with alcoholics and obese patients being treated in primary care (personal communication).

Comments

Although only presented recently, the DUFSS is worth consideration as a measure of limited aspects of social support. There are good grounds for focusing attention on the quality of support rather than amount. However, it should be remembered that important dimensions of social support are not covered in measures of confidant and affective support. The limited evidence of reliability and validity currently available is encouraging, but we would recommend that any intending user of the DUFSS should mount further studies designed to establish reliability and validity for the specific population being studied. There is also scope for further development work on those dimensions of functional social support not covered in the existing eight-item questionnaire.

References

1. Broadhead, W. E., Gehlbach, S. H., De Gruy F. V., and Kaplan, B. H. (1988). The Duke–UNC Functional Social Support Questionnaire: measurement of social support in family medicine patients. *Medical Care*, **26**, 709–23.
2. Broadhead, W. E., Gehlbach, S. H., De Gruy, F. V., and Kaplan, B. H. (1989). Functional versus structural social support and health care utilisation in a family medicine outpatient practice. *Medical Care*, **27**, 221–33.

Norbeck Social Support Questionnaire (NSSQ) (Norbeck and colleagues 1981)

Purpose

The NSSQ is intended to measure multiple dimensions of social support. It is a research tool designed for use in clinical research concerned with health outcome.[8]

Background

The NSSQ is based on Kahn's definition of social support – 'interpersonal transactions that include one or more of the following: the expression of positive affect of one person towards another; the affirmation or endorsement of another person's behaviours, perceptions or expressed views; the giving of symbolic or material aid to another.'[3] Jane Norbeck and her colleagues at the University of California, San Francisco, designed the NSSQ to measure the dimensions of affect, affirmation and aid for the whole of the individual's social network. They wanted to devise a questionnaire which would permit the presentation of a complex task in a simplified way to respondents.[8]

Description

The questionnaire consists of a series of half pages so that questions can be aligned with the respondents' personal network list (Exhibit 6.6). Respondents first list each significant person in their lives (using first names or

---

Exhibit 6.6 Norbeck Social Support Questionnaire

Adapted with permission from Norbeck, J. S., Lindseq, A. M., and Carrieri, V. L. (1981). The development of an instrument to measure social support. *Nursing Research*, **30**, 264–9)

For each person you listed, please answer the following questions by writing in the number that applies.

Number _____
Date   _____

1 = not at all
2 = a little
3 = moderately
4 = quite a bit
5 = a great deal

Question 1:	*Question 2:*	*Personal network*
How much does this person make you feel liked or loved?	How much does this person make you feel respected or admired?	List each significant person in your life on the right. Consider all the persons who provide personal support for you and who are important to you.

		First name	*Relationship*
1. _____	1. _____	1. _____	1. _____
2. _____	2. _____	2. _____	2. _____
3. _____	3. _____	3. _____	3. _____
20. _____	20. _____	20. _____	20.

Questions for rating network members

1. How much does this person make you feel liked or loved? [affect]
2. How much does this person make you feel respected or admired? [affect]
3. How much can you confide in the person? [affirmation]
4. How much does this person agree with or support your actions or thoughts? [affirmation]
5. If you needed to borrow $10, a ride to the doctor, or some other immediate help, how much could this person usually help? [aid—short term]
6. If you were confined to bed for several weeks, how much could this person help you? [aid—long term]
7. How long have you known this person? [duration of the relationship]
8. How frequently do you usually have contact with this person? (phone calls, visits or letters) [Frequency of contact]
9. During the past year, have you lost any important relationship due to moving, a job change, divorce or separation, death, or some other reason? [Recent loss]
   9a. If YES check the category(s) of persons who are no longer available to you [9 categories listed]
   9b. How much support did this person (or persons) provide for you during the past six months?

Exhibit 6.6 (continued)

Scoring

Ratings are based on a five-point rating scale specified for each question. Questions 1 to 6 and 9b ranged from 1 = not at all to 5 = a great deal; question 7 ranged from 1 = less than 6 months to 5 = more than 5 years; and question 8 ranged from 1 = once a year or less to 5 = daily.

initials) and specify the category of relationship (spouse or partner, family or relatives, friends, work or school associates, neighbours, health care providers, counsellor or therapist, minister, priest or rabbi, other). Up to 20 network members are listed in this way. Respondents then turn the first half page to reveal two questions which are answered for each member of the network. Each of the dimensions of social support is tapped by two questions. The properties of the network are measured by its size, the duration of relationships, and the frequency of contacts. The final question which appears on a separate full page deals with recent losses of important relationships.

In the original presentation of the NSSQ it was recommended that, for each of the first eight questions, the respondent's ratings for each network member on a given question should be added to determine the score for that question. This scoring system has been criticized for making the error of confounding the size of the network with the assessment of content.[2] Using the suggested scoring system, the measures are largely a function of the number of persons in the network. Unfortunately, the problem of confounding network size and quality of support is an inherent feature of inventory type instruments. If scores are summed they will reflect the size of the network, but if they are averaged they will tend to penalize those respondents who list larger networks including some individuals who provide lower quality support. Norbeck argues that a combined score is more valid than an average, because in real life the quantity and quality of support combine to produce an overall level (personal communication). Nevertheless, it is possible using the NSSQ to present these components separately in multivariate models in which averaged scores are used. Question 9 concerning recent losses is scored as a yes/no response and the quantity of loss is determined by the number of categories checked in question 9a. The quality of losses is scored on a five-point rating scale of responses to question 9b.

Administration and acceptability

The NSSQ is a relatively brief and simple self-administered questionnaire. This is one of its main advantages when compared with alternatives. It takes approximately 15 minutes to complete and no problems of understanding or acceptability have been reported. It should, however, be noted that testing was carried out on graduate nurses. However, no problems with response rates or acceptability have been reported in subsequent studies which have used the NSSQ.

Reliability and validity

Evidence of reliability is limited. Although Norbeck's original study was based on a small atypical group (135 nursing students, including only seven males and very few non-Caucasians), it showed good test–retest reliability over a one-week period and high internal consistency.[8] However, it should be noted that the scoring system used virtually guarantees high intercorrelations between items, because all scores are a function of the same number of people in the network.

NSSQ scores were correlated with scores on a social desirability scale to determine whether responses were likely to reflect subjects' perceptions of socially desirable responses, rather than an accurate reflection of levels of social support.[8] None of the NSSQ items were related to the social desirability scale.

Evidence of validity is also derived from studies of somewhat narrow populations, but is encouraging. Concurrent validity was assessed by comparisons with an alternative measure of social support in graduate nursing students. This produced significant but moderate correlations.[8,9] Construct validity was assessed in a study of 136 employees at a University medical centre.[9] NSSQ sub-scales were shown to relate to interpersonal constructs such as 'need for inclusion' and 'need for affection' as hypothesized. A study of the relationships between negative life events, social support, and negative mood provided limited evidence of a stress buffering role for social support.[9] Although Norbeck's original work showed that NSSQ scores were largely unrelated to mood, a subsequent study of depression in women with chronic illness suggested that particular supports were associated with both the presence and severity of depression.[10]

The issue of sensitivity to change has been addressed in a follow-up study of 44 Master's degree nursing students.[8] Seven months after entering graduate school, the NSSQ showed changes in network composition, but not in the level of support. Considerably more evidence would be required in order to form any judgement about the sensitivity to change of the NSSQ.

Populations/service settings

Although developed and tested on a population of student nurses, the NSSQ has subsequently been used with women with chronic illness,[10] young mothers,[4] pregnant women,[6,7] post-mastectomy patients,[1] and elderly people in institutional care.[5] It is clearly not intended as an instrument for use in routine clinical practice, although the fact that it is self completed suggests that it could be completed by patients attending primary care services. However, it is likely that respondents would require some supervision and help.

Comments

The NSSQ is convenient to use, and has a clear conceptual basis, and encouraging evidence of reliability and validity. It is particularly useful in allowing support levels from different sources (e.g. partner, mother, friends) to be analysed separately. With careful attention to the method of scoring and analysis, we consider it a good candidate for research applications in which measurement of both quantitative and qualitative dimensions of social support is required. However, there is a need for further evidence of reliability and validity based on more varied populations than those so far used.

References

1. Feather B. L. and Wainstock J. M. (1989). Perceptions of post mastectomy patients. Part 1, the relationship between social support and network providers. *Cancer Nursing*, **12**, 293–300.
2. House J. S. and Kahn R. L. (1985). Measures and concepts of social support. In *Social support and health*, (ed. S. Cohen and S. L. Syme), pp. 83–108. Academic Press, Orlando.
3. Kahn R. L. and Antonucci T. C. (1981). Convoys of social support: a life course approach. In *Aging: Social Change*, (ed. S. B. Kiesler, J. N. Morgan, and V. K. Oppenheimer), pp. 383–406. Academic Press, New York.
4. Koniak-Griffin D. (1988). The relationship between social support, self esteem and maternal-fetal attachment in adolescents. *Research in Nursing and Health*, **11**, 269–78.
5. Nelson, P. B. (1989). Social support, self-esteem and depression in the institutionalised elderly. *Issues in Mental Health Nursing*, **10**, 55–68.
6. Norbeck, J. S. and Anderson, N. J. (1989). Life stress, social support, and anxiety in mid- and late-pregnancy among low income women. *Research in Nursing & Health*, **12**, 281–7.
7. Norbeck, J. S. and Anderson, N. J. (1989). Psychosocial predictors of pregnancy outcomes in low-income black, Hispanic, and white women. *Nursing Research*, **38**, 204–9.
8. Norbeck J. S., Lindsey A. M., and Carrieri V. L. (1981). The development of an instrument to measure social support. *Nursing Research*, **30**, 264–69.
9. Norbeck, J., Lindsey, A., and Carieri, V. (1983). Further development of the Norbeck Social Support Questionnaire. Normative data and validity testing. *Nursing Research*, **32**, 4–9.
10. Primomo J., Yates B. C., and Woods N. F. (1990). Social support for women

during chronic illness: the relationship among sources and types of adjustment. *Research in Nursing and Health*, **13**, 153–61.

Conclusions

The four measures presented here provide an indication of the current state of development in this field. There is ample evidence of the importance of social support in health and illness. For this reason alone it seems essential that research concerned with needs for, and outcomes of, medical care should incorporate measures of social support. There is no shortage of measures, a wide selection of which are reviewed by House and Kahn[2] and by Heitzmann and Kaplan,[1] but the psychometric properties of these have not been convincingly documented. In particular, the reliability and validity of most social support scales have not been adequately tested. All four of the instruments presented in this chapter require further evidence of reliability and validity if they are to be used with confidence.

In terms of the content of measures, we have two areas of concern. Firstly, none of the measures we have reviewed provides a satisfactory balance between the sources and amount of social support on the one hand, and individuals' subjective evaluations of this support on the other. The adequacy of social support must be a result of both objective factors and how the individual experiences his or her situation. Our second concern is with the lack of emphasis in many measures on the practical components of social support. Only the Norbeck instrument of those reviewed here includes a measure of symbolic or material aid. There is a need for measures which describe the availability of practical support with activities of daily living. The growing importance of chronic illness and associated disability in the health problems dealt with by primary health care makes the need for such measures particularly important.

References

1. Heitzmann, C. A. and Kaplan, R. M. (1988). Assessment of methods for measuring social support. *Health Psychology*, **7**, 75–109.
2. House, J. S. and Kahn, R. L. (1985). Measures and concepts of social support. In *Social Support and Health* (ed. S. Cohen and S. L. Syme), pp. 83–108. Academic Press, London.

7 Multidimensional measures

Introduction

In Chapters 4 to 6 we have dealt with instruments which have been developed to measure particular dimensions of health. It is of course possible to select a number of different instruments to assess physical function, mental health/illness, and social support or well-being. Indeed the measures devised for the Rand Health Insurance Experiment were designed with the intention of being incorporated into the same questionnaire. However, in recent years researchers in the field of health status measurement have devoted considerable efforts to the development of multidimensional measures that incorporate physical, psychological, and social components in a single instrument. Some of these have been developed for specific diseases, and we deal with a small selection of these in Chapter 8, but many have been designed for general use. Most of these general-purpose measures of health status have been developed initially in response to the needs of health policy, service planning, and resource allocation, but they have found increasing applications in the evaluation of specific services and clinical research. Most recently, some clinicians and other health professionals have begun to look to multidimensional measures of health status as aids to monitoring patients in clinical practice.

There have been two broad approaches to the development of general health status measures, profiles and indexes. Instruments which adopt the profile approach summarize information about levels of function and well-being within discrete areas, but do not attempt to combine these to create an overall health status index. These measures can be seen as the next logical step from employing separate measures in each of the broad areas of physical, psychological, and social functioning. They have the advantage that the methods used and the results obtained are the same in each of the areas. Health profiles are essentially descriptive measures which permit the user to identify specific areas of need or outcomes. In some cases construction of an overall score may be possible, but this is not the main purpose of the profile approach.

Health indexes, in contrast to profiles, are specifically designed to provide a single scale of health states. They employ methods of scaling which permit measurement at an interval or metric level (see Chapter 3). All health states, including death, can be incorporated into the measure, thus permitting comparisons across disease states and allowing for all possible outcomes. Scaling of health indexes is accomplished by the application of values to each health state, so that decisions about who should undertake the valuation are vitally important. The choice of judges can be seen as essentially a political decision. The final stage in the development of health indexes is to incorporate into the model transition probabilities or prognoses. The truly comprehensive index must incorporate not only a description of current state, but also the likelihood that the individual will get better, stay the same, or get worse. This inclusion of a time component provides the basis for the assessment of health outcomes in quality adjusted life years, which has become increasingly popular as a method of informing decisions about resource allocation. Although health indexes have been mainly applied at the level of service evaluation, planning, and resource allocation, they are increasingly used alongside other measures in clinical trials.

The measures included in this chapter fall into three general groups. The first five (Sickness Impact Profile, Nottingham Health Profile, McMaster Health Index, and the MOS Short-Form Health Survey Measures) are general purpose health profile measures. The Duke–UNC Health Profile, the Functional Status Questionnaire and the Coop Function Charts are health profiles developed specifically for use in primary health care. Lastly, Rosser's classification of illness states and the Quality of Wellbeing Scale are attempts to devise global health indexes which can be used in service planning and resource allocation as well as in the evaluation of services and treatments.

The Sickness Impact Profile (SIP)/Functional Limitations Profile (FLP) (Bergner and colleagues 1976; Patrick and colleagues 1982)

Purpose

SIP is a measure of sickness-related behavioural dysfunction as judged by the individual's perception of the impact of sickness on usual daily activities. It was developed in the USA with the intention of fulfilling a variety of different needs for a measure of perceived health, including outcomes of care, health surveys, programme planning, policy formulation, and monitoring patient progress. It was designed to be applicable across types and severities of illness and with demographic and cultural subgroups. The authors set out to create a general-purpose measure of the impact of disease.

The FLP is a British version of the original SIP, developed specifically for the purposes of longitudinal studies of disability. However, it has the same range of potential applications as the SIP.

Background

Work on the SIP began in 1972 and the first version was produced in 1976.[1] Continued development work resulted in a revised version which has become one of the most widely used general measures of the effects of illness.[2] The concept of sickness, which denotes the individual's experience of illness through its effects on everyday life and feelings, is contrasted with the medical model of disease, which denotes a professional or provider definition based on clinical observation.[10] Since the aim of most health care is to reduce sickness or modify its effects on the individual, needs for, and outcomes of, health care interventions should be measured in these terms.

Given a focus on the individual's experience of illness, the content of a measure can focus on behaviour or feelings, or a mixture of both. The authors of the SIP decided to concentrate on behaviour, which it is argued can be reliably reported and which can be verified by observation. Feelings in contrast are, by their very nature, subjective and thus not amenable to external validation. It was also felt that behavioural reports would be less prone to cultural bias than reports of feelings.[1] Aspects of behaviour included in the profile were selected because they represented 'universal patterns' of limitations that may be affected by any sickness, regardless of specific conditions, treatment, individual characteristics, or prognosis.

An initial pool of statements describing aspects of behaviour was derived from professionals, interviews with healthy and ill people, and a review of literature. Extensive field trials of 312 statements grouped into 14 categories provided the basis for reducing the number of items to be included in the final version. Weights for individual items were devised using equal-appearing interval scaling procedures. Twenty five judges rated each item on a 15 point scale ranging from minimally dysfunctional to maximally dysfunctional.[4] Judges included both consumers and professionals. Weights are intended to represent the relative severity of limitation on behaviour implied by each statement.

The authors of the FLP took all of the items included in the SIP and reviewed their relevance to British people. Some items were reworded and the weighting exercise repeated using British judges.[19]

Description

The final versions of both the SIP and the FLP contain 136 statements in 12 categories; sleep and rest, eating, work, home management, recreation and pastimes, ambulation, mobility, body care and movement, social interaction, and communication. Exhibit 7.1 shows the items included in three categories of the FLP. Apart from the wording of items there are also some differences between the FLP and SIP in the order in which categories are presented. However, the number of items and the basic content is exactly the same. It is not possible for reasons of space to present all 136 items. Copies of the schedules and instructions are available for both the SIP[11] and FLP.[17]

Subjects are asked to endorse only those statements which describe them on a given day and are related to their health. The wording of items and instructions focuses on performance rather than capacity. Respondents are

Exhibit 7.1   Sample categories from the Functional Limitations Profile

(From Patrick, D. L. and Peach, H. (1989). *Disablement in the Community*. Oxford University Press, Oxford with permission)

Body care and movement items (maximum possible score = 1927)

The following statements describe how you move about, bath, go to the toilet, dress yourself today. If 'AGREE', PROBE: Is this due to your health?

13. I make difficult movements with help; for example, getting in or out of the bath or a car. –(082)
14. I do not get in and out of bed or chairs without the help of a person or mechanical aid. –(100)
15. I only stand for short periods of time. –(067)
16. I do not keep my balance. –(093)
17. I move my hands or fingers with some difficulty or limitation. –(066)
18. I only stand up with someone's help. –(093)
19. I kneel, stoop, or bend down only by holding on to something. –(061)
20. I am in a restricted position all the time. –(124)
21. I am very clumsy. –(047)
22. I get in and out of bed or chairs by grasping something for support or by using a stick or walking frame. –(079)
23. I stay lying down most of the time. –(120)
24. I change position frequently. –(053)
25. I hold on to something to move myself around in bed. –(082)
26. I do not bathe myself completely; for example, I need help with bathing. –(085)
27. I do not bathe myself at all, but am bathed by someone else. –(100)
28. I use a bedpan with help. –(107)
29. I have trouble putting on my shoes, socks, or stockings. –(054)
30. I do not have control of my bladder. –(122)
31. I do not fasten my clothing; for example, I require assistance with buttons, zips, or shoelaces. –(068)
32. I spend most of the time partly dressed or in pyjamas. –(075)
33. I do not have control of my bowels. –(124)
34. I dress myself, but do so very slowly. –(043)
35. I only get dressed with someone's help. –(082)

Mobility items (maximum possible score = 0727)

These next statements describe how you get about the house and outside. If 'AGREE' PROBE: Is this due to your health?

36. I only get about in one building. –(076)

Exhibit 7.1 (continued)

37. I stay in one room.   -(101)
38. I stay in bed more.   -(091)
39. I stay in bed most of the time.   -(114)
40. I do not use public transport now.   -(052)
41. I stay at home most of the time.   -(079)
42. I only go out if there is a lavatory nearby.   -(064)
43. I do not go into town.   -(047)
44. I only stay away from home for short periods.   -(046)
45. I do not get about in the dark or in places that are not lit unless I
    have someone to help.   -(057)

Emotion items (maximum possible score = 0693)

The next statements describe your feelings and behaviour. Again think of yourself today. If 'AGREE' PROBE: Is this due to your health?

84. I say how bad or useless I am; for example, that I am a burden to
    others.   -(089)
85. I laugh or cry suddenly.   -(058)
86. I often moan and groan because of pain or discomfort.   -(067)
87. I have attempted suicide.   -(141)
88. I behave nervously or restlessly.   -(048)
89. I keep rubbing or holding areas of my body that hurt or are
    uncomfortable.   -(059)
90. I am irritable and impatient with myself; for example, I run myself
    down, I swear at myself, I blame myself for things that happen.   -(079)
91. I talk hopelessly about the future.   -(096)
92. I get sudden frights.   -(056)

---

asked to describe actual behaviour, rather than to make judgements about what they could do. However, they are asked to make a judgement about whether the limitation on behaviour is related to their health, and this might sometimes present difficulties.

The distribution of items between categories is shown in Exhibit 7.2. Scores are calculated using the item weights, which represent the relative severity of limitation imposed by that item. The respondent scores the item weight for any item endorsed. Percentage scores are calculated for categories by simply adding item values for each item endorsed, dividing by the maximum possible score for that category and multiplying by 100. The authors of both the SIP and the FLP recommend the calculation of dimension scores representing physical and psychosocial dimensions, but there are slight variations in the categories included (see Exhibit 7.2). The grouping of categories in each case was based on analyses of survey data.[5,11] Dimension scores are calculated in the same way as category scores by adding item values, dividing by the maximum possible score for that dimension, and multiplying by 100.

Exhibit 7.2	SIP/FLP categories and dimensions

Category	Number of items	Physical dimension		Psychosocial dimension	
		SIP	FLP	SIP	FLP
Ambulation	12	*	*		
Body care and movement	23	*	*		
Mobility	10	*	*		
Household management	10		*		
Recreation and pastimes	8				*
Social interaction	20			*	*
Emotion	9			*	*
Alertness	10			*	*
Sleep and rest	7				*
Eating	9				
Communication	9			*	
Work	9				

Administration and acceptability

Three different methods of administration have been used for the SIP and FLP: interviewer administered, interviewer administered self-completion, and postal self-completion. Respondents seem to have little difficulty in completing the SIP or FLP and the areas of questioning do not appear to generate any resistance. They are longer than many instruments in this book and take between 20 and 30 minutes to complete. They are therefore unlikely to be suitable for use in the course of a normal consultation. One study has reported the use of the SIP in routine practice with older chronically ill patients in primary care.[12] However, the instrument was administered by a research assistant and patients were paid $5 to participate. Although the physicians found it useful, they were unanimous in their view that it was too long for use in routine practice. The SIP/FLP might also be considered too long for use in situations where a general health status measure is required to supplement more detailed disease-specific measures. They would also be rather lengthy for inclusion in surveys requiring a health status measure to supplement more detailed questioning in other areas.

Reliability and validity

The authors of the SIP have conducted extensive trials of reliability and validity, and there has been confirmation of some of their findings in other studies. Test–retest reliability has been shown to be consistently high for both interviewer administered and self-administered versions.[2,20,7] Internal consistency has also been examined, both for the instrument as a whole and for each category.[2] Test-retest reliability and inter-rater reliability have also been examined for the FLP.[5,17] The authors concluded that individual items should not be used independently.

The development procedures employed in the SIP ensure good content validity. Subsequent tests of validity have included comparisons with clinical assessments, other functional assessment instruments, and subjective ratings made by respondents. Initial validation against clinical assessments included patients suffering from arthritis and hyperthyroidism, and patients who had a hip replacement.[2] These showed good correlations between SIP scores and clinical assessments of functioning, although a study by Deyo and colleagues reported lower levels of correlation between clinicians' functional assessment and the SIP physical dimension, and very low correlation with the psychosocial dimension.[7] However, to the extent that the SIP goes beyond the criteria applied in normal clinical assessments, one might not expect high levels of correlation. In a primary care study, patients reported twice as many disabilities as were reported by physicians, but the physicians regarded the SIP as helpful in identifying problems that might otherwise have gone unrecognized.[12] Comparisons with other measures of function (e.g. Katz IADL and National Health Interviews Survey) have yielded good correlations.[2] Validation against clinical measures of function has been reported with patients suffering from rheumatoid arthritis,[21] inflammatory bowel disease[8] and chronic airflow limitation.[14] As with clinical judgements, the correlations are not very high, but this reflects the fact that the SIP is measuring the impact of the disease process on everyday life, which is unlikely to show a simple linear relationship with clinical criteria. There is some evidence that total SIP scores might be significantly affected by coexisting psychological problems.[9] A recent systematic study of the impact of psychological factors on SIP scores in patients with medical and psychiatric problems showed that the SIP does discriminate between physical and psychosocial dimensions of function, but that a major portion of the variance in scores is explained by depression.[3]

Little attention was paid in early development work to the ability of the SIP to detect change. Although it has been used in clinical trials across a wide range of conditions, Jette has criticized it for its lack of measurement sensitivity.[13] Whether or not it is sufficiently responsive to clinically significant change will depend to some extent on the particular circumstances. Liang in a comparison of five instruments for orthopedic evaluation showed that it was as good or better than the other instruments in detecting improvements over three months and one year following joint replacement.[16] In contrast, in a randomized placebo-controlled heart failure trial the SIP was unable to detect differences between treatment groups which were detected by Spitzer's Quality of Life Index[22] (see p. 204).

The authors of the FLP have devoted considerable attention to the validity of the global indexes of physical and psychosocial dimensions, the remaining independent categories (eating, communication and work) and overall FLP scores.[5] As mentioned above, their analyses produced slightly different groupings of categories than the SIP. However, in analyses of service use, they showed that both categories and global scores were equally poor predictors of service use.[5] This may be due to lack of measurement sensitivity, but it might also be that disability is in fact a poor predictor of overall service use.

Although the FLP uses weights derived from British judges, in a comparison of results from Britain and the USA, there was a striking similarity in the valuations placed upon health states by the judges.[19] Consequently the FLP item weights are only marginally different from those employed in the SIP.

Populations/client groups

The SIP has been used with a wide variety of populations and client groups, but it has been particularly useful in studies of patients suffering from chronic illness. A Medline search for the three-year period 1988–90 yielded more than 40 papers reporting studies which have used the SIP. Most studies have been carried out in the USA and these have included studies of patients suffering from chronic pain, arthritis, cancer, angina, heart failure, fatigue, and chronic lung disease. It was designed to be broadly applicable across demographic and cultural sub-groups. Although development work was carried out in the USA the SIP has been used in a number of other countries and is claimed to be as free as possible of cultural biases. Original development work was carried out with samples drawn from a pre-paid group practice, including both random samples and samples of consulters. Many of the studies which have used the SIP have been carried out in hospital settings, but the measure has also been used with both general population samples and people consulting primary care physicians.[12,15] However, the length of the SIP and therefore the time necessary to complete it, suggests that its use in primary care will be limited to research applications.

The FLP has not yet been employed in a similarly wide range of British studies because it was only recently published. Its use to date has been in surveys of disabled people[17] and people with chronic respiratory disorders.[24] There seems, however, to be no reason that it should not have a similar range of applications as the SIP. It is worth noting that developmental work on the FLP was carried out using patients drawn from a general medical practice.[18]

Comments

The SIP is one of the best multipurpose measures of the impact of disease currently available. It is well documented and has been widely used, particularly in the USA. It is likely to be useful in a wide variety of clinical and survey research settings, particularly those dealing with chronic illness. Although the FLP is more recent and has thus not been widely used, its very close similarity to the SIP suggests that much of the evidence for validity and usefulness in different clinical settings will be equally relevant.

Two important reservations should be borne in mind when considering use of the SIP. Firstly, its length may make it impractical for use in many situations. Secondly, because it is a general purpose measure and designed to be reliable and valid across a wide variety of groups, it may not be very responsive to clinically significant change over time in the same individuals. One approach to these problems of length, specificity, and responsiveness is to develop sections for specific applications. A number of researchers have begun to explore these possibilities,[6,23] and the authors of the FLP have questioned whether the number of items in the overall measure could not be reduced without loss of precision.[5]

References

1. Bergner, M., Bobbitt, R.A., Kressel, A., Pollard, W.E., Gilson, B.S., and Morris, J.R. (1976). The Sickness Impact Profile: conceptual formulation and methodology for the development of a health status measure. *International Journal of Health Services*, **6**, 393–415.
2. Bergner, M., Bobbitt, R.A., Carter, W.B., and Gilson, B.S. (1981). The Sickness Impact Profile: development and final revision of a health status measure. *Medical Care*, **19**, 787–805.
3. Brooks, W.B., Jordan, J.S., Divine, G.W., Smith, K.S., and Neelon, F.A. (1990). The impact of psychologic factors on measurement of functional status. *Medical Care*, **28**, 793–804.
4. Carter, W., Bobbitt, R., Bergner, M., and Gilson, B. (1976). Validation of an interval scaling: the Sickness Impact Profile. *Health Service Research*, **11**, 516–28.
5. Charlton, J.R.H., Patrick, D.L., and Peach, H. (1983). Use of multi-variate measures of disability in health surveys. *Journal of Epidemiology & Community Health*, **37**, 296–304.
6. Deyo, R. (1986). Comparative validity of the Sickness Impact Profile and shorter scales for functional assessment in low back pain. *Spine*, **11**, 951–4.
7. Deyo, R.A., Inui, T.S., Leininger, J.D., and Overman, S.S. (1983). Measuring functional outcomes in chronic disease: a comparison of traditional scales and a self administered health status questionnaire in patients with rheumatoid arthritis. *Medical Care*, **21**, 180–92.
8. Drossman, D.A., Patrick, D.L., Mitchell, C.M., Zagami, E.A., and Appelbaum, M.I. (1989). Health-related quality of life in inflammatory bowel

disease. Functional status and patient worries and concerns. *Digestive Diseases and Sciences*, **34**(9), 1379–86.

9. Follick, M. H., Smith, T. W., and Ahern, D. K. (1985). The Sickness Impact Profile: a global measure of disability in chronic low back pain. *Pain*, **21**, 67–76.
10. Gilson, B. S., Gilson, J. S., Bergner, M., Bobbitt, R. A., Kressel, S., Pollard, W. E., and Vesselago, M. (1975). The Sickness Impact Profile: development of an outcome measure of health care. *American Journal of Public Health*, **65**, 1304–10.
11. Gilson, B. S., Bergner, M., Bobbitt, R. A., and Carter, W. B. (1979). *The Sickness Impact Profile: final development and testing 1975–1978*. University of Washington Department of Health Services, Seattle.
12. Goldsmith, G. and Brodwick, M. (1989). Assessing the functional status of older patients with chronic illness. *Family Medicine*, **21**, 38–41.
13. Jette, A. M. (1980). Health status indicators: their utility in chronic disease evaluation research. *Journal of Chronic Diseases*, **33**, 567–79.
14. Jones, P. W., Baveystock, C. M., and Littlejohns, P. (1989). Relationships between general health measured with the Sickness Impact Profile and respiratory symptoms, physiological measures, and mood in patients with chronic airflow limitation. *American Review of Respiratory Diseases*, **140**(6), 1538–43.
15. Kroenke, K., Wood, D. R., Mangelsdorff, A. D., Meier, N. J., and Powell, J. B. (1988). Chronic fatigue in primary care. Prevalence, patient characteristics, and outcome. *Journal of the American Medical Association*, **260**, 929–34.
16. Liang, M. H., Fossel, A. H., and Larson, M. G. (1990). Comparisons of five health status instruments for orthopedic evaluation. *Medical Care*, **28**, 632–42.
17. Patrick, D. L., and Peach, H. (1989). *Disablement in the community*. Oxford University Press, Oxford.
18. Patrick, D. L., Peach, H., and Gregg, I. (1982). Disablement and care: a comparison of patient views and general practitioner knowledge. *Journal of the Royal College of General Practitioners*, **32**, 429–34.
19. Patrick, D. L., Sittampalam, Y., Sommerville, S. M., Carter, W. B. and Bergner, M. (1985). A cross cultural comparison of health status values. *American Journal of Public Health*, **75**, 1402–7.
20. Pollard, W. E., Bobbitt, R. A., Bergner, M., Martin, D. P., and Gilson, B. S. (1976). The Sickness Impact Profile: reliability of a health status measure. *Medical Care*, **14**, 146–55.
21. Sullivan, M., Ahlmen, M., and Bjelle, A. (1990). Health status assessment in rheumatoid arthritis. I. Further work on the validity of the Sickness Impact Profile. *Journal of Rheumatology*, **17**, 439–47.
22. Tandon, P. K., Stander, H., and Schwarz, R. P. Jr. (1989). Analysis of quality of life data from a randomized, placebo-controlled heart-failure trial. *Journal of Clinical Epidemiology,* **42**, 955–62.
23. Temkin, N. R., Dikmen, S., Machamer, J., and McLean, A. (1989). General v disease specific measures: further work on the Sickness Impact Profile for head injury. *Medical Care*, **27**, 544–53.
24. Williams, S. J., and Bury, M. R. (1989). 'Breathtaking': the consequences of chronic respiratory disorder. *International Disability Studies*, **11**, 114–20.

Nottingham Health Profile (NHP) (Hunt, and colleagues 1980)[1]

Purpose

The NHP measures levels of self-reported distress, including both distress caused by pathological changes and that resulting from adverse social and/or environmental conditions. It was intended to: provide an assessment of needs for care which is not based on purely medical criteria, enable subsequent evaluation of the care provided for people in need and make a start on the development of an indicator for use in population health status surveys.[11] The authors also suggest that it may be a useful adjunct to clinical interviews as a means of improving the quality of doctor–patient communication.[3] It provides a tool for examining the relationships between observed pathologies and subjective responses to these.

Background

The authors set out to develop a measure of health that utilized patients' perceptions and language rather than medical judgements and categories. The NHP is similar to the Sickness Impact Profile in its focus on the impact of disease on the individual, but whereas the SIP focuses on the behavioural consequences, the NHP asks about feelings and emotional states directly.

Statements concerning aspects of ill health were derived from interviews with 768 patients suffering from a variety of acute and chronic ailments. These provided the basis for the first version of the NHP.[10] Between 1978 and 1981 a second team of researchers, working on the same set of statements, developed a different version of the scale and conducted tests of reliability and validity.[4] They also devised a system of weights for individual items using Thurstone's method of paired comparisons. Groups of patients and non-patients were asked to compare statements and make judgements as to which was worse. This later version of the NHP has become the most well known and widely used, and the remainder of this section refers to this version.

Description

The NHP consists of two parts which can be used independently. Part I, which is most commonly used, consists of 38 statements grouped into six sections (The sections are physical mobility, pain, sleep, social isolation, emotional reaction, and energy). A copy of this has appeared in *Quality of life: assessment and application*.[11] The number of statements in each section ranges from three for energy to nine for emotional reactions. Respondents are asked to indicate for each statement whether they experience the problem at the moment. All statements are simply constructed, for example 'I'm in constant pain', 'I'm tired all the time'. None exceeds 10 words in length although two are extended by examples (for instance 'I find it hard to stand for long e.g. at the kitchen sink, waiting for a bus'). Permission to reproduce the scale has been denied by the authors who require written applications for use.† A slight variation in the wording asks whether respondents consider statements to be true for them in general.[9] In neither case is any clear guidance given as to the time period to be considered when answering, although the two versions 'at the moment' and 'in general' might be interpreted quite differently by respondents.

Item scoring is straightforward, zero for a no response and one for a yes. Scores are presented in terms of a profile rather than an overall score. The authors do not recommend the construction of overall scores and no work has been reported on the validity of combining scores on different sections. Scores for each section are calculated by applying a weight to each item and summing the item scores for that section.[4] All scores range between 0 and 100, but it should be remembered that the range of possible scores is very limited. On a section such as energy, which consists of only three statements, only eight scores are possible. It is also important, from the point of view of analysing and interpreting data from the NHP, to note that scores are heavily skewed in relatively healthy populations. The majority of respondents score zero on each section. Indeed, in a recent population survey, just under half of all respondents answered 'no' to all 38 items.[8] The modal response for all items and categories is zero. For this reason, some users of the NHP have used a simple distribution between zero and non-zero scores, in preference to calculating weighted scores that might imply a spurious sense of precision. It has been suggested that mean category scores should be calculated only for those making one or more positive responses.[8]

Part II of the NHP asks respondents to indicate whether or not their state of health affects activity in seven areas of everyday life: job of work, looking after the home, social life, home life, sex life, interests and hobbies, and holidays. Responses are coded as a simple yes/no, and no weighting is provided for different items, although the authors did explore this possibility.[4] Part II has been used less extensively than Part I and deals with a very different conceptual area.

Administration and acceptability

The NHP is self-administered and can be used as a postal questionnaire. It can also be completed in the presence of an interviewer or in a waiting room or other similar location. Most respondents can complete it in about five minutes and the authors report that it is acceptable to and easily understood by most respondents. Some respondents do, however, have difficulty with

† Galen Research & Consultancy, 2 Finney Drive, Chorlton Green, Manchester M21 IDS, UK.

simple yes/no responses to statements, and with defining a suitable time period. It is not clear whether 'at the moment' should be treated literally, and, if not, what time period does it represent?

Reliability and validity

Two studies of test–retest reliability have been carried out on patients with osteoarthritis and peripheral vascular disease, using repeat testing after a gap of four weeks.[2] High correlations between scores on each administration were achieved. Other forms of reliability testing have not been used, because they were considered inappropriate.[11] However, although the authors considered measures of internal consistency inappropriate, Kind and Carr-Hill have shown both a lack of homogeneity within categories and significant correlations between category scores and between items in different categories.[8] In particular, there is substantial intercorrelation between the mobility and pain dimensions.

Extensive tests of the validity of Part I of the NHP have been mounted using a variety of populations. Content validity is claimed through the method of development, using statements generated by a large sample of patients. It is not, however, clear how items were grouped into categories. The various studies of validity are summarized by the authors,[4,11] and include studies of both criterion and construct validity with elderly people, GP consulters and non-consulters, fit workers, pregnant women, patients suffering from chronic illnesses, and general population samples. NHP scores have been shown to be related to sex, age, and social class, to differentiate between well and ill people and between consulters and non-consulters of general practitioners, and to be sensitive to improvements in health in patients recovering from fracture. The authors conclude that the NHP has been shown to be a highly satisfactory measure of subjective health status.

Despite the evidence of validity produced by the authors, the NHP has been criticized by Kind and Carr-Hill.[8,7] They have questioned the legitimacy of item weights, the claim that each category measures only one dimension and the utility of a measure whose modal value in the general population is zero, either as a screening tool or for evaluative purposes.

There does seem to be good evidence that the NHP is capable of identifying people suffering from chronic conditions and distinguishing between those suffering from different conditions.[4] Comparisons of patients suffering from rheumatoid arthritis and migraine showed marked differences, and the authors concluded that the NHP may be used to assess the impact of illness on sufferers' lives.[6,5] Nevertheless, in this study the weakness of the pain dimension seemed to be confirmed, in that migraine sufferers reported no more pain than samples from the general population.

There is some evidence from clinical trials of heart/lung transplants[12] and anti-hypertensive medication[1] that the NHP is able to detect changes resulting from specific treatments. In other trials, however, the NHP has failed to detect change. Without systematic evaluation of its responsiveness to clinically significant change, including comparisons with other instruments, it is impossible to assess how useful the NHP is as an outcome measure in clinical trials.

Populations/service settings

The NHP is suitable for use with individuals or groups of people over the age of 16 years. Studies have demonstrated its applicability to populations of elderly people, fit, and ill people, as well as to general population samples. In general populations or those with only minor health problems most respondents will score zero on most items. Because of the extensive development work it has been possible to develop population norms for a variety of age, sex, and patient groups,[4] although the small numbers on which some of these are based suggests a need for caution in using these. Despite the fact that it has been widely used in population surveys, the content of the items and the distribution of scores suggest that its main applications will be with people suffering from chronic illness. Recent studies report its use with patients who have undergone heart transplants, those suffering from angina, rheumatoid arthritis, migraine, hypertension, Parkinson's disease, irritable bowel syndrome, and multiple sclerosis. It has become one of the most commonly used health status measures in Britain. Its brevity and acceptability to respondents make it easy to use in primary medical care.

Comments

The NHP is shorter than other measures such as the Sickness Impact Profile. It attempts a compromise between comprehensiveness and sensitivity on the one hand, and brevity and economy on the other. For these reasons it is likely to be attractive to both clinicians and researchers. However, it is at least questionable whether it succeeds in achieving this compromise without losing out on both counts. It suffers from a number of weaknesses that should be borne in mind when contemplating its use. Firstly, it is not a measure of health, but a measure of the distress caused by ill health. Its content seems more suited to people suffering from chronic illnesses than to general populations or those suffering minor health problems which cause discomfort. Secondly, the method of development and testing has concentrated on its ability to discriminate between groups, rather than to respond to clinically significant changes in the same individuals over time. It may therefore lack sensitivity or responsiveness. This is obviously the case for any respondent who scores zero on any section at first administration. Subsequent improvement cannot be measured. Thirdly, criticisms have been made of the method of weighting items in each section, the construction of category scores and the lack of evidence concerning operating characteristics. Lastly, the profile presentation of results can make analysis cumbersome and interpretation difficult.

It should be noted that unlike all other instruments in this chapter, the authors do make a charge for its use.

References

1. De Lame, P. A., Droussin, A. M., Thomson, M., Verhaest, L., and Wallace, S. (1989). The effects of enalapril on hypertension and quality of life. A large multicenter study in Belgium. *Acta Cardiologica*, **44**, 289–302.
2. Hunt, S. M., McKenna, S. P. and Williams, J. (1981). Reliability of a population survey tool for measuring perceived health problems: a study of patients with osteo arthrosis. *Journal of Epidemiology and Community Health*, **35**, 297–300.
3. Hunt, S. M., McEwen, J., and McKenna, S. P. (1985). Measuring health status: a new tool for clinicians and epidemiologists. *Journal of the Royal College of General Practitioners*, **35**, 185–8.
4. Hunt, S. M., McEwen, J., and McKenna, S. P. (1986). *Measuring health status.* Croom Helm, London.
5. Jenkinson, C. and Fitzpatrick, R. (1990). Measurement of health status in patients with chronic illness: comparison of the Nottingham Health Profile and the General Health Questionnaire. *Family Practice*, **7**, 121–4.
6. Jenkinson, C., Fitzpatrick, R., and Argyle, M. (1988). The Nottingham Health Profile: an analysis of its sensitivity in differentiating illness groups. *Social Science and Medicine*, **27(12)**, 1411–14.
7. Kind, P. (1982). A comparison of two models for scaling health indicators. *International Journal of Epidemiology*, **11**, 271–5.
8. Kind, P. and Carr-Hill, R. (1978). The Nottingham Health Profile: A useful tool for epidemiologists? *Social Science and Medicine*, **25**, 905–10.
9. McDowell, I. W. and Newell, C. (1987). *Measuring health: a guide to rating scales and questionnaires.* Oxford University Press, New York.
10. McDowell, I. W., Martini C. J. M., and Waugh, W. (1978). A method for self assessment of disability before and after hip replacement operations. *British Medical Journal*, **2**, 957–9.
11. McEwen, J. (1988). The Nottingham Health Profile. In *Quality of life: assessment and application* (ed. S. R. Walker and R. M. Rosser), pp. 95–111 MTP, Lancaster.
12. O'Brien, B. J., Banner, N. R., Gibson, S., and Yacoub, M. H. (1988). The Nottingham Health Profile as a measure of quality of life following combined heart and lung transplantation. *Journal of Epidemiology and Community Health*, **42**, 232–4.

McMaster Health Index Questionnaire (MHIQ) (Chambers 1976)

Purpose

The MHIQ is a measure of global health status in terms of physical, emotional, and social functioning. It is designed to be sufficiently flexible to be used with people suffering a wide range of health problems. It is intended to be a general measure of quality of life for use in health service evaluation and clinical trials, rather than an instrument for use in individual patients as part of normal clinical practice.

Background

Chambers and his colleagues began developing the MHIQ in 1970 because they recognized the need for a general health index which provided more information than routine health statistics (e.g. mortality and morbidity), and which could be used to supplement the sort of highly specific outcome measures used in clinical trials of specific therapeutic or preventive procedures.[8] They set out to develop a measure which would be credible to both clinicians and administrators and would meet the following criteria: comprehensiveness, positive orientation, general applicability, sensitivity, simplicity, precision, and amenability to index construction. Rather than seeking a single global index, the authors adopted the WHO definition of health and sought to develop separate indexes of physical, emotional, and social functioning.

Using the WHO definition as a conceptual foundation, an initial pool of 172 items was generated from a review of existing instruments and from discussions with a wide variety of clinicians, social scientists and other professionals. Items in the physical function section were derived from Garrad and Bennett's Disability and Impairment Interview Schedule[7] and from Katz's Index of ADL (see p. 43). Items in the emotional function section were also adopted from a number of existing measures.[2] The social function items were based on an extensive review of available measures, but did not draw directly on particular instruments.[3] The items were selected from the initial pool by assessing their responsiveness to changes in function and their ability to predict family physician's global assessments of physical, emotional, and social function.

Description

The MHIQ consists of 68 items which are presented in questionnaire format. Three broad sections deal with physical, emotional, and social functions. The questionnaire is too long to reproduce here, but Exhibit 7.3 shows examples of questions and response categories under each of the three headings (the full questionnaire is published in a recent paper).[2] Physical function items cover physical activities, mobility, self-care, and communication. Emotional function items cover self esteem, personal relationships, thoughts about the future, and critical life events. Social function items cover general well-being, work, social role performance, material welfare, family participation, and friendships. Each section also includes a global assessment of function.

Exhibit 7.3 Sample items from the McMaster Health Index Questionnaire

(Adapted with permission, from Chambers, L. W. (1988). The McMaster Health Index Questionnaire: an update. In *Quality of Life: Assessment and Application* (ed. S. R. Walker and R. M. Rosser). MPT, Lancaster)

Section A: Physical function items

1. Today, are you physically able to run a short distance, say 300 feet, if you are in a hurry?
   (This is about the length of a football field or soccer pitch.)
   1. NO
   2. YES

2. Today, do you (or would you) have any physical difficulty at all with:

	DIFFICULTY	NO DIFFICULTY
a. walking as far as a mile?	1	2
b. climbing up two flights of stairs?	1	2
c. standing up from and/or sitting down on a chair	1	2
d. feeding yourself?	1	2
e. undressing?	1	2
f. washing (face and hands), shaving (men),and/or combing hair?	1	2
g. shopping?	1	2
h. cooking?	1	2
i. dusting and/or light housework?	1	2
j. cleaning floors?	1	2

3. Today, are you physically able to take part in any sports (hockey, swimming, bowling, golf, and so forth) or exercise regularly?
   1. NO
   2. YES

Section B: Emotional function items

Often people's health affects the way they feel about life. For these next questions, please circle the choice that is closest to the way you feel about each statement.
   If you: **STRONGLY AGREE**, circle 1; **AGREE**, circle 2,; if you are **NEUTRAL**, circle 3; if you: **DISAGREE**, circle 4; **STRONGLY DISAGREE**, circle 5.

	STRONGLY AGREE				STRONGLY DISAGREE
10. I sometimes feel that my life is not very useful	1	2	3	4	5

Exhibit 7.3 (continued)

11. Everyone should have someone in his life whose happiness means as much to him as his own	1	2	3	4	5
12. I am a useful person to have around	1	2	3	4	5
13. I am inclined to feel that I'm a failure	1	2	3	4	5
14. Many people are unhappy because they do not know what they want out of life	1	2	3	4	5
15. In a society where almost everyone is out for himself, people soon come to distrust each other	1	2	3	4	5

Section C: Social function items

This section contains some questions on general health and on your social activities.

29. How would you say your health is today? Would you say your health is (Circle your answer)
     1 VERY GOOD
     2 PRETTY GOOD
     3 NOT TOO GOOD

29. Taking all things together, how would you say things are today? Would you say you are:
     1 VERY HAPPY
     2 PRETTY HAPPY
     3 NOT TOO HAPPY

30. In general, how satisfying do you find the way your're spending your life today? Would you call it
     1 COMPLETELY SATISFYING
     2 PRETTY SATISFYING
     3 NOT VERY SATISFYING

41. How long has it been since you last had a holiday?
     (Write in number '0' if presently on holidays)
     _____ MONTHS _____ YEARS

42. During the last year, have any of the following things happened to you?
     a. separation from your spouse?
        1 YES
        2 NO
     b. divorce?
        1 NO
        2 YES
     c. going on welfare during the last year?
        1 NO
        2 YES

Exhibit 7.3 (continued)

---

    d. trouble getting along with
       friends/relatives during the last year?
       1 NO
       2 YES
    e. retired from work during the last year?
       1 NO
       2 YES
    f. some other problem or change in your
       life? (please specify)

Physical function items relate to the day on which the MHIQ is administered, emotional function items to the present or recent past, and social function items to various specified time periods (e.g. today, past week, past year). All questions are designed to elicit information about performance rather than capacity, so that they ask respondents to describe what they do, rather than estimate what they could do. No attempt is made to establish whether respondents have any help with activities or how difficult they find them.

Response categories range from simple yes/no dichotomies to five point scales. Some are ordinally scaled but many are nominal categories. Despite the fact that Chambers and others have published a substantial number of both methodological and empirical papers on the MHIQ, the scoring system has not been published in an easily accessible form. Since all of the papers employ the same scoring system this seems an unfortunate omission. Even the most recent paper,[2] which reproduces the questionnaire, does not describe the scoring system, which seems to be available only in a research report.[1] Scores for each section are calculated by converting all responses to dichotomies, which are scored 0 for poor health and 1 for good health. Thus, for example, responses to the statement 'people feel affectionate towards me' are scored as follows: strongly agree, agree, $= 1$; strongly disagree, disagree neutral, no answer $= 0$. This procedure produces some odd classifications, so that watching television for between one and two hours per day scores 0 (poor social function), whilst watching less than one hour per day but more than three hours per week scores 1 (good social function). Section scores are calculated by adding the scores for all items in the section and dividing by the number of items. Twenty four items are used for the physical function score, and 25 each for the emotional and social function scores. However, a number of items are combined in the physical section to give a total of 19 for scoring purposes. Six items are included in both the emotional and social function sections for the purposes of scoring. Since scores on each section are not combined to produce a grand total, this does not present any difficulty.

Administration and acceptability

Three methods of administration have been tested: self completion, telephone interview and personal interview. The mode of administration has little effect on reliability and the choice between different methods can be made on grounds of convenience, acceptability, and expected response rates. Unfortunately, response rates for different methods are not reported, although it is to be expected that use of the self-completed version as a postal questionnaire would produce a lower response rate than other methods. Self-completion of the questionnaire takes about 20 minutes and no problems of acceptability have been reported.

Reliability and validity

Evidence from a number of studies of reliability and validity is summarized in a recent review of work on the MHIQ.[2] Test–retest reliability has been established with physiotherapy and psychiatry out-patients over a one-week period.[1] Less attention seems to have been devoted to assessing internal consistency, but a study of physiotherapy patients showed acceptable levels of internal consistency for group comparisons.[1] Comparisons of different methods of administration (self-completion, telephone interview, personal interview) demonstrated acceptable levels of reliability.[5] Overall, the evidence of reliability seems limited but satisfactory for group comparisons, although not sufficient to justify using the MHIQ for individual assessment.

Although the method of generating items for the MHIQ seemed to be intended to ensure content validity, no systematic appraisal of content validity has been undertaken. However, considerable attention has been devoted to establishing criterion and construct validity. The MHIQ scores have been shown to correlate with global assessments by health professionals.[6,8] Physical function scores reflect actual physical performance, assessments by therapists, and clinical measures of function in patients suffering from rheumatoid arthritis.[4] Studies of a variety of different patient groups show that the different sections are able to discriminate between patients with different problems. Thus, for example, family practice patients were shown to have better physical function scores but worse emotional function scores than patients attending a physiotherapy clinic, those suffering chronic respiratory disease, and insulin dependent diabetic patients.[2] Scores also confirmed the hypothesis that chronic respiratory disease and diabetic patients would have lower social function scores.

In the study of physiotherapy patients MHIQ physical function scores were shown to be responsive to clinically significant change.[5] There was no change in scores one week after starting treatment, but a significant improvement on discharge. In a study of methotrexate in rheumatoid arthritis, the MHIQ showed statistically significant but modest improvements in all three dimensions,[9] but it was much less sensitive to change than a disease-specific patient preference questionnaire.

Populations/service settings

The MHIQ is a general-purpose measure suitable for use in a wide variety of service settings. It can be used with healthy people in the community, patients attending primary health care, and hospital out-patients and in-patients. It is sufficiently reliable and sensitive for group comparisons but not suitable for assessing individuals over time. It is suitable for use with patients suffering from a wide range of conditions, as reported above, but Chambers recommends that it be used in conjunction with more focused measures in disease-specific studies. It has not, however, been widely used by other researchers. A literature search for the period 1988–90 yielded references to only four papers reporting use of the MHIQ.

Comments

The development and testing of the MHIQ has continued over a period of nearly twenty years. When it was first developed there were few multidimensional measures of health status available. Alongside the range of measures currently available the MHIQ has a number of weaknesses. It is not based on patients' experiences or preferences, it is relatively cumbersome to administer, the scoring system is somewhat arbitrary and questionable, levels of reliability are no more than satisfactory, and evidence of validity is limited. Chambers has suggested either that further develop-ment would be desirable or alternative instruments might yield better results.[2] Nevertheless, the MHIQ may be worth considering in association with disease specific measures for studies involving group comparisons in the evaluation of health services or specific therapeutic interventions.

References

1. Chambers, L.W. (1982). *The McMaster Health Index Questionnaire: methodologic documentation and report of the second generation of investigations*. Department of Clinical Epidemiology and Biostatistics, McMaster University, Hamilton, Ontario.
2. Chambers, L.W. (1988). The McMaster Health Index Questionnaire: an update. In *Quality of Life: Assessment and Application* (ed. S.R. Walker and R.M. Rosser) pp. 113–31. MTP, Lancaster.
3. Chambers, L.W., Sackett, D.L., Goldsmith, C.H., Macpherson, A.S., and McAuley, R.G. (1976). Development and application of an index of social function. *Health Service Research*, **11**, 430–41.
4. Chambers, L.W., MacDonald, L.A., Tugwell, P., Buchanan, W.W., and Kraag, G. (1982). The McMaster Health Index Questionnaire as a measure of quality of life for patients with rheumatoid disease. *Journal of Rheumatology*, **9**, 780–4.
5. Chambers, L.W., Haight, M., Norman, G., and MacDonald, L. (1987). Sensitivity to change and the effect of mode of administration on health status measurement. *Medical Care*, **25**, 470–9.
6. Fortin, F., and Kerouac, S. (1977). Validation of questionnaires on physical function. *Nursing Research*, **26**, 128–35.
7. Garrad, J. and Bennett, A.E. (1971). A validated interview schedule for use in population surveys of chronic disease and disability. *British Journal of Preventive and Social Medicine*, **25**, 97–104.
8. Sackett, D.L., Chambers, L.W., Macpherson, A.S., Goldsmith, C.H., and McAuley, R.G. (1977). The development and application of indices of health: General methods and summary of results. *American Journal of Public Health*, **67**, 423–8.
9. Tugwell, P., Bombardier, C., Buchanan, W.W., Goldsmith, C., Grace, E., Bennett, K.J., *et al* (1990). Methotrexate in rheumatoid arthritis. Impact on quality of life assessed by traditional standard-item and individualized patient preference health status questionnaires. *Archives of Internal Medicine*, **150**, 59–62.

MOS Short-Form General Health Survey measures (MOS SF-20, RAND 36-Item Health Survey 1.0 and SF-36) (Ware, Stewart, and colleagues, 1988 to 1992)

Purpose

The time needed to complete many of the longer health status measures restricts the circumstances and settings in which they can be used. The authors of the MOS short-forms set out to develop general health survey measures which would be comprehen-sive and psychometrically sound, yet short enough to be practical for use in large-scale studies of general populations and patients in practice settings. They were also intended to have applications in health policy research to evaluate the effects of health care and in clinical trials. Two versions have been widely tested and used: the 20-item short-form (SF-20) and the newer 36-item version. A third, based on six single-item measures, has been less thoroughly evaluated.

Background

The MOS short-forms have their origins in the Medical Outcomes Study, a large-scale observational study of variations in physician styles and patient outcomes in different systems of care. The MOS researchers developed a comprehensive general health survey instrument consisting of 149 items (35 scales and 8 summary indices) referred to as the Functioning and Well-being Profile. This drew heavily upon existing measures, particularly those selected or developed for the RAND Health Insurance Experiment (HIE) (some of which are covered in earlier chapters). However, they also introduced substantial improvements affecting conceptualization, reliability, validity, and efficiency. Subsequently, a core subset of 113 items (20 scales and 4 summary indices) was derived from this. Details of the full range of MOS measures have recently been published.[16] A scoring manual for the core subset is also available.[7]

The SF-20 was also based on original HIE instruments and was developed and tested as part of the Medical Outcomes Study. Item selection was based on Ware's criteria for a comprehensive health measure.[17] Six health concepts are represented with between one and six items for each dimension. The SF-20 answered two problems: the impracticality in clinical settings of using existing measures taking up to 45 minutes to complete, and the poorer precision and reliability of single-item measures which limit their value in group comparisons on multiple health dimensions. Stewart and her colleagues tested and reliability and validity of the SF-20 on more than 11000 patients consulting in a variety of settings and on a general population sample of over 2000 adults with very encouraging results.[15, 19]

The 36-item measure is a more recent development. It is based on the full MOS battery and reflects the authors' accumulated experience in constructing, evaluating, and improving the precision of short-form scales. Items have been selected to reproduce the parent scales as much as possible. A degree of comparability with the SF-20 is retained, but eight health concepts are covered with between two and 10 items for each dimension, and changes in scales and the number of levels within them have been incorporated.[18] Two versions of this measure exist, containing identical items but using different scoring systems. One, known as the MOS SF-36, was published by Ware and Sherbourne[18] and is under the Medical Outcomes Study Trust copyright. The other, known as the RAND 36-item Health Survey 1.0, is under the copyright of RAND. Both organizations have indicated their desire to ensure free access to their instrument. An anglicized version (under the copyright of the New England Medical Center Hospitals) and normative data for Britain are available.[2, 4] Free access to the anglicized version is routinely granted by the copyright holder. Further development work is planned within the framework of the Medical Outcomes Study.[18]

Description

The six health concepts represented in the SF-20 are physical, role, and social functioning, mental health, current health perceptions, and pain. The 36-item measure includes the additional concept of energy/fatigue, and separates role functioning into two separate scales to reflect the effects of physical and emotional problems. The emphasis on health perceptions is also changed from a current to a general perspective. Exhibit 7.4 shows the anglicized text[2] which, for instance, substitutes miles/yards for blocks walked, feeling low for feeling blue, etc. Question 2 is not included in the eight dimensions, nor is it scored. Items which also appear in the SF-20 have been marked, and variations between the two versions have been noted. For instance, physical functioning in the SF-20 has six items with responses based on duration of limitation, resulting in seven scale levels. In the SF-36 physical functioning has 10 items with responses based on severity of limitation, resulting in 21 scale levels.

Scores are constructed for each dimension by adding the scores for each item within that dimension. Generally, higher scores indicate better functioning or health, and the response categories for some items are thus reversed. For the MOS SF-36, many questions are scored simply by assigning the value '1' to the first (or last) listed response category and increasing the score by one for each succeeding (or preceding) category. However, questions 1, 7, and 8 are somewhat more complex, with values reflecting unequal intervals between response categories or the cumulative effect of more than one problem. Once again, scales are constructed by adding together the scores for all questions within a dimension. However, this raw scale score is then transformed into a value between zero and 100 by deducting from it the lowest possible scale score, dividing the result by the potential range of scores, and multiplying the product by 100. For example, the lowest possible scale score for physical functioning is 10 and the potential range is 20 (i.e. between 10 and 30). A raw score of 21 thus converts as follows: $[(21–10)/20] \times 100 = 55$. Full details of the MOS SF-36 scoring system as used in their publications[9, 8] can be obtained from John Ware at the Health Institute, New England Medical Center Hospitals, 750 Washington Street, NEMC No. 345, 750 Washington Street, Boston, MA 02111, USA. Two manuals, one of which includes a floppy diskette containing scoring algorithms and a test data set with results, are available free of charge.[11, 12]

The RAND scoring procedures involve assigning values to response categories of between zero and 100 at equal intervals, dependent upon the number of possible responses. Thus, a question with six response categories may be scored 0, 20, 40, 60, 80, or 100, whilst one with three categories is scored 0, 50, or 100. Scales are constructed by adding together the scores for all questions within a dimension and averaging them across the number of questions included. A detailed description of this scoring system is available from R. Hays or C. Sherbourne at RAND, 1700 Main Street, P.O. Box 2138, Santa Monica, CA 90407, USA.

Scoring procedures for the SF-20 are more complex and have been reproduced elsewhere.[19] Current evidence suggests that the 36-item measure will become the more widely used short-form measure in the future.

Administration and acceptability

The SF-20 takes three to four minutes to complete; the 36-item measure takes between five and 10 minutes. Both are suitable for postal, telephone, or on-site administration. No problems of acceptability have been reported with either. Response rates are generally high. In the MOS study, the SF-20 achieved rates of at least 65 per cent.[15] One US study reported rates of over 85 per cent[10] and a British study achieved 73 per cent.[1] For the 36-item measure, two British studies, both postal surveys, have reported rates of 72 per cent and 83 per cent,[2, 4] and the incidence of missing data appears to be low (0.5 to 4 per cent on each dimension). However, problems with higher levels of missing data have been reported among populations aged 65 and over.[2]

Reliability and validity

The SF-20 has achieved levels of internal consistency on multi-item dimensions which are only marginally lower than those obtained from the corresponding full-length MOS measures, and in all cases are acceptable for group comparisons.[1, 15, 16, 19] The reliability of single-item dimensions (pain and social function) is more questionable. The 36-item measure apparently outperforms the SF-20, achieving marginally lower levels than the parent measures for consistency on pain and mental health, but

Exhibit 7.4   MOS 36-ITEM Short-form General Health Survey (SF-36)

SF-20
Code

*   1. In general, would you say your health is:

*   Excellent   Very good   Good   Fair   Poor

–   2. *Compared to one year ago* how would you rate your health in general *now*?

Much better...   Somewhat better...   About the same...   Somewhat worse...   Much worse...

1   3. The following questions are about activities you might do during a typical day. Does *your health now limit you* in these activities? If so, how much?

*   a) **Vigorous activities**, such as running, lifting heavy objects, participating in strenuous sports
1   b) **Moderate activities**, such as moving a table, pushing a vacuum cleaner, bowling or playing golf
1   c) Lifting or carrying groceries
1   d) Climbing **several** flights of stairs
–   e) Climbing **one** flight of stairs
1   f) Bending, kneeling or stooping
–   g) Walking **more than one mile**
–   h) Walking **half a mile**
1   i) Walking **one hundred yards**
1   j) Bathing or dressing yourself

2   Yes, limited a lot.   Yes, limited a little.   No, not limited at all

–   4. During the *past 4 weeks* have you had any of the following problems with your work or other regular daily activities *as a result of your physical health*?

a) Cut down on the **amount of time** you spent on work or other activities
b) **Accomplished less** than you would like
c) Were limited in the **kind** of work or other activities
d) Had **difficulty** performing the work or other activities (for example, it took extra effort)

Yes   No

–   5. During the *past 4 weeks* have you had any of the following problems with your work or other regular daily activities *as a result of any emotional problems* (such as feeling depressed or anxious)?

a) Cut down on the **amount of time** you spent on work or other activities
b) **Accomplished less** than you would like
c) Didn't do work or other activities as **carefully** as usual

Yes   No

–   6. During the *past 4 weeks*, to what extent has your physical health or emotional problems interfered with your normal social activities with family, friends, neighbours, or groups?

Not at all   Slightly   Moderately   Quite a bit   Extremely

Exhibit 7.4 (continued)

*   7. How much *bodily* pain have you had during the *past 4 weeks*?

    None   Very mild   Mild   Moderate   Severe   Very severe

–   8. During the *past 4 weeks*, how much did *pain* interfere with your normal work (including both work outside the home and housework)?

    Not at all   A little bit   Moderately   Quite a bit   Extremely

1   9. These questions are about how you feel and how things have been with you *during the past 4 weeks*. For each question, please give the one answer that comes closest to the way you have been feeling. How much of the time during the *past 4 weeks*

–   a) did you feel full of life?
*   b) have you been a very nervous person?
*   c) have you felt so down in the dumps that nothing could cheer you up?
*   d) have you felt calm and peaceful?
–   e) did you have a lot of energy?
*   f) have you felt downhearted and low?
–   g) did you feel worn out?
*   h) have you been a happy person?
–   i) did you feel tired?

*   All of the time   Most of the time   A good bit of time   Some of the time   A little of the time   None of the time

1   10. During the *past 4 weeks*, how much of the time has your *physical health or emotional problems* interfered with your social activities (like visiting with friends, relatives, etc.)?

2   All of the time   Most of the time   Some of the time   A little of the time   None of the time

1   11. How TRUE or FALSE is *each* of the following statements for you?

–   a) I seem to get ill a little more easily than other people
*   b) I am as healthy as anybody I know
–   c) I expect my health to get worse
*   d) My health is excellent

*   Definitely true   Mostly true   Dont know   Mostly false   Definitely false

---

SF-20 codes:
- not included in SF-20
* Appears in similar form to SF-36 item
1. Concept remains but changes in wording and/or presentation
2. Changed scale categories.

---

matching them for physical and role functioning, and exceeding them for social function in one US Study.[9] (The parent measure of social function has recognized limitations.) General health perceptions performed less well, but still within acceptable limits. British studies[2,4] have also reported acceptable levels of internal consistency for all dimensions, though the two-item social functioning scale apparently retains the limitations experienced with the parent measure.

No reports on test–retest reliability have been found for the SF-20. However, recent British work on the SF-36[2] found that the mean of the differences did not exceed one point on a 100 point scale, making it clinically insignificant.

The construct validity of both the SF-20 and the 36-item measure is supported by correlations within the measures, comparisons between general and patient populations, and correlations with sociodemographic characteristics.[2,4,15,14,18]

Evidence of the SF-20's discriminant validity has been reported in studies comparing patient scores across several chronic conditions and between these conditions and depression.[10, 20] Unique score profiles have been generated by groups with different conditions, and groups with multiple problems have scored less highly than those with a single condition. However, the advent of the 36-item measure has shifted attention to establishing the validity of this instrument.

SF-36 scores have been shown to correlate well with health service utilization and the existence of long-standing illness.[2, 4] The instrument has been shown to discriminate well between renal dialysis, diabetic, and hypertensive patients.[6] In a comparison with the Nottingham Health Profile (p. 142), scores were less skewed and it proved more sensitive to minor deviations from good health on five of its eight dimensions.[2] Its ability to distinguish between groups with known different problems and clinically defined levels of severity has been reported to approach that of its MOS parent measures.[9] In comparison with COOP charts (p. 159), which also discriminate well, it offers an assessment of severity which appears to be less influenced by psychological distress.[9]

A recent study compared the use of SIP (p. 133), FSQ (p. 165), AIMS (p. 208), HAQ (p. 215), and the SF-36 on a small sample of patients before and after total hip arthroplasty.[5] All instruments were able to detect significant improvements in health status over time but the sample size was too small to detect significant differences between the measures in sensitivity. The creation of a composite score across dimensions for the SF-36 in this study is somewhat dubious.

As the authors of the SF-20 and the 36-item measure recognize,[16,18] there remains a considerable amount of work to do in establishing evidence of reliability, validity, and sensitivity. Studies should evaluate further how well the instruments discriminate between groups, how effective they are in predicting future health and health service utilization, and the responsiveness of different dimensions to clinically significant change in individuals. The King's Fund is supporting a number of British validation studies on the SF-36. Its central role in an Outcomes Management System,[3] currently used by over 70 organizations in North America,[13] should ensure that a growing body of literature on its reliability and validity emanates from the United States.

Populations/Service Settings

These instruments are designed to be used with all adults, though in common with other self-report measures, a higher incidence of missing data among elderly respondents has been noted.[2] They have been tested on general population samples and patients attending a variety of health professionals. They are appropriate for use in a busy clinical practice where there will be little time for completing a longer instrument. As part of the OMS,[3] the SF-36 is now in regular use with patients suffering from a wide range of conditions. A three-year programme of international research, the International Quality of Life Assessment (IQOLA) project has been launched to adapt culturally, translate, validate, and norm the SF-36 for use in 15 countries. Normative data is already available for Britain[4] based on a general population of nearly 10 000 and broken down by age, sex, social class, longstanding illness, and recent consulting.

Comments

Although these instruments, particularly the 36-item measures, are relatively new and further evidence of their reliability and validity is needed, they are largely derived from existing RAND Health Insurance Experiment measures, which have been extensively tested for reliability and validity. Their development and testing is characterized by the same attention to conceptual clarity and rigorous testing. However, we should like to see more evidence of their ability to discriminate in terms of disease groups and severity, to predict health service use and outcomes, and to measure small changes in health status over time.

We have illustrated the 36-item measure rather than the SF-20 because it offers a potentially more sensitive measure which, though longer than the SF-20, is still short enough to be incorporated into the normal routine of clinical practice. It is likely to be particularly useful where a general health measure is required to supplement disease specific measures, or as part of a wider ranging survey.

At the time of writing, there remain outstanding issues concerning title and copyright. However, it appears to be the wish of all concerned that the instrument should be widely and freely used, subject only to signing a User Agreement. We recommend that those intending to use the SF-36 should contact both John Ware and RAND at the addresses provided above.

Despite a developing pedigree, the SF-36 should not be seen as a 'gold standard', appropriate to all studies and all circumstances. Many longer-established instruments offer more extensive evidence on reliability, validity, and sensitivity and have also been widely used. The publication of the complete range of measures employed in the Medical Outcome Study marks a substantial advance in the field.[16] For many research purposes one of the longer instruments or sections of it may be more appropriate than the short-form instruments.

References

1. Anderson, J. StC., Sullivan, F., and Usherwood, T. P. (1990). The Medical Outcomes Study Instrument (MOSI) — use of a new health status measure in Britain. *Family Practice*, 7, 205–18.
2. Brazier, J. E., Harper, R., Jones, N. M. B., O'Cathain, A., Thomas, K. J., Usherwood, T., and Westlake, L. (1992). Validating the SF-36 health survey questionnaire: new outcome measure for primary care. *British Medical Journal*, 305, 160–4.
3. Ellwood, P. M. (1988). Outcomes management: a technology of patient experience. *New England Journal of Medicine*, 318, 721–7.
4. Jenkinson, C., Coulter, A., and Wright, L. (1993). The SF-36 Health Survey Questionnaire: normative data from a large random sample of working age adults. *British Medical Journal*, (in press).
5. Katz, J. N., Larson, M. G., Phillips, C. B., Fossel, A. H. and Liang, M. H. (1992). Comparative measurement sensitivity of short and longer health status instruments. *Medical Care*, 30, 917–25.
6. Kurtin, P. S., Davies, A. R., Meyer, K. B., deGiacomo, J. M., and Kantz, M. E. (1992). Patient-based health status measures in outpatient dialysis: early experiences in developing an outcomes assessment program. *Medical Care*, 30, MS136–49.
7. Mays, R. D., Sherbourne, C. D., and Mazel, E. (In press). *User's manual for the Medical Outcomes Study (MOS). Measures of health related quality of life*. RAND, Santa Monica, CA.
8. McHorney, C. A., Ware, J. E., and Raczek, A. E. (1993). The MOS 36-item Short-form Health Survey (SF-36): II. Psychometric and clinical tests of validity in measuring physical and mental health constructs. *Medical Care*, 31: (in press).
9. McHorney, C. A., Ware, J. E., Rogers, W., Raczek, A. E., and Lu, J. F. R. (1992). The validity and relative precision of MOS short and long-form health status scales and Dartmouth COOP charts. *Medical Care*, 30, MS253–65.
10. Nerenz, D. R., Repasky, D. P., Whitehouse, F. W., and Kahkonen, D. M. (1992). Ongoing assessment of health status in patients with diabetes mellitus. *Medical Care*, 30, MS112–23.

11. New England Medical Center Hospitals (1992). *How to score the MOS 36-item Short-form Health Survey (SF-36)*. New England Medical Center Hospitals, Boston, MA.
12. New England Medical Center Hospitals (1992). *Scoring exercise for the MOS SF-36 Health Survey including SF-36 test dataset on diskette*. New England Medical Center Hospitals, Boston, MA.
13. Outcome Management System (1992). *OMS Update*, 3, 1-4.
14. Stewart, A.L., Greenfield, S., Hays, R.D., Wells, K., Rogers, W.H., Berry, S.D., *et al.* (1989). Functional status and well-being of patients with chronic conditions. Results from the Medical Outcomes Study. *Journal of the American Medical Association*, **262**, 907-13.
15. Stewart, A.L., Hays, R.D., and Ware, J.E. (1988). The MOS short-form general health survey. *Medical Care*, **26**, 724-35.
16. Stewart, A.L., Ware, J.E. (ed.) (1992). *Measuring functioning and well-being: the Medical Outcomes Study approach*. Duke University Press, Durham, NC, and London.
17. Ware, J.E. (1987). Standard for validating health measures: definition and content. *Journal of Chronic Disease*, **40**, 473-80.
18. Ware, J.E. and Sherbourne, C.D. (1992). The MOS 36-item short form health survey (SF-36). 1. Conceptual framework and item selection. *Medical Care*, **30**, 473-81.
19. Ware, J.E., Sherbourne, C.D., and Davies, A.R. (1992). Developing and testing the MOS 20-Item Short-form Health Survey: A general population application. *Measuring functioning and well-being: the Medical Outcomes Study Approach*, In (ed. A.L. Stewart and J.E. Ware), Ch. 15. Duke University Press, Durham, NC, and London.
20. Wells, K.B., Stewart, A., Hay, R., Burnham, A., Rodgers, W., Daniels, M., *et al.* (1989). The functioning and well-being of depressed patients: results from the Medical Outcomes Study. *Journal of the American Medical Association*, **262**, 914-19.

The Coop Function Charts (Nelson and colleagues 1987)

Purpose

Unlike most of the measures in this book, the Dartmouth Coop Charts were developed specifically for use in clinical practice. They are intended to provide clinicians in primary health care with an efficient system for screening, assessing, monitoring, and maintaining patient function in routine office practice. It is claimed that they improve doctor–patient communication by identifying topics which may otherwise go unnoticed, and can be used to trigger changes in patient management. The charts can also be used in surveys to assess needs and to provide a measure of outcome in clinical research.

Background

The authors argued that the emphasis in medical care has expanded from a disease-specific, organ-based approach to encompass global physical, mental, and social function. This requires the physician to be able to measure the important functional parameters. However, although the authors identified many measures appropriate for this purpose, they considered none of them suitable for daily use in the office. Existing measures contained large numbers of questions, required staff to ask a detailed set of questions, and/or required complicated scoring. They set out to develop alternative measures which would produce reliable and valid data on core functional dimensions, fit easily into routine office practice, be applicable to a wide range of problems, possess face validity and acceptability to clinicians and patients, yield easily interpretable scores, and provide clinically useful information on patients' functional status.[4]

The charts were developed using three sources of information: existing literature and instruments, consultations with health measurement experts, and discussions with practising clinicians. Three 'core' measures of function were initially developed and these were then supplemented by six further charts.[5] Although each chart went through a number of versions, the authors do not provide much information about how the final versions were arrived at.

Description

There are nine charts (8.5" × 14") measuring function, general health status, and quality of life without reference to any specific disease (Exhibit 7.5). Each chart is a single item measure of a particular dimension of health status. Respondents are asked to rate themselves according to how they have felt over the past four weeks, although a one-week version has also been used.[7] Physical function is equated with gross motor activity, emotional function with symptoms of anxiety and depression, role function with daily work activities, and social function with normal social activities. It should be noted that physical function focuses on cardio-vascular function, rather than disabilities associated with other conditions such as arthritis, and it fails to classify severe disability, such as being confined to a chair. Although role function focuses on daily activities, there is potential for confusion with physical condition. Also, since there is no means of describing what constitutes normal daily activity, this will be relative to the individual.[6] Thus, for example, 'no difficulty' will have very different meanings for a construction worker and an office worker. General health status is covered in three items dealing with overall condition, change in the past four weeks, and the experience of pain. With the addition of illustrations, the overall condition item is similar to many such questions used in omnibus surveys such as the British General Household Survey. Lastly, two items deal with quality of life in terms of patients' perceptions and levels of social support.

For the purposes of routine practice it is assumed that only some of the charts will be used for selected patients, although the authors do not suggest which charts would be most useful with which categories of patient. In a Dutch study only the four charts dealing with physical function, emotional

Exhibit 7.5 Dartmouth Coop Function Charts

(Reproduced, with permission, from Nelson, E. C., Landgraf, J. M., Hays, R. D., Kirk, J. W., Wasson, J. H., Keller, A., and Zubkoff, M. (1990). *Functional Status Measurement in Primary Care*, WONCA Classification Committee. New York, Springer)

PHYSICAL CONDITION

During the past 4 weeks...
What was the most strenuous level of physical activity you could do for at least 2 minutes?

Very heavy, e.g. Run, fast pace / Carry heavy bag of groceries upstairs		1
Heavy, e.g. Jog, slow pace / Climb stairs at moderate pace		2
Moderate, e.g. Walk, fast pace / Garden, easy digging / Carry heavy bag of groceries		3
Light, e.g. Walk, regular pace / Golf or vaccum / Carry light bag of groceries		4
Very light, e.g. Walk, slow pace / Drive car / Wash dishes		5

EMOTIONAL CONDITION

During the past 4 weeks...
How much have you been bothered by emotional problems such as feeling unhappy, anxious, depressed, irritable?

Not at all		1
Slightly		2
Moderately		3
Quite a bit		4
Extremely		5

DAILY WORK

During the past 4 weeks...
How much difficulty did you have doing your daily work, both inside and outside the house, because of your physical health or emotional problems?

No difficulty at all		1
A little bit of difficulty		2
Some difficulty		3
Much difficulty		4
Could not do		5

SOCIAL ACTIVITIES

During the past 4 weeks...
To what extent has your physical health or emotional problems interfered with your normal social activities with family, friends, neighbours or groups?

Not at all		1
Slightly		2
Moderately		3
Quite a bit		4
Extremely		5

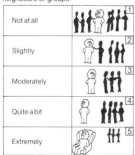

PAIN

During the past 4 weeks...
How much bodily pain have you generally had?

No pain		1
Very mild pain		2
Mild pain		3
Moderate pain		4
Severe pain		5

CHANGE IN CONDITION

How would you rate your physical health and emotional condition now compared to 4 weeks ago?

Much better	++	1
A little better	+	2
About the same	±	3
A little worse	−	4
Much worse	−−	5

OVERALL CONDITION

During the past 4 weeks...
How would you rate your overall physical health and emotional condition?

Excellent		1
Very good		2
Good		3
Fair		4
Poor		5

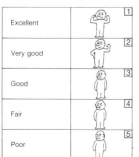

SOCIAL SUPPORT

During the past 4 weeks...
Was someone available to help you if you needed and wanted help? For example if you
—felt very nervous, lonely, or blue
—got sick and had to stay in bed
—needed someone to talk to
—needed help with daily chores
—needed help just taking care of yourself

Yes, as much as I wanted		1
Yes, quite a bit		2
Yes, some		3
Yes, a little		4
No, not at all		5

QUALITY OF LIFE

How has the quality of your life been during the past 4 weeks? i.e. How have things been going for you?

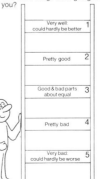

Very well: could hardly be better	1
Pretty good	2
Good & bad parts about equal	3
Pretty bad	4
Very bad: could hardly be worse	5

function, role function, and social function were used, and wording and illustrations were changed.[2]

Scoring is very simple, each item being rated one to five on a five point ordinal scale. Scores are not combined in any way to produce either section totals or overall scores. The authors do not claim anything more than ordinal measurement properties for each of the items. However, there is a temptation to produce average scores on each item for different patient groups, which is of questionable validity. The authors suggest that one application of the charts is to use them as a screen in conjunction with more sophisticated instruments which might permit more precise measurement of function.

Administration and acceptability

Concern with the costs of administering lengthy assessment instruments in clinical practice was a major factor in the development of the Coop Function Charts. They are designed to be administered by a doctor, nurse or patient self administered. Where they are administered by a professional the patient is shown the card and the professional records the response. All nine charts can be administered in three to five minutes. However, Palmer has pointed out that the question of who administers the charts should be given careful consideration.[6] She argues that the results obtained, the interpretation placed on them, and their usefulness will differ according to who administers them.

Both doctors and patients found the content of the charts acceptable. Doctors and nurses found them not difficult to incorporate into the normal routine, and reported no effect or positive effect on communication in 98 per cent of consultations.[5] Patients had no difficulty understanding the charts and the vast majority (89 per cent) enjoyed completing them.[1]

Reliability and validity

In developing the Coop charts the authors have drawn on data from over 3000 patients in a variety of clinical settings.[3,5] Test–retest reliability appears to be excellent for time periods between administration of one hour and over two weeks. Inter-rater reliability was generally good, although the authors suggest that care should be taken to ensure that different raters are using the charts in the same way.

The authors have conducted extensive tests of the validity of the charts with encouraging results.[3,5] Construct validity was demonstrated both in terms of relationships between chart scores and indicator variables (e.g. age, disease status) and in terms of convergent and discriminant validity. Criterion validity has been assessed using the Rand Health Status Scales as a 'quasi gold standard'. The charts showed a high correlation with the much longer Rand measures and were as sensitive to the impact of disease on functioning. Moderate correlations were also achieved with clinical indicators (symptom score, medicines). At least as important as these more usual valida-tion criteria, for an instrument designed to aid clinical practice, is their perceived value to the clinicians using them. In 59 per cent of 22 case studies, clinicians reported that the charts improved communication and in 41 per cent that they resulted in a modified physical plan.[1] The case studies illustrate very well the ways in which clinicians were able to make use of the chart information.

In addition to the initial development work reported by the authors, four of the charts have been compared with the General Health Questionnaire and the Nottingham Health Profile[2] (see pp. 94 and 142). Although this study also provided evidence of both criterion and construct validity, it questioned the independence of the Coop Chart items, and suggested that there might be grounds for treating the four charts (physical, emotional, role, and social function) as measuring a single health construct.

There is considerable scope for further testing of the validity and reliability of the charts, particularly in the area of their sensitivity to change over time.[6] If they are to be useful in clinical practice, further evidence of their ability to detect clinically significant change is essential. However, initial results are encouraging.

Populations/service settings

The Coop Function Charts are explicitly designed for use in clinical practice in ambulatory/primary medical care. They can be used with all adults regard-less of condition. Although no problems have been reported in use with elderly people, it might be anticipated that the items on physical activity and daily work would be less appropriate than for adults of working age. The charts have been mainly employed in medical settings, but there seems no reason why they shouldn't be used by other primary care professionals, such as community nurses or physiotherapists.

Comments

Although developed only recently, the Dartmouth Coop Function Charts offer one of the most promising prospects for measures of need and outcome which are useful in busy clinical practice. The authors recognize that more developmental work and testing is necessary, and this may result in changes to the content of the charts. However, there is already good evidence of reliability and validity. There is a need for evidence on the responsiveness of the charts to clinically significant change, but reports from clinicians on their utility in clinical practice are encouraging.

One of the most refreshing features of the Coop Function Charts is their 'user friendly' presentation. The advantages of pictorial presentation are obvious, but there are also potential disadvantages, and these require more investigation.[6] Nevertheless, the authors have devoted more attention, at both design and testing stages, to professional and patient views than is the case for any other measure in this book. It is all too rare for the authors of instruments to ask potential users and respondents for their views. Certainly, if systematic measures of need and outcome are to become a part of routine practice as well as research, this is absolutely essential.

References

1. Landgraf, J.M., Nelson, E.C., Hays, R.D., Wasson, J.H., and Kirk, J.W. (1990). Assessing function: Does it really make a difference? A preliminary evaluation of the acceptability and utility of the Coop Function Charts. In *Functional status measurement in primary care* (WONCA Classification Committee), pp. 150–65. Springer, New York.
2. Meyboom-de Jong, B. and Smith, R.J.A. (1990). Studies with the Dartmouth Coop Charts in general practice: comparison with the Nottingham Health Profile and the General Health Questionnaire. In *Functional status measurement in primary care* (WONCA Classification Committee), pp. 132–49. Springer, New York.
3. Nelson, E.C., Landgraf, J.M., Hays, R.D., Kirk, J.W., Wasson, J.H., Keller, A., and Zubkoff, M. (1987). *Dartmouth Coop proposal to develop and demonstrate a system to assess functional health status in physicians' offices. Final version.* Dartmouth Medical School, Hanover.
4. Nelson, E., Wasson, J., Kirk, J., Keller, A., Clark, D., Dietrich, A., Stewart, A., and Zubkoff, M. (1987). Assessment of function in routine clinical practice: description of the Coop Chart method and preliminary findings. *Journal of Chronic Disease*, **40** Suppl, 55S–63S.
5. Nelson, E.C., Landgraf, J.M., Hays, R.D., Kirk, J.W., Wasson, J.H., and Zubkoff, M. (1990). The Coop Function Charts: a system to measure patient function in physicians' offices. In *Functional status measurement in primary care* (WONCA Classification Committee), pp. 97–131. Springer, New York.
6. Palmer, H.R. (1987). Commentary: assessment of function in routine clinical practice. *Journal of Chronic Disease*, **40** Suppl, 65S–9S.
7. Westbury, R.C. (1990). Use of the Dartmouth Coop Charts in a Calgary practice. In *Functional status measurement in primary care* (WONCA Classification Committee), pp. 166–80. Springer, New York.

Functional Status Questionnaire (FSQ)
(Jette and colleagues 1986)

Purpose

The FSQ is designed to provide a comprehensive assessment of physical, psychological, social, and role function in ambulatory patients. It is intended to screen for disability and monitor clinically meaningful change in function as part of routine clinical practice in primary care.

Background

The authors of the FSQ argued that existing instruments for measuring functional status were inappropriate for use in routine clinical practice.[5] They tend to focus on only one or two dimensions and thus lack the comprehensiveness needed for clinical use. Although more comprehensive multidimensional instruments are available, the time required to complete them or the requirement for a trained interviewer may make them unsuitable for use in a clinical setting. The authors therefore developed the FSQ. Little information is provided concerning the selection and wording of items, other than that it was adapted from existing instruments, including the Functional Status Index (p. 56), the Sickness Impact Profile (p. 133), and the Rand Functional Status Indexes (p. 65).

Description

The FSQ consists of a 34-item questionnaire covering physical function, psychological function, social/role function, restriction due to illness, sexual function, and satisfaction with health (Exhibit 7.6). Most of the questions

---

Exhibit 7.6   Functional Status Questionnaire

(Adapted, with permission, from Jette, A. M., Davies, A. R., Cleary, P. D. Calteins, D. R., Rubenstein, L. V., Fink, A., Kosecoff, J., Young, R. T., Brook, R. H., and Delbonco, T. L. (1986). The Functional Status Questionnaire: reliability and validity when used in primary care. *Journal of General and Internal Medicine*, 1, 143–9)

Category	Item
Physical Function	During the past month have you had difficulty:
Basic activities of daily living	Taking care of yourself, that is, eating, dressing, or bathing?
	Moving in and out of a bed or chair?
	Walking indoors, such as around your home?
Intermediate activies of daily living	Walking several blocks?
	Walking one block or climbing one flight of stairs?
	Doing work around the house, such as cleaning, light yard work, home maintenance?
	Doing errands, such as grocery shopping?
	Driving a car or using public transportation?
	Doing vigorous activities, such as running, lifting heavy objects, or participating in strenuous sports?

Exhibit 7.6 (continued)

Responses: Usually did with no difficulty (4); usually did with some difficulty (3); usually did with much difficulty (2); usually did not do because of health (1); usualy did not do for other reasons (0)

Psychological function During the past month:
Mental Health

Have you been a very nervous person?
Have you felt calm and peaceful?*
Have you felt downhearted and blue?
Were you a happy person?*
Did you feel so 'down in the dumps' that nothing could cheer you up?

Responses: All of the time (1); most of the time (2); a good bit of the time (3); a little of the time (5); none of the time (6)

Social-role function During the past month have you:
Work performance
(for those employed during
the previous month)

Done as much work as others in similar jobs?
Worked for short periods of time or taken frequent rests because of your health?
Worked your regular number of hours?*
Done your job as carefully and accurately as others with similar jobs?*
Worked at your usual job, but with some changes because of your health?
Feared losing your job because of your health?

Responses: All of the time (1); most of the time (2); some of the time (3); none of the time (4)

Social activity During the past month have you had difficulty:
Visiting with relatives or friends?
Participating in community activities, such as religious services, social activities, or volunteer work?
Taking care of other people, such as family members?

Responses: Usually did with no difficulty (4); usually did with some difficulty (2); usually did not do because of health (1); usually did not do for other reasons (0)

Quality of interaction During the past month did you:
Isolate yourself from people around you?
Act affectionate toward others?*
Act irritable toward those around you?
Make unreasonable demands on your family and friends?
Get along well with other people?*

Responses: All of the time (1); most of the time (2); a good bit of the time (3); some of the time (4); a little of the time (5) none of the time (6)

Single-item questions:
Which of the following statements best describes your work situation during the past month?
Responses: working full-time; working part time; unemployed; looking for work; unemployed because of my health; retired because of my health; retired for some other reason.

Exhibit 7.6 (continued)

During the past month, how many days did you cut down on the things you usually do for one-half day or more because of your illness or injury? *Responses*: 0–31 days.

During the past month, how satisfied were you with your sexual relationships? *Responses*: Very satisfied; satisfied; not sure; dissatisfied; very dissatisfied; did not have any sexual relationships.

How do you feel about your own health? *Responses*: very satisfied; satisfied; not sure; dissatisfied; very dissatisfied.

During the past month, about how often did you socialize with friends or relatives, that is, go out together, visit in each other's homes, or talk on the telephone? *Responses*: Every day; several times a week; about once a week; two or three times a month; about once a month; not at all.

*Indicates that scores are reversed.

are standard response categories which are scored on ordinal scales from 1 to 4 or 1 to 6. Activity restrictions which are not due to health problems are not scored and are treated as invalid responses. In addition to the scale items there are six single-item questions. Standardized scores are calculated for each of six sub-scales using the formula shown in Exhibit 7.7. It should be noted that the original published formula[4,5] and a subsequently published

Exhibit 7.7   Scoring the Functional Status Questionnaire

Scales scores are calculated as follows:

$$SS = \frac{\sum_{i=1}^{n} (yi) - n \times 100}{k}$$

where
SS = transformed FSQ scale score
yi = individual questionnaire response score
n = number of questions in the scale for which valid information is available
k = maximum minus minimum *valid* response score

Scale values range between 0 and 100 with a score of 100 indicating maximum functional ability.

NOTE: Valid responses range between 1 and 4 or 6 depending on the scale. Code 0 is invalid.

correction are wrong. The formula shown here will produce scores ranging between 0 and 100 making allowance for any non-valid items. Scores of 100 indicate maximum functional ability.

Since it was intended that the FSQ should be used in clinical practice, a computerized scoring and presentational system was developed at the same time.[5] The software for IBM PCs was designed to produce graphical individual patient profiles. These included defined 'warning zones' for each scale to alert clinicians to important losses in functional ability. Warning zones were determined through consultation with a panel of experienced clinicians. However, values for their warning zones have not been published.

Administration and acceptability

The FSQ is self-administered and can be administered either in a clinical setting or in the patient's own home. Although it is claimed to be brief, the authors estimate that it takes 15 minutes to complete, which compares unfavourably with some other short measures. The questionnaire summarized in Exhibit 7.7 would need to be suitably presented for self-completion. No problems with acceptability to patients have been reported, but the question on sexual relationships might be expected to offend some patients.

Reliability and validity

Evidence on the reliability and validity of the FSQ comes from a single study of 1153 ambulatory care patients.[4,5] Patients were recruited to the study and assessed using the FSQ if they reported difficulty in one or more of the activities included in the scales. Internal consistency of the six scale scores was good, with the ADL and mental health scales achieving the highest values. Test–retest reliability has not been assessed.

Construct validity for the scales is claimed on the basis of analyses of the interrelationships between scale scores and between scale scores and responses to single-item questions. Correlations between sub-scales followed the hypothesized patterns, so that high correlations were reported between ADL scores and social activity, and low correlations between ADL scores and mental health.[4] Correlations between scale scores and single items such as number of bed days, restricted activity days and satisfaction with health were all in the predicted directions, but the correlations were in most cases only weak.

No evidence of responsiveness to clinically significant change is reported by the authors, which seems somewhat unfortunate in a measure specifically designed to monitor clinically meaningful change. However, a more recent study with elderly patients suffering from heart disease, showed the FSQ to be more sensitive to change than the commonly used New York Heart Association Classification.[7]

Brief reports of a study designed to assess the impact of providing clinicians with FSQ summaries showed no differences in patient outcomes for physicians given the scores and those who did not have the information.[1,6] However, it should be noted that both groups carried out FSQ assessments on their patients.

Populations/service settings

The FSQ was originally designed for and used in hospital-based ambulatory care. It is likely to be most useful as a means of assessing disability and monitoring change, but may not be appropriate for non-disabled populations. It has subsequently been used with older patients suffering from heart disease,[7] polio,[2] and in a survey of poor patients.[3] It would be adaptable for use in routine primary medical care, although a completion time of 15 minutes may be problematic.

Comments

The FSQ is included here because it is one of the few instruments designed for clinical applications in primary care. The basic idea of a routine monitoring system generating individualized reports is attractive and the instrument is certainly comprehensive in its coverage. Evidence of reliability, validity, and responsiveness to change is, however, severely limited at present. We would recommend its use only after further work in this area.

References

1. Calkins, D.R., Rubenstein, L.V., Cleary, P.D., Jette, A.M., Brook, R.H., and Delbanco, T.L. (1986). The Functional Status Questionnaire: a controlled trial in a hospital-based practice. *Clinical Research*, **34**, 359A.
2. Einersson, G., and Grimby, G. (1990). Disability and handicap in late poliomyelitis. *Scandanavian Journal of Rehabilitation Medicine*, **22**, 113-21.
3. Hubbell, F.A., Waitzkin, H., and Rodriguez, F.I. (1990). Functional status and financial barriers to medical care among the poor. *South Medical Journal*, **83**, 548-50.
4. Jette, A.M., and Cleary, P.D. (1987). Functional disability assessment. *Physical Therapy*, **67**, 1854-9.
5. Jette, A.M., Davies, A.R., Cleary, P.D., Calkine, D.R., Rubenstein, L.V., Fink, A., *et al.* (1986). The Functional Status Questionnaire: reliability and validity when used in primary care. *Journal of General Internal Medicine*, **1**, 143-9.
6. Rubenstein, L.V., Calkins, D.R., Young, R.T., Fink, A., Delbanco, T.L., and Brook, R.H. (1986). Improving patient functional status: can questionnaires help? *Clinical Research*, **34**, 835A.
7. Tedesco, C., Manning, S., Lindsay, R., Alexander, C., Owen, R., and Smucker, M.L. (1990). Functional assessment of elderly patients after percutaneous aortic

balloon valvuloplasty: New York Heart Association classification versus Functional Status Questionnaire. *Heart Lung*, **19**, 118–25.

Duke–UNC Health Profile (DUHP)/Duke Health Profile (Parkerson and colleagues 1981, 1990)

Purpose

The DUHP is a health status measure for adults. Its principal application is to assess the effect of primary medical care services on the self-reported functional status and feelings of patients. It is intended to be brief and easily understood by a broad cross section of patients in primary health care. It is designed for use both in research and clinical assessment. The Duke Health Profile is a shorter version of the same instrument, designed as a measure of health outcomes for purposes of research, health promotion, and clinical applicability.

Background

The research team at Duke University and the University of North Carolina set out to develop a measure which would meet the particular needs of applications in primary health care.[7] Items from a number of other instruments (e.g. SIP, MHI, OARS, SDS) were reviewed and adapted for the DUHP. Four dimensions were used: symptom status, physical function, emotional function, and social function. Symptom status was conceptualized as a separate dimension despite its overlap with other areas, because of its importance in primary care. Two general strategies were used in the selection of items. Firstly, the most critical subcomponents of each of the four dimensions for an ambulatory population were identified from literature and clinical experience, avoiding items that occur only infrequently in primary care. Secondly, general categories of functioning were used rather than questions about specific activities, so as to ensure applicability across a wide range of populations.

Conceptualization of the four dimensions is somewhat limited. Symptoms are seen as the natural expression of dysfunction in body and mind, and of particular importance in primary health care. Physical function is defined in terms of disability days, ambulation, and use of upper extremities. Emotional function is defined in terms of self-esteem, and social function in terms of the individual's ability to perform his or her role in society.

The authors have recognized problems in the conceptualization of the DUHP. In particular the fact that the symptom dimension does not accord with the conceptualization of health in terms of physical, mental and social well-being was seen as a major problem. They were also concerned that the length of the original version made it unsuitable for use in primary care settings. The Duke Health Profile is therefore designed to overcome these problems by conceptualizing health in terms of physical, mental, and social dimensions.[6]

Description

The original 74-item version of the DUHP was reduced to 63 items by deleting 11 which failed to meet reliability criteria. The final 63-item version is shown in Exhibit 7.8. It should be noted that this version varies slightly in the order and wording of items compared to the original published version. Twenty-six items deal with symptoms, 9 with physical function, 23 with emotional function, and 5 with social function. All questions, except those on

---

Exhibit 7.8   Duke—UNC Health Profile

(Adapted with permission, from Parkerson G. R., Gehlbach, S. H., Wagner, E. H., James, S. A., Clapp, N. E. (1981). The Duke–UNC Health Profile: an adult health status instrument for primary care. *Medical Care*, **19**, 806–28.)

Here are a number of questions about your health and feelings. Please read each question carefully and give your best answer. You should answer the questions in your own way. There are no right or wrong answers.

[Symptom Status]

During the *past week*, how much trouble have you had with:

1. Eyesight	10. Moving your bowels	*17. Getting tired easily
2. Hearing	11. Passing water/urinating	18. Fainting
3. Talking	12. Headache	19. Poor memory
4. Tasting food	*13. Hurting or aching in any	20. Weakness in any part
5. Appetite	part of your body	of your body
6. Chewing	14. Itching in any part	*21. Feeling depressed or sad
7. Swallowing	of your body	*22. Nervousness
8. Breathing	15. Indigestion	
*9. Sleeping	16. Fever	

During the *past month* how much trouble have you had with:

23. Undesired weight loss	25. Unusual bleeding
24. Undesired weight gain	26. Sexual performance (having sex)

Response categories items 1–26: none; some; a lot

[Physical Function]

During the *past week:*

*32. How many days did you stay *in your home* because of sickness, injury, or health problems?

 33. How many days were you *in bed* most of the day because of sickness, injury, or health problems?

Response categories: none; 1–4 days; 5–7 days

Exhibit 7.8 (continued)

Today would you have any physical trouble or difficulty:

34. Peeling an apple
35. Combing your hair
36. Walking to the bathroom
*37. Walking up a flight of stairs

*38. Running the length of a football field (100 yards)
39. Running a mile
40. Running five miles

Response categories: none; some; a lot.

[Emotional Function]

Here are some statements you could use to describe how you feel about yourself. Please read each statement carefully and place a check in the blank that best fits how the statement describes you.

Here is an example:
I like TV soap operas

Describes me exactly		Somewhat describes me		Doesn't describe me at all
___	___ X ___	___	___	___

If you put an 'x' where we have, it means that liking TV soap operas describes you more than 'somewhat' but not 'exactly'.

Answer each item as best you can. Remember, there are no right or wrong answers.

41. I am a pleasant person
42. I don't feel useful
43. I get on well with people of the opposite sex
44. My family doesn't understand me
*45. I like who I am
46. I feel hopeful about the future
47. I try to look my best
48. I am a clumsy person
49. I have difficulty making decisions
50. I like meeting new people
52. I'm a failure at everything I try to do
51. I'm not an easy person to get along with

*53. I'm basically a health person
54. I wish I had more sex appeal
*55. I give up too easily
56. I like the way I look
57. I'm not as smart as most people
*58. I have difficulty concentrating
59. I'm satisfied with my sexual relationships
*60. I'm happy with my family relationships
61. I don't treat other people well
*62. I am comfortable being around other people
63. I can take care of myself in most situations

[Social Function]

During the *past week* how often did you:

27. Do your usual work (either inside or outside the home)
28. Get your work done as carefully and accurately as usual
*29. Socialise with other people (talk or visit with friends or relatives)
*30. Take part in social, religious or recreation activities (club meetings, movies, dancing, sports, parties, church)
31. Care for yourself (bathe, dress, feed yourself)
Response categories: 5-7 days; 1-4 days; not at all

physical activity, seek reports of actual performance of activities or feelings. The physical activity items are phrased in terms of capacity (i.e. '*would* you have difficulty?' rather than '*did* you?') Symptoms, physical function, and social function items all provide three response categories, phrased in terms of either frequency or degree of difficulty or trouble. Emotional function items are rated on a five point scale. Separate scores are calculated for each dimension by adding item scores (response reflecting worst health is scored 0) and dividing by the maximum possible score for that dimension. Items are not weighted in any way to reflect different contributions to the dimension, so that difficulty peeling an apple carries the same weight as difficulty running five miles.

The item content of the different dimensions seems somewhat unusual. Symptom status items, although fairly comprehensive, include a number of items which seem more concerned with function (e.g. talking, hearing, sexual performance) than with symptoms. Emotional function items are explicitly concerned with self-perception, rather than emotional function, and social function items include self care, which is more usually regarded as part of basic ADL skills. The problems inherent in attempting to assess capacity for physical activities were mentioned in Chapter 3, but an additional problem here is that there is no category which allows respondents to say that they are unable to perform the activity. Lastly it should be noted that the time period covered varies from 'today' to the 'past month' for symptom status, physical function, and social function, whilst emotional function provides no time frame.

Although Parkerson did not advocate constructing composite scores by combining the different dimensions, this has been tried in a study of adults with high psychosocial risk.[2] Blake and his colleagues simply summed item scores regardless of the number of items in each dimension and divided by the total possible score for all items answered. There appears to be no theoretical or conceptual foundation for constructing a composite score in this way.

The 17-item Duke Health Profile includes only those items indicated with an asterisk in Exhibit 7.10. Items were selected to represent the dimensions of physical, mental, and social health. The selection of items was based on face validity and psychometric considerations. These 17 items are used to construct three dimension scores, and a general health score. They are also used in varying combinations to generate scores for perceived health, self esteem, anxiety, depression, pain, and disability. However, it should be noted that perceived health, pain, and disability are based on single items. Full details of the Duke Health Profile and recommended scoring procedures are published in a recent article by Parkerson and his colleagues.[6]

Administration and acceptability

The DUHP questionnaire is designed for self-completion, but can be completed by an interviewer.[7] Self-completion takes about 10 minutes and interviewer completion about 30 minutes. The authors do not report any problems in administration, but they do not indicate the response rate achieved in their study of reliability and validity, merely that acceptance by patients was 'excellent'.

The Duke Health Profile has only been used as a free standing instrument in one, as yet unpublished, study.[6] There is therefore no information on length of time taken to complete, although it will clearly take less time than the DUHP.

Reliability and validity

The original paper in which the DUHP is presented is concerned with its reliability and validity and uses results based on trials in a family medical centre.[7] Internal consistency was assessed only for the emotional function dimension, on the grounds that this was the only unidimensional construct. Guttman scalogram analysis was applied to the ambulation items of the physical function dimension. All dimensions were assessed in terms of test–retest reliability and further evidence of test–retest reliability over 15 months was reported by Blake.[2] This somewhat limited strategy for assessing reliability produced encouraging results, although test–retest reliabilities for social function and a number of individual items in other dimensions were quite low. Further testing of reliability, particularly for the symptom status dimension, is essential.

The authors have not addressed directly the issue of content validity, which seems particularly important for the symptom status dimension. Evidence of construct validity is derived from correlations with demographic variables, correlations with other instruments (including SIP and Zung's SDS) and multi-trait, multi-method correlations.[7] Most correlations were in the expected directions, but some correlations were lower than might have been expected. Symptom status scores correlated well with overall SIP scores and emotional function scores with an alternative measure of self-perception. In the only other study of validity, DUHP dimension scores and composite scores were shown to correlate with whether or not patients were under the care of a physician and alternative measures of morbidity (bed days, hospital days, illness restricted days, and physician visits).[2] Nevertheless, as with reliability, further work on the validity of the DUHP seems essential.

Evidence for the reliability and validity of the Duke Health Profile is drawn from the same studies as for the DUHP.[6] It is important to note that the new instrument has not been tested independently of its parent instrument. Internal consistency of the different dimensions was moderate, although not as good as achieved by some other short instruments. Test-retest reliability on 55 patients was acceptable in most cases, but poor for pain and disability. Duke dimension scores correlate appropriately with relevant scores derived from the larger DUHP. Construct validity was established in terms of correlations with socio-demographic variables and convergent/discriminant validity in terms of correlations with dimension scores on the Sickness Impact Profile, Tennessee Self Concept Scale, and Zung SDS. Although each of these latter correlated appropriately with the relevant Duke dimensions, there was also substantial correlation with other dimensions. Lastly, the Duke was shown to be capable of discriminating between patients with and without health problems.

Despite the authors' wish to develop an instrument which is intended as an outcome measure for primary health care, and which focuses on the individual as the basic unit of study, they have not attempted to establish the responsiveness of either the DUHP or the Duke Health Profile to change.

Populations/service settings

Both instruments were designed specifically for use in primary health care with adults attending for treatment. They are suitable for use in ordinary clinical practice, although the shorter instrument is likely to be more practicable. However, it has not yet been widely used in studies of outcomes in primary health care. Apart from studies also conducted at Duke University,[3,4] use of the DUHP has been reported in only two other studies.[1,5] The Duke Health Profile has only very recently been published. The authors report its use in only one study as part of a health promotion programme for medical students.[6]

Comments

The DUHP and Duke Health Profile warrant their place in this review because they are addressed specifically to the needs of primary health care. The DUHP is one of the few instruments to tackle the problem of developing an index of symptoms. However, its deficiencies probably outweigh these advantages when compared with some of the other multidimensional measures included in this section. Nevertheless, we believe that the approach adopted by its authors does recognize some of the important differences between the concerns of primary health care and those of hospital-based specialist care. In particular, we feel that there is a need for more work on general measures of symptoms, as opposed to the concentration on the ways in which disease affects performance of activities. Many patients seeking primary health care are not limited in their activities, but do experience symptoms.

The Duke Health Profile abandons the emphasis on symptoms for a more conventional approach to the measurement of health status. Although this makes it more practicable for use in routine clinical practice, it is not clear that it has any advantages over alternative short instruments such as the MOS Short Form or the Coop Function Charts. In any case, further testing of this shortened instrument separately from the parent instrument is essential before its use could be recommended.

References

1. Blake, R. L. Jr. and Vandiver, T. A. (1988). The association of health with stressful life changes, social supports, and coping. *Family Practice Research Journal*, **7**, 205–18.
2. Blake, R. L. Jr. Vandiver, T. A., Zweig, S. C., and Brent E. E. (1986). Evaluation of a health status measure in adults with high psychosocial risk. *Family Practice Research Journal*, **5**, 158–66.
3. Broadhead, W. E., Gehlbach, S. H., De Gruy, F. V., and Kaplan, B. H. (1988). The Duke–UNC Functional Social Support Questionnaire. *Medical Care*, **26**, 709–23.
4. Broadhead, W. E., Gehlbach, S. H., De Gruy, F. V., and Kaplan, B. H. (1989). Functional versus structural social support and health care utilization in a family medicine outpatient practice. *Medical Care*, **27**, 221–33.
5. Burckhardt, C. S., Woods, S. L., Schultz, A. A., and Ziebarth, D. M. (1989). Quality of life of adults with chronic illness: a psychometric study. *Research in Nursing and Health*, **12**, 347–54.
6. Parkerson, G. R., Broadhead, W. E., and Tse, C. K. J. (1990). The Duke Health Profile: A 17 item measure of health and disfunction. *Medical Care*, **28**, 1056–72.
7. Parkerson, G. R., Gehlbach, S. H., Wagner, E. H., James, S. A., Clapp, N. E., and Muhlbaier, L. H. (1981). The Duke–UNC Health Profile: an adult health status instrument for primary care. *Medical Care*, **19**, 806–28.

The OARS Multidimensional Functional Assessment Questionnaire (MFAQ) (Older Americans Resources and Services, Duke University 1975)

Purpose

The MFAQ was designed to assess overall functional capacity and utilization of services, and the links between them, for older people (aged 55 years and over) living at home. It is intended to be used to assess current needs for services and predict future outcomes as a result of specific interventions in people with differing functional capacities. The instrument was developed as part of a service evaluation programme and resource allocation model.

Background

The Older Americans Resources and Services Programme (OARS) is part of the Duke University Center for the Study of Aging and Human Development. The OARS programme was established in 1972 to evaluate alternatives to institutional care for older people. A large multi-disciplinary team was involved in developing a model which would not only address the specific issue of institutionalization, but also would facilitate programme evaluation and resource allocation more generally. There are three critical elements to this model: (1) assessment of individual functional status so that classes of functionally equivalent persons can be formed (2) disaggregation of services and reaggregation according to actual use, and (3) a matrix tying these together and permitting a prediction of future outcome as a result of specific intervention.[3]

The authors considered a new measure of function necessary because, although several excellent measures of particular aspects of functioning were available, none of these was sufficiently comprehensive. Information was felt to be necessary on five dimensions: social resources, economic resources, mental health, physical health and activities of daily living. The items used in the functional assessment were partly derived from other instruments and partly developed specifically for the MFAQ. After initial testing, those items which failed to discriminate between different levels of functioning were discarded. Questions dealing with service utilization were developed specifically for this questionnaire.

Description

The MFAQ is divided into two parts; Part A is a functional assessment and Part B a services assessment. The services assessment is not dealt with here as it is beyond the scope of this volume. Even Part A is too long to reproduce here. Exhibit 7.9 shows the sections included in the assessment of functioning, and a brief description of the content of each section. The six dimensions of functioning are covered in 65 questions, although if sub-sections are counted there are 120 questions in all. A further 10 questions are asked of a reliable informant. Minor revisions to the questionnaire have been introduced in the latest version.[6]

After completing the questionnaire, respondents are rated on each of the five sections (social resources, economic resources, mental health, physical health, activities of daily living) on a six point scale. Definitions of rating categories vary for each section, but have the same underlying definition; 1 = excellent to 6 = totally impaired. Information from these ratings can be handled in a variety of ways; as a profile, summed to produce a cumulative impairment score, a count of the number of sections on which the subject shows significant impairment (scores of 4 or more), and dichotomized into impaired (scores 1 to 3) or not impaired (scores 4 to 6).[3,6]

Exhibit 7.9   OARS Multidimensional Functional Assessment Questionnaire: subjects covered, part A

(From Centre for the Study of Aging and Human Development (1978). *Multidimensional Functional Assessement: The OARS Methodology, (2nd edn)*. Duke University Medical Center, North Carolina, with permission.)

Part A: Assessment of individual functioning

Part A is divided into seven major sections. These sections, in order, with a listing of the number of primary questions (some questions include several items) and a description of their content, are:

Section	No. of questions	Content
Basic demographic	11	Address; date; interviewer; informant; place of interview; duration; sex; race; age; education; telephone number.
Social resources	9	Marital status; resident companions; extent and type of contact with others; availability of confidante; perception of loneliness; availability, duration, and source of help.
Economic resources	15	Employment status; major occupation of self (and of spouse, if married); source and amount of income; number of dependents; home ownership or rental, and cost; source and adequacy of financial resources; health insurance; subjectively assessed adequacy of income.
Mental health	6	Short Portable Mental Status Questionnaire (SPMSQ), a ten-item test of organicity; extent of worry, satisfaction and interest in life; assessment of present mental status and change in the past five years; fifteen-item Short Psychiatric Evaluation Schedule.
Physical health	16	Physician visits, days sick, in hospital and/or nursing home in past six months; medications in past month; current illnesses and their extent of interference; physical, visual, and hearing disabilities; alcoholism; participation in vigorous exercise; self-assessment of health.

Exhibit 7.9 (continued)

Activities of daily living	15	Extent of capacity to: telephone, travel, shop, cook, do housework, take medicine, handle money, feed self, dress, groom, walk, transfer, bathe, and control bladder and bowels. Also presence of another to help with ADL tasks.
Informant assessments	10	Information on the focal person's level of functioning on each of the five dimensions is sought from a knowledgeable informant. Specifically: Social: capacity to get along with others; availability, duration, and source of help in time of need. Economic: extent to which income meets basic self-maintenance requirements. Mental: ability to make sound judgements, cope, interest in life; comparison with peers; change in past five years. Physical: assessment of health; extent of interference of health problems.
Interviewer section		
(a)	4	Sources of information; reliability of responses.
(b)	15	Social: availability and duration of help when needed; adequacy of social relationships. Economic: assessed adequacy of income; presence of reserves; extent to which basic needs are met. Mental: ability to make sound judgements, cope; interest in life; behaviour during interview. Physical: whether obese or malnourished. Rating scales: five six-point scales, one for each dimension.

Administration and acceptability

In its original version the MFAQ is designed for interviewer administration. Detailed guidance on administration is provided in the manual,[3] although the authors recommend that interviewers should receive training. The complete schedule takes between 45 and 60 minutes to administer, and Part A (individual functioning) about 30 minutes. Where the MFAQ is the only, or the main, instrument being used, administration time may not be a problem, but it could be excessive in studies where functioning is only one aspect of questioning. However, the subjects covered are extremely wide ranging, which may make it unnecessary to include other measures. Although the MFAQ was originally designed only for administration by trained interviewers, self-completed postal versions and telephone administration have now been used, although sections of the mental health questions cannot be administered in these ways.[6] These methods will clearly be less costly than using trained interviewers. On the other hand, response rates are likely to be higher for interviewer administration than for self-completion, and for elderly, frail people the advantages of personal contact may outweigh the increased costs.

Apart from the time taken to complete the MFAQ, the areas of questioning are unlikely to present any major problems. The manual provides a very useful guide to many practical issues of administration, including selection of interviewers, follow-up procedures, and how to handle questions that might seem sensitive or pointless. Summary ratings originally depended on having trained interviewers, but the most recent manual provides computer programs to calculate these ratings.[6]

Reliability and validity

Extensive testing of reliability was undertaken in the development of OARS methodology,[3,7] and numerous studies conducted subsequently have contributed further evidence, often related to specific populations or particular sections of the instrument. Inter-rater reliability is particularly important for the MFAQ because of the need for the interviewer to make an overall rating on each section of the questionnaire. The authors have been careful to emphasize the importance of interviewer training as a means of ensuring reliability. With appropriate training, they reported complete agreement between 11 raters on 30 patients for 74 per cent of ratings.[7] Test–retest reliability seemed to be good for the sections on activities of daily living, but less satisfactory in areas such as life satisfaction and mental health.[3]

Content validity is claimed for the MFAQ on the grounds that only those items which experts agreed should be present were included. Various studies have been conducted of criterion validity, using both alternative interview data and clinical examination as the criteria.[3,7] These have shown high correlations between MFAQ ratings and the criterion measures for physical and mental health and self-care capacity. Comparisons of elderly people in different care settings have been presented to show the ability of the instrument to discriminate.[11,12,15] The mental health section has been validated against a psychiatric interview.[1] A short 15-item version achieved moderate sensitivity and high specificity, but the balance between sensitivity and specificity can be improved by further reducing the number of items to six. In a separate study of the mental health section, factor analysis showed that in addition to the second-order construct of mental health there were four first-order factors: life satisfaction, psychosomatic symptomatology, alienation, and cognitive deficit.[10]

Despite the authors' emphasis on the usefulness of the measure for longitudinal evaluation research by examining transitions between functional classes,[5] the validation studies do not include an examination of its responsiveness to clinically significant change. We would like to see studies which compare the OARS instrument with other available measures of function in terms of their ability to detect change in response to medical care.

Populations/service settings

The MFAQ was developed as part of a programme of studies on elderly people, although the authors are not specific about the age range covered. However, it is also suggested that MFAQ is appropriate for adults in general.[3] Whilst it may be useful for the assessment of disability and the effects of chronic illness in other age groups, we are not aware of published studies of this type, and we feel that further testing of reliability and validity would be essential. The method was developed primarily for use in service evaluation and planning. It has been used in studies concerned with allocation of resources between health and social care.[2,4,11] It has also been used for a variety of other purposes in different settings,[8] including family medicine.[13]

The questionnaire is designed specifically for use with people living in their own homes and is thus well suited to use in a primary care setting. It can also be used with people living in institutions, since questions on activities all deal with capacity rather than performance (i.e. 'Can you . . .?' rather than 'Do you . . .?'). Nevertheless, we feel that it is better suited to a community setting.

Comments

Part A of the MFAQ is one of the best multidimensional assessments of functioning in older people currently available. It is well researched and has been widely used in the USA. With minor modifications in use of language it should be readily applicable in other countries. The use of a variety of different methods of expressing scores for different purposes seems very sensible, and the emphasis on the relationship between functioning and services makes it particularly appropriate as a measure of need. Transitions between functional categories may provide a measure of outcome, but clear evidence of the instrument's responsiveness to change is necessary before we could recommend its use in this way. In the meantime it is more likely to find application as a measure of needs for a wide variety of service inputs.

The main criticism of the MFAQ is that it is, perhaps, unnecessarily long and complicated. Other reviewers have suggested that it might be amenable to streamlining,[9] and this has been attempted with some success.[14] Certainly for the purposes of everyday clinical practice the original version is far too time consuming. Nevertheless, it is worthy of consideration as a research tool if resources are available.

References

1. Blay, S. L., Ramos, L. R., and Mari J. de J. (1988). Validity of a Brazilian version of the Older Americans Resources and Services (OARS) Mental Health Screening Questionnaire. *Journal of the American Geriatric Society*, **36**, 687-92.
2. Burton, R. M. and Dellinger, D. C. (1980). Planning the care of the elderly: the Duke OARS experience. In *Operational research applied to health services* (ed. D. Boldy) pp. 129-58. Croom Helm, London.
3. Center for the Study of Aging and Human Development (1978). *Multidimensional functional assessment: the OARS methodology*, (2nd edn). Duke University Medical Center, North Carolina.
4. Coulton, C. and Frost, A. K. (1982). Use of social and health services by the elderly. *Journal of Health and Social Behaviour*, **23**, 330-9.
5. Fillenbaum, G. G. (1985). *The wellbeing of the elderly: approaches to multidimensional assessment*. World Health Organization, Geneva.
6. Fillenbaum, G. G. (1988). *Multidimensional functional assessment of older adults: The Duke Older Americans Resources and Services Procedures*. Erlbaum, New Jersey.
7. Fillenbaum, G. G. and Smyer, M. A. (1981). The development, validity and reliability of the OARS Multidimensional Functional Assessment Questionnaire. *Journal of Gerontology*, **36**, 428-34.
8. George, L. K. and Fillenbaum, G. G. (1985). OARS methodology: a decade of experience in geriatric assessment. *Journal of the American Geriatric Society*, **33**, 607-15.
9. Kane, R. A. and Kane, R. L. (1981). *Assessing the elderly: a practical guide to measurement*. Lexington Books, Lexington.
10. Liang, J., Levin, J. S., and Krause, N. M. (1989). Dimensions of the OARS mental health measures. *Journal of Gerontology*, **44**, 127-38.
11. Maddox, G. L. (1981). Assessment of individual functional status in a programme evaluation and resource allocation model. In *Ageing: a challenge to science and society*, Volume 2, Part II: Social sciences and social policy (ed. W. W. Holland pp. 221-30). Oxford University Press, Oxford.
12. Milligan, W. L., Powell, D. A., and Furchtgott, E. (1988). The Older Americans Resources and Services interview and the medically disabled elderly. *Journal of Geriatric Psychiatry and Neurology*, **1**, 77-83.
13. Moore, J. T. and Fillenbaum, G. G. (1981). Change in functional disability of geriatric patients in a family medicine programme: implications for medical care. *Journal of Family Practice*, **12**, 59-66.
14. Pearlman, R. A. (1987). Development of a functional assessment questionnaire for geriatric patients. The Comprehensive Older Persons' Evaluation (COPE). *Journal of Chronic Diseases*, **40** Suppl 1, 855-945.

15. Pfeiffer, E., Johnson, T.M., and Chiofolo, R.C. (1981). Functional assessment of elderly subjects in four service settings. *Journal of the American Geriatric Society*, **29**, 433–7.

Disability/Distress Scale (Rosser 1972)

Purpose

Rosser's description of illness states was initially developed for use in measuring hospital output, but has subsequently been applied as a more general measure of health output. It was designed to place in perspective the magnitude of change achieved in particular clinical trials, rather than to provide a clinically sensitive measure of outcome. It has been used to provide the basis for calculating Quality Adjusted Life Years which can then be applied to decisions about health service policies.[9] Thus, like the Quality of Wellbeing Scale (QWB) (p. 188), the disability/distress scale can be seen as part of a general health service decision model.

Background

In developing descriptions of illness states Rosser and her colleagues developed a set of descriptions by asking 60 doctors to identify the characteristics which they took into account in assessing the severity of illness in their patients.[5] They were instructed to ignore prognosis or any information which might relate to patients' future state of health. Two descriptive dimensions emerged from these discussions: disability or objective dysfunction, and distress or subjective experience. The reliability and comprehensiveness of this classification was tested in a number of hospitals. Although these states were useful as a means of describing the distribution of patients' health status, they provided no information about the magnitude of differences or any changes which might be detected. The researchers explored a number of different approaches to placing relative values on each of the illness states described in the classification.[5] Seventy subjects, including medical and psychiatric patients, doctors, nurses, and healthy volunteers were asked to rank marker states drawn from the full range of descriptions and to estimate relative severity. The remaining states were then placed within this framework, with a zero being assigned to a state to which it would be reasonable to restore any ill person. Subjects were also asked to locate death within this set of valuations.

Description

The description of illness states developed from discussions with doctors is shown in Exhibit 7.10. The two-dimensional system yields 29 possible com-

Exhibit 7.10 Rosser's classification of illness states

(Reproduced, with permission, from: Rosser, R. M. (1976). Recent studies using a global approach to measuring illness. *Medical Care*, **16** Suppl, 138-47.)

Disability		Distress
I. No disability.	A	None
II. Slight social disability.	B	Mild
III. Severe social disability and/or slight impairment of performance at work.	C	Moderate
Able to do all housework except very heavy tasks.	D	Severe
IV. Choice of work or performance at work very severely limited.		
Housewives and old people able to do light housework only but able to go out shopping.		
V. Unable to undertake any paid employment.		
Unable to continue any education.		
Old people confined to home except for escorted outings and short walks and unable to do shopping.		
Housewives able only to perform a few simple tasks.		
VI. Confined to chair or to wheelchair or able to move around in the house only with support from assistant.		
VII. Confined to bed.		
VIII. Unconscious.		

binations or states. For obvious reasons, unconsciousness is not rated in terms of subjective distress. Rosser points out that both dimensions are complex and amenable to further subdivisions.[5] Disability subsumes mobility and social function, whilst distress subsumes pain and other types of subjective distress, especially endogenous or reactive disturbances of mood and reactions to symptoms such as breathlessness and to disability. Classification of individuals can be carried out on the basis of observation, from secondary sources of information (e.g. using information from other health status assessments), or by conducting an assessment specifically for the purpose of classification. Rosser has not published a set of questions for undertaking the classification, but Williams[9] has published a simple questionnaire and instructions for converting response categories to the illness states defined by Rosser.

Having classified individuals in terms of disability and distress, a valuation matrix can be used to derive a value for each state. Exhibit 7.11 shows the valuations applicable to all 29 states based on the valuations provided by all of Rosser's judges. The convention used in this index is that a state of

Exhibit 7.11   Rosser's valuation matrix

(Reproduced with permission, from: Rosser, R. M. (1978). A health index and output measure. In *Quality of Life: Assessment and Application*, (ed. S. R. Walker and R. M. Rosser). MTP, Lancaster.)

Disability rating	Distress rating			
	A	B	C	D
I.	1.000	0.995	0.990	0.967
II.	0.990	0.986	0.973	0.932
III.	0.980	0.972	0.956	0.912
IV.	0.964	0.956	0.942	0.870
V.	0.946	0.935	0.900	0.700
VI.	0.875	0.845	0.680	0.000
VII.	0.677	0.564	0.000	− 1.486
VIII.	− 1.028			

optimum health/no illness is rated 1 and that being dead is rated 0. It allows for the possibility of states worse than death which receive a negative valuation. It should be remembered that the valuations shown in Exhibit 7.12 were derived from only 70 respondents and that these were not a representative sample of the population. Rosser and her colleagues have examined differences between sub-groups of these respondents in terms of the valuations placed on different states[3,7] and explored a variety of alternative scaling models.[2] They have shown considerable variation between, for example, psychiatric patients and medical patients in the valuations placed on different states. Williams points out that the decision about whose valuations to use is essentially a political decision as to whose values shall count.[9]

Further development of the classification system is continuing. In particular, the distress component has been divided into two sets of descriptions, one dealing with pain and the other with mental disturbance, yielding a possible 175 states.[5] Rosser also reports work on the development of a more elaborate instrument, the Index of Health Related Quality of Life (IHQL) with more than a hundred descriptors which subsume the original classification of disability, pain, and distress.[6]

Administration and acceptability

When conducted as part of normal clinical routine, classifications can be accomplished in ten seconds by staff who are experienced in its use.[5] It is therefore amenable to use in a busy clinical environment. It does not require additional questions to be asked of the patient and therefore poses no problems of acceptability. No information is available concerning the administration of the self-completed questionnaire proposed by Williams.[9]

Reliability and validity

In the original trials of the classification of illness states the reliability of classification by clinicians was examined.[8] Clinicians were asked to rate disability and distress and were given notes on the definition of these terms. The level of agreement between clinicians was high and classifications were shown to be repeatable by the same doctor. In another study, ward nurses were also shown to be able to conduct classifications reliably.[1] Whilst these results are encouraging, further evidence of inter-rater and test–retest reliability under varying conditions would be desirable. There is no evidence as to the reliability of assessments conducted using the sort of questionnaire advocated by Williams.[9] Limited evidence concerning test–retest reliability of the valuations placed on illness states by judges is available.[7]

Little attention seems to have been given to the formal validation of the classification system. Rosser has argued that what was needed was a standard set of descriptions which can be used reliably and which might be substantially modified in the light of experiences.[4] Whilst substantive studies using the classification are suggestive of its ability to discriminate between groups and to detect changes occurring during episodes of hospital care, more formal validation would make it possible to compare this scale with others currently available. Although content validity might be argued on the basis of the method of generating scale descriptions (clinicians' assessments of which factors were important in establishing severity) this seems very limited. In particular, the distress category clearly incorporates a number of different and potentially conflicting dimensions, although the latest versions which separate pain and mental disturbance go some way to overcoming this problem. The responsiveness of the scale to clinically significant change has not been examined. Indeed, it should be noted that it was explicitly *not* designed to provide a sensitive outcome measure for clinical trials.

Populations/service settings

The classification and associated weights have been used primarily in hospital settings where episodes of care are more easily defined, but Rosser has suggested that it would be applicable to community care, in which case an episode might be defined as one year of operation of a service.[5] The scale is applicable to adults regardless of condition or whether they are undergoing treatment. The method is currently being incorporated into a computerized management and evaluation package for use in primary health care, but at the time of writing details of this have not been published.

Comments

Like the QWB, Rosser's classification of illness states possesses the advantage of permitting comparisons across disease categories, but the disadvantage of sacrificing detailed information about important aspects of health. Its principal applications are likely to be in the area of informing policy decisions, but these need to be taken at all levels of health care, including primary health care. The classification may be most useful in conjunction with other disease specific or more comprehensive general measures by providing a basis for setting findings in a wider context.

Development work on the classification and on valuations of illness states is continuing, including eliciting utilities assigned to disability and distress among a random sample of the population and obtaining further descriptions. The research team is currently using more comprehensive descriptions of distress which distinguish between pain and mental disturbance.

Although in its current form the system is unlikely to find many applications in primary health care, this type of model is likely to find increasing applications in policy decisions, through the use of the concept of the quality adjusted life year. Williams shows how it can be used to evaluate alternative treatments by incorporating a time variable.[9] This approach, whilst unfamiliar to most clinicians in primary health care, is likely to play an increasingly important part in resource allocation in the future.

References

1. Benson, T. J. R. (1978). Classification of disability and distress by ward nurses. A reliability study. *International Journal of Epidemiology*, **7**, 359-61.
2. Kind, P. and Rosser, R. (1988). The quantification of health. *European Journal of Social Psychology*, **18**, 63-77.
3. Kind, P., Rosser, R. M., and Williams, A. (1982). Valuation of quality of life: some psychometric evidence. In *The value of life and safety* (ed. M. W. Jones-Lee) pp. 159-70. North Holland Publishing, Amsterdam.
4. Rosser, R. M. (1983). Issues of measurement in the design of health indicators: a review. In *Health Indicators* (ed. A. J. Culyer), pp. 34-81. Martin Robertson, Oxford.
5. Rosser, R. M. (1988). A health index and output measure. In *Quality of life: assessment and application* (ed. S. R. Walker and R. M. Rosser), pp. 133-60. MTP, Lancaster.
6. Rosser, R. (1990). From health indicators to quality adjusted life years. In *Measuring the outcomes of medical care* (ed. A. Hopkins and D. Costain), pp. 1-17. Royal College of Physicians, London.
7. Rosser, R. M. and Kind, P. (1978). A scale of valuations of states of illness – Is there a social consensus? *International Journal of Epidemiology*, **7**, 347-58.
8. Rosser, R. M. and Watts, V. C. (1972). The measurement of hospital output. *International Journal of Epidemiology*, **1**, 361-8.

9. Williams, A. (1988). Applications in management. In *Measuring health: a practical approach* (ed. G. Teeling-Smith), pp. 225–43. Wiley, Chichester.

Quality of Wellbeing Scale (QWB) (Bush, Anderson, Kaplan and others 1970 onwards)

Purpose

The QWB is the measurement system for a General Health Policy Model which is designed to express the benefits of medical care in terms of well years or quality adjusted life years. It summarizes current well-being and prognosis, and is intended to be used both as a measure of needs for care and an outcome measure for health programme evaluation.

Background

The General Health Policy Model was developed out of substantive theory in economics, psychology, medicine, and public health.[3] The authors recognized the limitations of mortality as an evaluative criterion for health care, but noted that measures of morbidity in terms of function, role performance, pain, etc. failed to incorporate mortality. The effect of this in terms of evaluating care is that deaths among the most seriously ill paradoxically produce apparent improvements in group health status scores. They therefore developed a model which would combine morbidity and mortality in the same index.

Kaplan and Anderson outline five steps which are necessary to build a general model for the evaluation of health policy alternatives: defining a functional status classification; classifying symptoms and problems; applying preference weights to functional states and symptoms; calculating the probability of transitions to other states; estimating the benefit–cost/utility ratio.[4] Bush and colleagues initially reviewed multiple sources to determine all the ways in which diseases and disabilities can affect function.[12,13] The items generated were grouped into scales representing mobility, physical activity, and social activity. Since function alone was felt to be insufficient as a health outcome measure, a set of symptoms and problems was also generated. Using several random samples from a metropolitan community, preference weights were assigned to functional levels and symptom/problem complexes. Calculation of the probabilities of transition to other states (i.e. prognosis) has been based on empirical evidence for specific conditions. The authors, not surprisingly, have not attempted a comprehensive classification of prognosis for all diseases.

Description

The QWB, previously known as the Index of Wellbeing, consists of two sections. The first provides a series of descriptions of functional states in the areas of mobility, physical activity and social activity, and the second is a list of symptom/problem complexes (Exhibit 7.12). In the functional classification, mobility and physical activity have only three levels, although more levels were used in earlier versions, and social activity has five levels. The 21 complexes of symptoms and problems are intended to represent all possible symptomatic complaints which might inhibit function.

The functional states have been used as a simple classification of outcome without the application of weights,[14] but they are intended to be used in conjunction with the symptom/problem complexes and the preference weights. These weights describe the relative desirability of all the functional states and symptom/problem complexes on a scale from 0 (death) to 1 (asymptomatic optimal function).[6,8] They represent the judgements of population samples on case descriptions. Although death is scored as 0, the authors recognize that states worse than death are possible.[5] The QWB score for any individual is obtained by adding the values associated with his or her functional state and symptoms as shown in Exhibit 7.12. A simple formula can be used to express the well-being of a group or population.[4]

Administration and acceptability

There were originally two versions of the questionnaire used to classify respondents: interviewer-administered and self-administered. However, the self-administered version is no longer used. Copies of the interviewer-administered questionnaire are available only from Professor Kaplan at the Department of Community and Family Medicine, University of California, San Diego. Questions were derived from a number of other instruments and are structured so that general screening questions lead to more specific questions about particular problems. An interviewer administered approach is recommended, since the self completed version resulted in considerable misclassification.[1] The interview takes between 10 and 15 minutes to administer, which may make it difficult to use in many service settings. However, it is argued that considerable probing is necessary in order to yield an accurate classification.

Reliability and validity

The reliability of the estimated preference weights has been examined in some detail with encouraging results[5,12] and weights obtained from different judges at different times showed only small variations.[7] The original preference weights were derived from general population samples, but a

Exhibit 7.12   Quality of Wellbeing Scale

(Adapted from Kaplan, R. M. and Anderson, J. P. (1988). The Quality of Wellbeing Scale: rationale for a single quality of life index. In *Quality of life: assessment and application*, (ed. S. R. Walker and R. M. Rosser). MTP, Lancaster).

A. Elements with calculating weights

Label	Step no.	Step definitions	Weights
Mobility	5	No limitation in driving or use of public transportation (bus, train, plane, subway) for health reasons.	– 0.000
	4,3	Did not drive a car or did not use public transportation, for health reasons (<age 16, did not ride in a car, or had more help to use public transportation than usual for age).	– 0.062
	2,1	In hospital (nursing home, hospice, home for the retarded, mental hospital, etc.) as a bed patient overnight.	– 0.090
	0	Death	– 0.090
Physical activity	4	No limitations for health reasons.	– 0.000
(PAC)	3,2	Found it difficult (or did not try) to lift, stoop, bend over, or use stairs or inclines, and/or limped, used a cane, crutches, or walker, or had any other physical limitation making it hard (or did not try) to walk as far or as fast as others of the same age, for health reasons, or in wheelchair, but controlled its movement without help.	– 0.060
	1	In bed, chair, or couch for most or all of the day (health related) or in wheelchair and did not control movement without help.	– 0.077
	0	Death	– 0.077

Exhibit 7.12 (continued)

Social activity (SAC)	5	Performed major role (work, home-making, school, retirement, etc.) and other (personal, community, religious, social, recreational) activities, with no limitations for health reasons.	– 0.000
	4,3,2	Limited in or did not perform major or other role activities for health reasons, but performed self-care (feeding, bathing, dressing, toilet).	– 0.061
	1	Did not perform self-care activities (or had more help than usual for age) for health reasons.	– 0.106
	0	Death	– 0.106

B. Symptom/problem complexes (CPX) with calculating weights

CPX no.	CPX description	Weights
1	Death (not on respondent's card)	– 0.727
2	Loss of consciousness such as seizure (fits), fainting, or coma (out cold or knocked out)	– 0.407
3	Burn over large areas of face, body, arms or legs	– 0.367
4	Pain, bleeding, itching or discharge (drainage) from sexual organs—does not include normal menstrual (monthly) bleeding.	– 0.349
5	Trouble learning, remembering, or thinking clearly	– 0.340
6	Any combination of one or more hands, feet, arms, or legs either missing, deformed, crooked, paralysed (unable to move), or broken—including wearing artificial limbs or braces	– 0.333
7	Pain, stiffness, weakness, numbness, or other discomfort in chest, stomach (including hernia or rupture), side, neck, back, hips, or any joints of hands, feet, arms or legs	– 0.299
8	Pain, burning, bleeding, itching, or other difficulty with rectum, bowel movements, or urination (passing water)	– 0.292
9	Sick or upset stomach, vomiting or loose bowel movements, with or without fever, chills, or aching all over	– 0.290
10	General tiredness, weakness, or weight loss	– 0.259
11	Cough, wheezing, or shortness of breath with or without fever, chills, or aching all over	– 0.257

Exhibit 7.12 (continued)

12	Spells of feeling upset, being depressed, or of crying	– 0.257
13	Headache, or dizziness, or ringing in ears, or spells of feeling hot, or nervous, or shaky	– 0.244
14	Burning or itching rash on large areas of face, body, arms, or legs	– 0.240
15	Trouble talking, such as lisp, stuttering, hoarseness, or being unable to speak	– 0.237
16	Pain or discomfort in one or both eyes (such as burning or itching) or any trouble seeing after correction	– 0.230
17	Overweight for age and height or skin defect of face, body, arms, or legs, such as scars, pimples, warts, bruises, or changes in colour	– 0.186
18	Pain in ear, tooth, jaw, throat, lips, tongue; several missing or crooked permanent teeth—including wearing bridges or false teeth; stuffy, runny nose; or any trouble hearing—including wearing a hearing aid	– 0.170 – 0.170
19	Taking medication or staying on a prescribed diet for health reasons	– 0.144
20	Wore eyeglasses or contact lenses	– 0.101
21	Breathing smog or unpleasant air	– 0.101
22	No symptoms or problems (not on respondent's card)	– 0.000
23	Standard symptom/problem (not on respondent's card)	– 0.257

C. Calculating formulae

Formula 1:   Point-in-time well-being score for an individual(W):
$$W = 1 + (CPXwt) = (MOBwt) = (PACwt) + (SACwt)$$

Where wt is the preference-weighted measure for each factor and CPX is symptom/problem complex. For example, the W score for a person with the following description profile may be calculated for one day as follows:

Quality of well-being element	Description	Weight
CPX-11	Cough, wheezing, shortness of breath, with or without fever, chill, or aching all over	– 0.257
MOB-5	No limitations	– 0.000
PAC-1	In bed, chair, or couch for most or all of the day, health-related	– 0.077
SAC-2	Performed no major role activity, health-related, but did perform self-care activities	– 0.061
	$W = 1 + (-0.257) + (-0.077) + (-0.061) = 0.605$	
Formula 2:	General Health Policy Model formula for well-years (WY) as an output measure $WY = [\text{No. of Persons} \times (CPXwt + MOBwt + PACwt + SACwt)] \times \text{Time}$	

study of patients with rheumatoid arthritis produced virtually identical weights.[3] Test–retest reliability was evaluated by correlating ratings made on one day with those made on eight subsequent days,[7] and by correlating ratings made retrospectively for consecutive days.[2] In both cases inter-day correlations were high. A comparison of interviewer administered with self-administered versions of the QWB showed the former to be considerably more reliable in its classification of individuals.[1]

Perhaps the strongest case for the content validity of the QWB can be made in terms of its incorporation of function, symptoms, and mortality into a single index. All three are central to a definition of health, but are rarely combined in proposed measures of health. Arguments for the content validity of the unweighted scale are advanced by Reynolds and colleagues,[14] and of the weighted scale by Kaplan and colleagues.[6] Further evidence of validity includes correlations with reported symptoms, chronic health problems and physician contact.[6] In a study of patients with cystic fibrosis, the QWB was shown to correlate well with commonly used pulmonary function measures.[11] Kaplan and Anderson argue that the QWB is responsive to relatively small changes because of its ability to make fine distinctions between health states.[4] They cite its ability to detect treatment effects, including adverse side effects in treatment trials with patients suffering from AIDS and arthritis.[9] However, the classifications used for both function and symptoms are extremely crude categories which may not be adequate to tap changes seen as significant by clinicans and patients. Liang, in a comparison of five health status instruments for orthopaedic evaluation, showed that although the QWB global scale was sensitive to change, the mobility and social scales were relatively insensitive.[10] However, Kaplan argues that because of multicolinearity in the preference weighting system, it is not appropriate to make separate interpretations of the sub-scales (personal communication). He also points out that more recent work in clinical trials for diabetic patients, outcomes for patients with HIV infection and stroke prevention in atrial fibrillation, the QWB has demonstrated its responsiveness to very small changes. Nevertheless, in a randomized placebo-controlled heart failure trial, the QWB was unable to detect any significant differences between treatment and placebo control groups, although differences were detected by other instruments.[15]

Populations/service settings

The QWB has been used primarily in its role as the measurement system for the General Health Policy Model. Its early use was therefore mainly in evaluation of service programmes, rather than in clinical trials. It has been used to evaluate preventive programmes for phenylketonuria, thyroid conditions and hypertension, tuberculin testing, oestrogen therapy, and pneumonia. It is equally applicable to any age group or disease category and can be applied in any service setting. Its great advantage for policy purposes is the ability to make comparisons across disease categories. More recently, it has been used in major clinical trials of auranofin treatment in rheumatoid arthritis, and coronary artery bypass grafts, and treatment of AIDS.

Clearly the QWB is a research instrument which would be inappropriate for use in routine clinical practice in primary care. However, there seems no reason why it should not be used in research concerned with policy planning and evaluation of primary care services.

Comments

The QWB and the associated General Health Policy Model has been influential in the development of many other measures. The ability to combine mortality and morbidity in a single index and to incorporate both benefits and side effects of treatment make it particularly attractive as a tool for policy decisions. However, its value in comparing disease states is dependent on being able to determine transition probabilities or prognosis. Only where this can be done with some degree of accuracy is it possible to calculate 'well years' accruing from different treatments.

Although the authors of the QWB have urged its use in clinical trials, and there are now a number of studies reporting its use, the evidence to date concerning its responsiveness to change is equivocal. Despite some evidence that it is sensitive to small changes, the key functional categories are very crude. Although it seems doubtful that the functional categories would be sufficiently responsive to many of the changes considered significant by patients or clinicians, the inclusion of changes in symptom status may account for the ability of the QWB to detect change. It may be worth considering in conjunction with disease-specific measures or more comprehensive health profiles, since the QWB permits comparisons to be made not only with other studies of the same treatment and condition, but also with other diseases and treatments. The ability to make such comparisons is essential to policy decisions at all levels of the health care system.

References

1. Anderson, J. P., Bush, J. W. and Berry, C. C. (1986). Classifying function for health outcome and quality of life evaluation. Self versus interviewer modes. *Medical Care*, **24**, 454–69.
2. Anderson, J. P., Kaplan, R. M., Berry, C. C., Bush, J. W., and Rumbaut, R. G. (1989). Interday reliability of function assessment for a health status measure. The Quality of Wellbeing Scale. *Medical Care*, **27**, 1076–83.
3. Balaban, D. J., Sagi, P. C., Goldfarb, N. I., and Nettler, S. (1986). Weights for scoring the Quality of Wellbeing Instrument among rheumatoid arthritics. *Medical Care*, **24**, 973–80.

3. Fanshel, S. and Bush, J. W. (1970). A health status index and its applications to health service outcomes. *Operational Research*, **18**, 1021–66.
4. Kaplan, R. M. and Anderson, J. P. (1988). The Quality of Wellbeing Scale: rationale for a single quality of life index. In *Quality of life: assessment and application* (ed. S. R. Walker and R. M. Rosser), pp. 51–77. MTP, Lancaster.
5. Kaplan, R. M. and Bush, J. W. (1982). Health related quality of life measurement for evaluation research and policy analysis. *Health Psychology*, **1**, 61–80.
6. Kaplan, R. M., Bush, J. W., and Berry, C. C. (1976). Health status: types of validity and the Index of Wellbeing. *Health Services Research*, **11**, 478–507.
7. Kaplan, R. M., Bush, J. W., and Berry, C. C. (1978). The reliability, stability and generalizability of a Health Status Index. *American Statistical Association Proceedings of the Social Statistics Section*, 704–9.
8. Kaplan, R. M., Bush, J. W., and Berry, C. C. (1979). Health Status Index: category rating versus magnitude estimation for measuring levels of wellbeing. *Medical Care*, **17**, 501–23.
9. Kaplan, R. M., Anderson, J. P., Wu, A. W., Mathews, W. C., Kozin, F., and Orenstein, D. (1989). The Quality of Wellbeing Scale. Applications in AIDS, cystic fibrosis and arthritis. *Medical Care*, **27** (3 Suppl.), S27–43.
10. Laing, M. H., Fossel, A. H., and Larson, M. G. (1990). Comparisons of five health status instruments for orthopedic evaluation. *Medical Care*, **28**, 632–42.
11. Orenstein, D. M., Nixon, P. A., Ross, E. A., and Kaplan, R. M. (1989). The quality of wellbeing in cystic fibrosis. *Chest*, **95**, 344–7.
12. Patrick, D. L., Bush, J. W., and Chen, M. M. (1973). Methods for measuring levels of wellbeing for a health status index. *Health Services Research*, **8**, 229–44.
13. Patrick, D. L., Bush, J. W., and Chen, M. M. (1973). Toward an operational definition of health. *Journal of Health and Social Behavior*, **14**, 6–21.
14. Reynolds, W. J., Rushing, W. A., and Miles, D. L. (1974). The validation of a function status index. *Journal of Health and Social Behavior*, **15**, 271–88.
15. Tandon, P. K., Stander, H., and Schwartz, R. P. Jr. (1989). Analysis of quality of life data from a randomized, placebo-controlled heart-failure trial. *Journal of Clinical Epidemiology*, **42**, 955–62.

Conclusions

We have included more measures in this chapter than any other, which is a reflection of the emphasis which has been placed in recent years on the development of multipurpose measures which cover a variety of dimensions of health. All nine measures are relatively recent in origin and, perhaps because of this, are founded on careful conceptualization and assessments of reliability and validity. Unlike many measures of specific dimensions of health, they have not developed out of clinical practice, but have been designed and tested to meet specified needs.

The primary focus of the authors of most of the multidimensional measures has been on broad epidemiological health policy, resource allocation, and service evaluation questions, rather than clinical research and practice. Nevertheless, all of the measures have found uses beyond the broad issues, and there is an increasing recognition that multidimensional measures of health status have an important part to play in clinical research, practice, and teaching.

A recent development has been the design and testing of a modular system of data collection instruments for use in outcomes management. A central generic health status questionnaire, the SF-36, based on the Medical Outcomes Study surveys (p. 153) is supplemented by a range of condition-specific, functional status and clinical data protocols. The Outcomes Management System (OMS) is being installed in a range of health service settings in the US, including group practices. Data from all users will be pooled in a national repository. Further information about this system is available from InterStudy, 5715 Christmas Lake Road, Excelsior, Minnesota, MN 55331–0458.

Despite the sophistication of existing measures, there remains considerable scope for further development. In addition to the need for more evidence of reliability and validity, particularly for use in specific situations, there may be scope for streamlining some of the longer instruments, and for exploring the possibilities of using sub-sections of instruments where the whole measure is not required. In some cases (e.g. physical function) the sub-scales from multidimensional measures may have advantages over existing instruments designed for specific dimensions.

Despite their origins in macro health service policy, planning, and resource allocation, multidimensional measures are likely to have increasing applications in primary health care. The very nature of primary health care is such that attention cannot be focused on narrow definitions of needs and outcomes. Physical, psychological, and social dimensions of health are intimately connected in the generation of needs for primary health care and in evaluating the impact of the service provided. It is thus encouraging to see new measures being developed specifically for use in primary health care and existing measures being adapted and tested for use in primary care settings.

8 Disease-specific measures

Introduction

The main focus of this review of measures of needs and outcomes has been on generic measures suitable for use across a wide variety of patient groups consulting primary health care providers. We have therefore excluded many excellent disease-specific measures. Indeed there are a sufficient number of these to warrant a separate volume. However, many disease-specific measures are unlikely to find widespread application in primary health care, either as aids to clinical practice or as research tools. Their main value is to specialists where the numbers of patients seen and the range of treatments offered warrants the use of instruments designed to gather detailed disease-specific assessments.

Despite our decision to exclude disease-specific measures from our review, there were a small number we felt were worth including. The distinction between generic and disease-specific measures is not always clear cut, so that some instruments, although developed to meet specialist needs, get adopted by others and applied to a wider range of conditions. Some of these have been included in earlier chapters because, despite their origins, they have become widely accepted in other specialties. However, we were left with a few instruments which did not fit easily into other chapters because of their emphasis on particular conditions, but which were, nevertheless, relevant to primary health care.

Of the measures presented here, two were developed in the field of the evaluation of cancer treatments, two in the management of arthritis, and the remainder were developed specifically for clinical trials with chronic respiratory disease, heart failure, and inflammatory bowel disease. Specialists in the treatment of cancer and arthritis have devoted considerable efforts to the problems of defining and measuring outcomes of treatment in the face of the inappropriateness of traditional indicators of mortality and morbidity. Karnofsky's measure of performance status (KPS) is now 40 years old, but remains in widespread use for both clinical and research purposes. It is one of the 'old style' instruments which were developed largely from clinical practice, with little regard for the niceties of psychometric techniques. Nevertheless, as with some other instruments with this background, the KPS has proved its value in its continued use by practitioners. Spitzer's Quality of Life Index represents a new generation of cancer treatment measures, in that it explicitly addresses the concept of quality of life. The two arthritis-specific measures, Meenan's Arthritis Impact Measurement Scale and Fries' Stanford Health Assessment Questionnaire, have both been developed to meet a need for outcome measures. They measure very similar dimensions and have achieved similar levels of reliability and validity. The final group of instruments are dealt with in one entry because they adopt a standard approach and emanate from the same authors. Gordon Guyatt and his colleagues at McMaster University have designed three instruments specifically for use in clinical trials with patients suffering from chronic respiratory disease, heart failure, and inflammatory bowel disease.

The Karnofsky Performance Status Scale (KPS) (Karnofsky and Burchenal 1949)

Purpose

The KPS was devised to assess the overall ability of cancer patients being treated with chemotherapeutic drugs to perform normal activities, and thus to estimate their needs for medical care. It has been widely used in both clinical practice and research as an indicator of prognosis, to predict ability to benefit from treatment, to select patients for treatment trials, to stratify patients in treatment trials, to measure the efficacy of treatment, and to measure the quality of survival.

Background

The KPS is the oldest measure included in this book. Karnofsky and Burchenal recognized the need for a measure which would enable them to quantify performance status as a means of evaluating the chemotherapeutic agents which were increasingly common in the treatment of cancer.[6] They designed the KPS on the basis of their clinical experience, paying little attention to formal assessment of reliability and validity. Over the following four decades it has been widely used in both clinical practice and research in the field of oncology. Various modifications to content and length have been made for particular purposes, but the original scale remains more or less intact in most studies.

Conceptually, the KPS represents a very limited and somewhat vague definition of performance. It is concerned with independence defined in terms of 'normal activity', which in turn is defined in terms of work and self-care. This narrow focus is perhaps more a reflection of prevailing medical attitudes at the time of its construction than any deliberate attempt on the part of the authors to restrict its scope.

Description

The KPS is a global assessment of function which allocates patients to one of three categories in terms of their ability to work, to undertake normal activities, and care for themselves. These three categories are subdivided into a further eleven as shown in Exhibit 8.1. There are no formal questions or specified procedure for assigning individuals to categories. In practice, determination of the most appropriate category is usually based on information from a variety of sources, including the patient, relatives, and clinical notes. Because of the dangers inherent in such a loosely structured approach some researchers have attempted to specify clearer criteria for making assessment.[4,9,15] Also shown in Exhibit 8.1 is a revised version of the KPS incorporating more explicit wording.

Exhibit 8.1   Karnofsky Performance Status Scale

(Reproduced from Karnofsky, D. A. and Burchenal, J. H. (1949). The clinical evaluation of chemotherapeutic agents in cancer. In *Evaluation of chemotherapeutic agents* (ed. C. M. MacLeod); Columbia Press, New York)

Original version

Condition	Percentage	Comments
A. Able to carry on normal activity and to work. No special care is needed	100	Normal, no complaints, no evidence of disease.
	90	Able to carry on normal activity, minor signs or symptoms of disease.
	80	Normal activity with effort, some signs or symptoms of disease.
B. Unable to work. Able to live at home and care for most personal needs. A varying degree of assistance is needed.	70	Cares for self. Unable to carry on normal activity or to do active work.
	60	Requires occasional assistance, but is able to care for most of own needs.
	50	Requires considerable assistance and frequent medical care.
C. Unable to care for self. Requires equivalent of institutional or hospital care. Disease may be progressing rapidly	40	Disabled, requires special care and assistance.
	30	Severely disabled, hospitalization is indicated although death not imminent.
	20	Hospitalization necessary, very sick, active supportive treatment necessary.

Exhibit 8.1 (continued)

10	Moribund, fatal processes progressing rapidly.
0	Dead.

Revised version

(Reproduced, with permission, from Grieco, A. and Long, C. J. (1984). Investigations of the Karnofsky Performance Status as a measure of quality of life. *Health Psychology*, 3, 129–42).

Elements:
A. Work–housekeeping, school, job activities, driving a car.
B. Social-communication, family and social relationships, marital, and sexual relationships.
C. Self-help skills—toileting, feeding, bathing, and dressing.

Percentage	Comments
100	Normal, no complaints, no evidence of disease or impairment. Does all activities as usual.
90	Does usual activities but minor signs or symptoms of disease or impairment. Work not adversely affected.
80	Does usual activities with effort, some signs or symptoms of disease or impairment. Work or social activities mildly impaired.
70	Self-help skills intact. May work part-time but does not work 40 hrs per week or does not carry on usual activities.
60	Self-help skills intact but does not work, attend school, or carry out routine housework. Social, family, and marital or sexual relationships may be impaired.
50	Self-help skills mildly impaired. Requires considerable assistance and frequent medical care. Ordinary social relationships may be prohibited or significantly impaired. Does a few chores beyond self-care, such as light housework.
40	Disabled, requires special care and assistance. One self-help skill is prohibited or significantly impaired.
30	Severely disabled, hospitalization or insititutionalization is indicated. More than one self-help skill prohibited or significantly impaired.
20	Hospitalization or institutionalization is necessary, very sick, active supportive treatment is necessary. Severely restricted behaviour. Poor awareness of environment.
10	Unconscious or in a stupor, near death. Little or no movement or awareness of surroundings.
0	Dead

The scale concentrates particularly on physical performance and motor functions. Although it seems to provide an overall indication of physical status, it neglects emotional state, pain, language, and cognitive function, except in so far as these are reflected in physical function. It might therefore be expected to correlate poorly with patients' own perceptions of their quality of life. Both the three- and eleven-point ratings are simple ordinal scales. The KPS reduces a complex multidimensional construct to a unidimensional scale, and it is this apparent simplicity which no doubt accounts for its continuing popularity, particularly in cancer research. There are no published instructions for scoring, and the percentage levels proposed by Karnofsky were recognized to be notional. From a psychometric point of view the scaling is therefore weak. There is no reason to suppose that the intervals between scores represent the same degree of dysfunction, although some researchers have treated scores as if they were derived from a ratio scale.

Administration and acceptability

The scale was originally designed for use by clinicians who would rate patients on the basis of their own observations and examinations. Considerable attention has been devoted in recent studies to the need to standardize assessment procedures for both clinicians and non-clinicians using the KPS.[4,5,9,11] Those studies which have shown good inter-rater reliability have only done so after careful training of raters and using standard procedures. Such precautions seem essential, particularly where ratings are likely to be carried out by more than one person.

Although the KPS is superficially a very simple and brief rating scale, accurate assessment can only be achieved with considerable knowledge about the individual. It is thus not a particularly economical measure, except where it is being used by professionals who, because they are caring for the patient, already possess the information necessary. Because the rating is conducted indirectly, it is unlikely to present any problems of acceptability to patients who may not be aware of the use of the scale.

Reliability and validity

For a scale which has been in widespread use for such a long period of time, it is surprising to find that attempts to assess its reliability and validity are relatively recent. Since the KPS is intended as a unidimensional ordinal scale, the question of internal item consistency does not arise. There appear to have been no attempts to assess test–retest reliability, because of the difficulty of mounting such studies with patients suffering from terminal illness. A number of studies have, however, looked at inter-rater reliability. The lack of clear questions, guidelines, or procedures makes this a particularly important issue for the KPS. Studies involving nurses, social workers, and non-physician interviewers have shown moderate to good inter-rater reliability where procedures are specified and training given.[1,4,9,15] However, other researchers have reported relatively poor correlations between physicians' ratings.[5,12] It seems likely that the level of agreement between raters will depend on the clarity of instructions and definitions used and the homogeneity of the patient group. The KPS is essentially a physician rating, but some studies have compared physician- and patient-rated scores.[1,3,12] They have shown only moderate correlations and argued that patient self-evaluation may be a more valid and reliable measure of quality of life.

The KPS seems to have achieved its popularity largely on the basis of its face validity to clinicians, but this is a very weak criterion of validity. Assessed against the more stringent criterion of content validity, the KPS seems deficient in a number of areas, particularly the lack of any reference to pain or emotional state. A number of recent studies have provided evidence of construct validity. Scores on the KPS are associated with ability to perform activities of daily living,[9] ambulation and activity,[14] self-care, daily activity, ability to work, and evidence of disease.[11] A comparison of KPS scores with scores on the Quality of Life Index (see p. 204) have shown good correlations between the two measures.[7] Grieco and Long, in a study of patients suffering from a variety of chronic conditions, showed positive correlations between KPS scores and those for the Quality of Wellbeing Scale and the Rand Health Perceptions Questionnaire (see pp. 188 and 262).[4] They also showed that KPS scores discriminated well between different patient groups. Perhaps most importantly, the KPS scores have been shown to be predictive of longevity in cancer patients[2,9,13] and to discriminate between groups of patients at varying time intervals prior to death.[10] In a comparison of a new Breast Cancer Chemotherapy Questionnaire and three existing instruments, only the new questionnaire and the KPS were able to demonstrate differences between treatment groups.[8] This ability to detect change may be the main strength of the scale, which has helped it to retain its appeal to clinicians over such a long period of time. However, the changes occurring in the weeks prior to death are often large, and it would be a very unresponsive instrument which failed to detect them.

Populations/service settings

The KPS is primarily an instrument designed for use with patients suffering from terminal illness, particularly cancer. It has, however, been used with some success on patients suffering from AIDS, strokes, chronic pain, and those on renal dialysis. Although its use in clinical practice and research has largely been confined to hospital-based medical care, it has been used in the community[15] and could be used in a primary health care setting. It remains one of the most commonly used instruments for assessing quality of life in cancer treatment trials. A MEDLINE search covering the period 1988–90 produced more than 150 references to studies using the KPS.

Comments

Although the KPS appears to lack the sophistication of many more recently developed measures, it has withstood the test of time. It continues to be used by both clinicians and researchers. However, we cannot ignore some of its more obvious weaknesses. It cannot be considered an adequate measure of quality of life, because it fails to include important aspects such as pain and emotional state. It provides no means of incorporating the patient's own perception of his or her condition. Lastly, the lack of clearly specified definitions and instructions makes it difficult to ensure reliability, although this can be achieved if proper precautions are taken. Despite these criticisms we believe that the KPS may have a worthwhile role in practice and research concerning chronically ill people, perhaps in conjunction with other measures.

References

1. Conill, C., Verger, E., and Salamero, M. (1990). Performance status assessment in cancer patients. *Cancer*, **65**, 1864–6.
2. Evans, C. and McCarthy, M. (1985). Prognostic uncertainty in terminal care: Can the Karnofsky Index help? *Lancet*, **i**, 1204–6.
3. Ganz, P. A., Schag, C. C., and Cheng, H. L. (1990). Assessing the quality of life–a study in newly-diagnosed breast cancer patients. *Journal of Clinical Epidemiology*, **43**, 75–86.
4. Grieco, A. and Long, C. J. (1984). Investigation of the Karnofsky Performance Status as a measure of quality of life. *Health Psychology*, **3**, 129–42.
5. Hutchinson, T. A., Boyd, N. F., Feinstein, A. R., Ganda, A., Hollomby, D., and Rowat, B. (1979). Scientific problems in clinical scales, as demonstrated in the Karnofsky Index of Performance Status. *Journal of Chronic Disease*, **32**, 661–6.
6. Karnofsky, D. A. and Burchenal, J. H. (1949). The clinical evaluation of chemotherapeutic agents in cancer. In *Evaluation of chemotherapeutic agents* (ed. C. M. MacLeod), pp. 191–205. Columbia, New York.
7. Koster, R., Gebeensleben, B., Stutzer, H., Salzburger, B., Ahrens, P., and Rohde, H. (1987). Quality of life in gastric cancer. *Scandinavian Journal of Gastroenterology*, **22**, 102–6.
8. Levine, M. N., Guyatt, G. H., Gent, M., De Pauw, S., Goodyear, M. D., Hryniuk, W. M., *et al.* (1988). Quality of life in stage II breast cancer: an instrument for clinical trials. *Journal of Clinical Oncology*, **6**, 1798–810.
9. Mor, V., Laliberte, L., Morris, T. N., and Wiermann, M. (1984). The Karnofsky Performance Status Scale: an examination of its reliability and validity in a research setting. *Cancer*, **53**, 2002–7.
10. Morris, J. N., Suissa, S., Sherwood, S., Wright, S. M., and Greer, D. (1986). Last days: a study of the quality of life of terminally ill cancer patients. *Journal of Chronic Disease*, **39**, 47–62.
11. Schag, C. C., Heinrich, R. L., and Ganz, P. A. (1984). Karnofsky Performance Status revisited: reliability, validity and guidelines. *Journal of Clinical Oncolology*, **2**, 187–93.

12. Slevin, M. L., Plant, H., Lynch, D., Drinkwater, J., and Gregory, W. M. (1988). Who should measure quality of life, the doctor or the patient. *British Journal of Cancer*, **57**, 109–12.
13. Stanley, K. E. (1980). Prognostic factors for survival in patients with inoperable lung cancer. *Journal of the National Cancer Institute*, **65**, 25–32.
14. Wood, C. A., Anderson, T., and Yates, J. W. (1981). Physical function assessment in patients with cancer. *Medical Pediatric Oncolology*, **9**, 129–32.
15. Yates, J. W., Chalmer, B., and McKegney, F. P. (1980). Evaluation of patients with advanced cancer using the Karnofsky Performance Status. *Cancer*, **45**, 2220–4.

Quality of Life (QL) Index (Spitzer 1981)

Purpose

The QL Index is intended to measure the general well-being of patients suffering from cancer. It has been used in research to evaluate specific treatments and supportive services in terms of patient outcomes.

Background

The QL Index was developed through collaboration between Australian and Canadian researchers who recognized a need for an easily administered scale which would encompass the various dimensions of quality of life. The authors felt that existing measures, such as the Karnofsky index of performance (see p. 198) were too narrow in scope and inadequately validated. In order to assess the relative benefits and risks of different treatments and/or support services it was necessary to develop a measure which encompassed physical, social, and emotional aspects of quality of life. A good quality of life should include a positive mood state and supportive relationships as well as the absence of physical or psychological distress. Possible themes for the Index were derived from panels containing cancer patients, their relatives, other chronically ill people, health professionals and well people.[7] The fourteen themes identified in this way were incorporated into two sets of questions for initial testing. Tests were carried out on 339 people, of whom 64 per cent were cancer patients. Correlation analysis of the results of these tests provided a basis for reducing the number of items to five for the final version. The final version was tested on healthy people and those suffering from chronic illnesses, including 105 cancer patients.

Description

The QL Index consists of five items (activity, daily living, health, support, and outlook) each of which is rated on a three-point scale (Exhibit 8.2). The

Exhibit 8.2   Quality of Life Index

(Adapted, with permission, from Spitzer, W. O., Dobson, A. J., Hall, J., Chesterman, E., Levi, J., Shepherd, R. *et al.* (1981). Measuring the quality of life of cancer patients: a concise QL-Index for use by physicians. *Journal of Chronic Disease*, 34, 591)

Score each heading 2,1, or 0 according to your most recent assessment of the patient.

Activity

During the last week, the patient:

Has been working or studying full-time or nearly so, in usual occupation; or managing own household; or participating in unpaid or voluntary activities, whether retired or not. 2

Has been working or studying in usual occupation or managing own household or participating in unpaid or voluntary activities; but requiring major assistance or a significant reduction in hours. 1

Has not been working or studying in any capacity and not managing own household. 0

Daily living

During the last week, the patient:

Has been self-reliant in eating, washing, toileting, and dressing, using public transport or driving own car. 2

Has been requiring assistance (another person or special equipment) for daily activities and transport but performing light tasks. 1

Has not been managing personal care nor light tasks/or not leaving own home or institution at all. 0

Health

During the last week, the patient:

Has been appearing to feel well or reporting feeling 'great' most of the time. 2

Has been lacking energy or not feeling entirely 'up to par' more than just occasionally. 1

Has been feeling very ill or 'lousy', seeming weak and washed out most of the time or was unconscious. 0

Support

During the last week:

The patient has been having good relationships with others and receiving strong support from at least one family member and/or friend. 2

Support received or perceived has been limited from family and friends and/or by the patient's condition. 1

Support from family and friends occurred infrequently or only when absolutely necessary or patient was unconscious. 0

Outlook

During the past week, the patient:

Has usually been appearing calm and positive in outlook, accepting and in control of personal circumstances, including surroundings. 2

Exhibit 8.2 (continued)

Has sometimes been troubled because not fully in control of personal circumstances or has been having periods of obvious anxiety or depression.	1
Has been seriously confused or very frightened or consistently anxious and depressed or unconscious.	0

QL-Index total: _____

How confident are you that your scoring of the preceding dimensions is accurate? Please ring (circle) the appropriate category.

Absolutely confident	Very confident	Quite confident	Not very confident	Very doubtful	Not at all confident
1	2	3	4	5	6

object is to assess the patient's functioning/experience over the preceding week by selecting the description which best describes the individual. Although the scaling of each item is only ordinal, scores are summed to provide a QL Index total. The authors found no evidence that any items were more important than any others, and therefore felt that equal weighting was justified. However, the construction of total scores from ordinal scales has been criticized.[2] For comparative purposes, Spitzer provides representative scores for well and ill populations, although it is not considered suitable as a measure of quality of life in healthy people. Two variants of the QL Index have been developed, but these do not seem to have been widely used. The Multiscale employs ten items selected from the original fourteen, and a single visual analogue scale, known as the Uniscale, was developed for self-administration or administration by a physician.[7]

Administration and acceptability

One of the greatest advantages of the QL Index is the ease with which it can be administered. It takes between one and two minutes to complete using information which would usually have been elicited in the course of a normal consultation. It is completed by a physician or other competent professional who knows the patient well, and does not therefore require patients to answer questions or fill out forms. Even the self-administered version is designed to be brief and easily completed by patients who may be very sick and/or anxious.

Reliability and validity

Evidence of internal consistency and inter-rater reliability is quite good, although based on fairly small studies by the original authors.[7] Although correlations between different physicians rating the same patients were reasonable, correlations between patient self-ratings and physician ratings were less satisfactory. Test–retest reliability is unfortunately not reported.

Validation of the QL Index is also rather limited. Content was assessed by asking patients, well people, doctors and researchers to judge the scope and content. The only other studies of validity were based on comparisons of different versions of the index. Thus the final five-item version was compared with the longer version and with the self-administered version.[7] The ability of the scale to discriminate between well people and various categories of patients has been established, but whether it is sufficiently sensitive to identify small but clinically significant changes is not clear. When used in a study of hospice patients, the QL Index did not demonstrate very good discriminatory power.[5] It is unfortunate that the QL Index has not been validated against more comprehensive measures of quality of life in cancer patients. However, the only comparative studies to date have shown moderate correlations with self administered linear analogue scales[1] and the Karnofsky Performance Index.[3] There is limited evidence that the QL Index is responsive to changes in treatment trials.[6,8] Indeed, in one heart-failure trial the QL Index showed a significant difference between treatment and placebo groups which was not detected by either the Sickness Impact Profile or the Quality of Wellbeing Scale (see pp. 133 and 188).[8]

Populations/service settings

The QL Index is intended primarily for patients suffering from cancer and is not suitable for use with relatively healthy populations. Although originally developed for use in the context of specialist hospital-based services, it could be used in primary health care, either as a supplement to normal clinical assessments or for research purposes to evaluate treatments or patterns of care for patients suffering from cancer and other terminal illnesses. Although it has been used in a study of patients with arthritis,[4] further validation of its applicability to other chronic conditions is essential before use.

Comments

The QL Index is an advance on measures of function and activities of daily living. The ease with which it can be incorporated into normal clinical practice will make it particularly attractive. However, when considering its use it should be remembered that the price paid for brevity is a loss of detail. Evidence of reliability and validity is satisfactory as far as it goes, but considerably more work is required to establish its validity as a measure of the complex concept of quality of life. In particular, evidence of the ability of the QL Index to identify relatively small improvements or deterioration would be desirable. Also, further work needs to be undertaken on the meaning of total scores constructed from ordinally scaled items.

References

1. Gough, I.R., Furnival, C.M., Schilder, L., and Grove, W. (1983). Assessment of the quality of life of patients with advanced cancer. *European Journal of Cancer and Clinical Oncology*, **19**, 1161–5.
2. Kind, P. (1988). Development of health indices. In *Measuring health: a practical approach* (ed. G. Teeling-Smith), pp. 23–43. Wiley, Chichester.
3. Koster, R., Gebeensleben, B., Stutzer, H., Salzburger, B., Ahrens, P., and Rohde, H. (1987). Quality of life in gastric cancer. *Scandinavian Journal of Gastroenterology*, **22** Suppl. 133, 102–6.
4. Liang, M., Partridge, A.J., Larsen, M.G., Gall, V., Taylor, J., Berkman, C., *et al.* (1984). Evaluation of comprehensive rehabilitation services for elderly homebound patients with arthritis and orthopaedic disability. *Arthritis and Rheumatism*, **27**, 258–66.
5. Morris, J.N., Suissa, S., Sherwood, S., Wright, S.M., and Greer, D. (1986). Last days: a study of the quality of life of terminally ill cancer patients. *Journal of Chronic Disease*, **39**, 47–62.
6. Paul, A., Vestweber, K.H., Bode, C., and Eypasch, E. (1987). Percutaneous endoscopic duodenostomy (PED). Case report. *Surgical Endoscopy*, **1**, 123–6.
7. Spitzer, W.O., Dobson, A.J., Hall, J., Chesterman, E., Levi, J., Shepherd, R., *et al.* (1981). Measuring the quality of life of cancer patients: a concise QL Index for use by physicians. *Journal of Chronic Disease*, **34**, 585–97.
8. Tandon, P.K., Stander, H., and Schwarz, R.P. Jr. (1989). Analysis of Quality of Life data from a randomized, placebo-controlled heart-failure trial. *Journal of Clinical Epidemiology*, **42**, 955–62.

The Arthritis Impact Measurement Scale (AIMS) (Meenan 1980)

Purpose

AIMS is designed to measure the health status component of patient outcome in the rheumatic diseases and has been used to evaluate various treatments and programmes in both clinical research and service evaluation. It has also been used as part of routine assessment in clinical practice.

Background

Meenan and his colleagues began work on the AIMS in 1978. They criticized traditional outcome measures on both conceptual and practical grounds, and argued that health status, incorporating the key dimensions included in the WHO definition, should constitute the criterion for outcome evaluation.[12] In developing a new measure the researchers decided to build on existing instruments, rather than developing an instrument from scratch. The Quality of Wellbeing Scale (p. 188) and the Rand measures of physical and mental health (p. 65) provided the core elements of AIMS, and new measures of dexterity, ADL, and pain were developed.[14] No further information is provided as to the procedures used to develop the scales, but good descriptions of subsequent testing are available.[13,14]

Description

The complete schedule (copies available from Dr Meenan) consists of 66 items, but only 45 of these are shown in Exhibit 8.3. The remaining 21 items consist of three general health questions, four health perception questions, one overall impact item (visual analogue scale), one estimation of medication use, three items dealing with co-morbidity, and nine demographic items. These 21 items do not constitute an integral part of the AIMS. The 45 items shown in the exhibit are broken down into nine scales of between four and seven items each. Items were selected for inclusion on the basis of Guttman analyses and are listed in descending order of difficulty, so that a respondent indicating disability on one item will tend to indicate disability on all

---

Exhibit 8.3   Arthritis Impact Measurement Scale: questionnaire items

(Adapted, with permission, from Meenan, R. F. (1984). *Arthritis impact measurement scales*. Boston University).

Mobility

4   Are you in bed or chair for most or all of the day because of your health?
3   Do you have to stay indoors most or all of the day because of your health?
2   When you travel around your community does someone have to assist you because of your health?
1   Are you able to use public transportation?

Physical Activity

5   Are you unable to walk unless you are assisted by another person or by a cane, crutches, artificial limbs, or braces?
4   Do you have any trouble either walking one block or climbing one flight of stairs because of your health?
3   Do you have any trouble either walking several blocks or climbing a few flights of stairs because of your health?
2   Do you have trouble bending, lifting, or stooping because of your health?
1   Does your health limit the kind of vigorous activities you can do such as running, lifting heavy objects, or participating in strenuous sports?

Exhibit 8.3 (continued)

Dexterity
5   Can you easily write with a pen or pencil?
4   Can you easily turn a key in a lock?
3   Can you easily tie a pair of shoes?
2   Can you easily button articles of clothing?
1   Can you easily open a jar of food?

Household activity
7   If you had a telephone, would you be able to use it?
6   If you had to take medicine, could you take all your own medicine?
5   Do you handle your own money?
4   If you had a kitchen, could you prepare your own meals?
3   If you had laundry facilities (washer, dryer, etc.), could you do your own laundry?
2   If you had the necessary transportation, could you go shopping for groceries or clothes?
1   If you had household tools and appliances (vacuum, mops, etc.) could you do your own housework?

Social activity
4   About how often were you on the telephone with close friends or relatives during the past month?
3   During the past month, about how often did you get together socially with friends or relatives?
2   During the past month, about how often have you had friends or relatives to your home?
1   During the past month, how often have you visited with friends or relatives at their homes?

Activities of daily living
4   How much help do you need to use the toilet?
3   How well are you able to move around?
2   How much help do you need in getting dressed?
1   When you bathe, either a sponge bath, tub, or shower, how much help do you need?

Pain
4   During the past month, how long has your morning stiffness usually lasted from the time you wake up?
3   During the past month, how often have you had pain in two or more joints at the same time?
2   During the past month, how often have you had severe pain from your arthritis?
1   During the past month, how would you describe the arthritis pain you usually have?

Depression
6   During the past month, how often did you feel that others would be better off if you were dead?

Exhibit 8.3 (continued)

5   How often during the past month have you felt so down in the dumps that nothing could cheer you up?

4   How much of the time during the past month have you felt downhearted and blue?

3   How often during the past month did you feel that nothing turned out for you the way you wanted it to?

2   During the past month, how much of the time have you been in low or very low spirits?

1   During the past month, how much of the time have you enjoyed the things you do?

Anxiety

6   How often during the past month did you find yourself having difficulty trying to calm down?

5   How much have you been bothered by nervousness, or your 'nerves' during the past month?

4   During the past month, how much of the time have you felt tense or 'high strung'?

3   How much of the time during the past month were you able to relax without difficulty?

2   How much of the time during the past month have you felt calm and peaceful?

1   How much of the time during the past month did you feel relaxed and free of tension?

Response categories:

Mobility, physical activity, dexterity: YES, NO

Household activity: Without help; with some help; completely unable.

Social activity: Every day; several days a week; about once a week; 2 or 3 times in the past month; once in the past month; not at all in the past month.

Activities of daily living: *Item 1*: No help at all; help with reaching some parts of the body; help in bathing more than one part of the body. *Item 2*: No help at all; only need help tying shoes; need help getting dressed. *Item 3*: Able to get in and out of bed or chairs without the help of another person; need help of another person; don't get out of bed. *Item 4*: No help at all; some help in getting to or using the toilet; not able to get to the bathroom at all.

Pain: *Item 1*: Very severe; severe; moderate; mild; very mild; none. *Item 2, 3*: Always; very often; fairly often; sometimes; almost never; never. *Item 4*: Over 4 hrs; 2 to 4 hrs; 1 to 2 hrs; 30 mins to 1 hr, less than 30 mins; do not have morning stiffness.

Depression and anxiety: *Items: 1,2,4, (depression), 1,2,3,4 (anxiety)*: All of the time; most of the time; a good bit of the time; some of the time; a little of the time; none of the time. *Items 3,5,6 (depression), 6 (anxiety)*: Always; very often; fairly often; sometimes; almost never; never. *Item 5 (anxiety)*: Extremely so; very much so; quite a bit; some; just a little bit; not bothered at all.

subsequent items in that section. Response categories range from simple yes/no responses in the first three sections to six point ratings of frequency and severity.

The AIMS produces a score for each section (e.g. mobility, dexterity, pain, etc.) by simply adding the scores on each item within the section. All items in a section have to be answered to calculate a score. Higher scores indicate greater disability, and it should be noted that where the phrasing of a question is reversed the scoring of response categories also has to be reversed. No item weights are used, so that each item within a section has an equal contribution to the total score. When raw scores have been calculated these can be converted to a standard range of 0 to 10 using simple standardization formulae provided in the AIMS users' guide.[2] A total health score can be calculated by adding together the values for six sections; mobility, physical and household activities, dexterity, pain, and depression. Scores for three separate components of health (physical function, psychological status, pain) can also be calculated. Lastly, a single page computer-generated summary of AIMS scores has been developed to facilitate multiple assessments over a period of time.[2]

A British version of the AIMS has been developed incorporating modifications to the terminology and spelling.[7] A shortened version, reducing the number of items to 18, has recently been developed and tested,[17] although it has not yet been widely used.

Administration and acceptability

The questionnaire is self-administered, either in the care setting (e.g. surgery, waiting room) or in the patient's own home. It takes between 15 and 20 minutes to complete, and respondents should not be given any assistance as this may bias results. A Research and Evaluation Support Care Unit at the Multipurpose Arthritis Centre in Boston is available to provide assistance with applications and data processing.[2] The authors report no major problems of comprehension during the testing of the instrument, and the questions are unlikely to generate antipathy in respondents since the areas of questioning are not particularly sensitive. British patients found the Anglicized version easier to complete than the original.[7]

Reliability and validity

In the development of the AIMS Meenan and his colleagues have conducted extensive tests which have established the reliability and validity of the scales, and a number of subsequent studies have confirmed their findings. Although the scales are not intended to be scored as Guttman scales, each section was developed as a cumulative unidimensional scale. The authors have shown that they do conform to Guttman criteria of scalability and reproducibility.[12,14] In the same studies, they have also shown high levels of internal consistency and of test–retest reliability for several diagnostic groups. Further evidence of test–retest reliability and internal consistency of the original version,[5] and the short version,[17] is available from more recent studies.

Evidence supporting the validity of the AIMS is extensive and has employed a variety of techniques. Scores have been shown to correlate predictably with age, patients' perceptions of general health, and recent disease activity.[14] Scores have also been validated against assessments derived from an occupational therapist's interview.[16] Concurrent validity has been examined in comparisons with a variety of other health status instruments.[3,7,9,17] Most commonly, the AIMS has been compared with the Stanford Health Assessment Questionnaire (HAQ) (see p. 215) and shown to produce high correlations for physical function and pain. Since the HAQ has no psychological component, the anxiety and depression scales have been independently validated against the Hospital Anxiety and Depression Scale[7] and the Beck Depression Inventory[6] (p. 90 and 80). However, Hagglund and colleagues conclude that the AIMS fails to discriminate between anxiety and depression in patients suffering from rheumatoid arthritis.[6] The short version was shown to correlate both with the full-length version and with a variety of alternative measures.[17]

Although the AIMS includes nine dimensions, a factor analytic study of data on 360 patients with rheumatoid arthritis identified five components of health status; lower extremity function, upper extremity function, affect, symptoms, and social interaction.[11]

Evidence concerning the responsiveness of the AIMS to change comes from a study comparing scale scores with standard clinical outcome measures in a trial of 'gold' against a placebo.[15] In a further trial, the AIMS was shown to be sensitive to short-term changes in response to treatment with non-steroidal anti-inflammatory drugs for both osteo- and rheumatoid arthritis.[1] A comparison of five instruments showed the AIMS to be responsive in relation to pain, mobility and global assessment, but relatively unresponsive as a measure of social function.[10]

Populations/service settings

The AIMS is limited to use with patients suffering from rheumatic diseases. Although large sections of the instrument may be applicable to patients suffering from other chronic illnesses, their use has been more or less confined to patients suffering from arthritis. Also it is not considered suitable for patients suffering from juvenile arthritis.

The AIMS seems particularly suited for use in primary health care settings and it has been used extensively in American ambulatory care. Although questions are phrased in such a way as to apply both to people living in their own homes and those in hospital or residential care (e.g. household activity section), they are likely to be most useful with people living in their own homes. A system of patient profiles suitable for use in clinical practice has recently been developed and tested.[8]

Comments

This is a well documented and carefully tested measure which is likely to be of particular value in studies of rheumatic diseases in general practice, or as a routine adjunct to clinical practice. It deserves serious consideration as an indicator of both needs for care and outcomes among arthritic patients.

Dr Meenan has informed us that he has recently completed a major revision of the AIMS which will be called AIMS2. This instrument differs from the original in three major ways. First, the nine original AIMS scales have been revised by adding, deleting or revising items, and by standardizing the number and phrasing of response options. Second, three new scales have been added to assess arm and shoulder function, work, and social support from family and friends. Third, three new sections have been added to assess satisfaction with function, the extent to which health status problems can be attributed to arthritis, and the respondent's top three priority areas for health status improvement. We recommend that readers considering using AIMS should contact Dr Meenan at The Arthritis Centre, Boston University Medical Centre, Conte Building, 80 East Concord Street, Boston, Massachusetts 02118-2394 for further information on AIMS2. Publication of AIMS2 and supporting evidence of reliability and validity is expected during 1991.

References

1. Anderson, J.J., Firschein, H.E., and Meenan, R.F. (1989). Sensitivity of a health status measure to short-term clinical changes in arthritis. *Arthritis and Rheumatism*, **32**, 844–50.
2. Boston University Multipurpose Arthritis Center (1984). *AIMS Users' Guide*. Boston University, Boston.
3. Brown, J.H., Kazis, L.E., Spitz, P.W., Gertman, P., Fries, J., and Meenan, R.F. (1984). The dimensions of health outcomes: a cross-validated examination of health status measurement. *Americal Journal of Public Health*, **74**, 159–61.
4. Deyo, R.A. (1988). Measuring the quality of life of patients with rheumatoid arthritis. In *Quality of life: assessment and application* (ed. S.R. Walker and R.M. Rosser), pp. 205–22. MTP, Lancaster.
5. Goeppinger, J., Doyle, M.A., Charlton, S.L., and Lorig, K. (1988). A nursing perspective on the assessment of function in persons with arthritis. *Research in Nursing and Health*, **11**, 321–31.
6. Hagglund, K.J., Roth, D.L., Haley, W.E., and Alarcon, G.S. (1989). Discrimi-

nant and convergent validity of self-report measures of affective distress in patients with rheumatoid arthritis. *Journal of Rheumatology*, **16**, 1428–32.

7. Hill, J., Bird, H. A., Lawton, C. W., and Wright, V. (1990). The Arthritis Impact Measurement Scales: an anglicized version to assess the outcome of British patients with rheumatoid arthritis. *British Journal of Rheumatology*, **29**, 193–6.

8. Kazis, L. E., Anderson, J. J., and Meenan, R. F. (1988). Health status information in clinical practice: the development and testing of patient profile reports. *Journal of Rheumatology*, **15**, 338–44.

9. Liang, M. H., Larson, M. G., Cullen, K. E., and Schwartz, J. A. (1985). Comparative measurement efficiency and sensitivity of five health status instruments for arthritis research. *Arthritis and Rheumatism*, **28**, 542–7.

10. Liang, M. H., Fossel, A. H., and Larson, M. G. (1990). Comparisons of five health status instruments for Orthopedic Evaluation. *Medical Care*, **28**, 632–42.

11. Mason, J. H., Anderson, J. J., and Meenan, R. F. (1988). A model of health status for rheumatoid arthritis. A factor analysis of the Arthritis Impact Measurement Scales. *Arthritis and Rheumatism*, **31**, 714–20.

12. Meenan, R. F. (1982). The AIMS approach to health status measurement: conceptual background and measurement properties. *Journal of Rheumatology*, **9**, 785–8.

13. Meenan, R. F. (1985). New approaches to outcome assessment: the AIMS questionnaire for arthritis. *Advances in Internal Medicine,* **31** 167–85.

14. Meenan, R. F., Gertman, P. M., and Mason, J. H. (1980). Measuring health status in arthritis: The Arthritis Impact Measurement Scales. *Arthritis and Rheumatism*, **23**, 146–52.

15. Meenan, R. F., Anderson, J. J., Kazis, L. E., Egger, M. J., Altz-Smith, M., and Samuelson, C. O. (1984). Outcome assessment in clinical trials: evidence for the sensitivity of a health status measure. *Arthritis and Rheumatism*, **27**, 1344–52.

16. Spiegel, J. S., Hirshfield, M. D., and Spiegel, T. M. (1985). Evaluating self care activities: comparisons of a self reported questionnaire with an occupational therapist interview. *British Journal of Rheumatology*, **24**, 357–61.

17. Wallston, K. A., Brown, G. K., Stein, M. J., and Dobbins, C. J. (1989). Comparing the short and long versions of the Arthritis Impact Measurement Scales. *Journal of Rheumatology*, **16**, 1105–9.

Stanford Health Assessment Questionnaire (HAQ) (Fries and others 1980)

Purpose

The HAQ is designed to assess four outcome dimensions in patients or normal subjects: disability, pain, drug side effects, and costs. It is intended to be of use in both clinical practice and research evaluation of the outcomes of medical care.

Background

Fries and his colleagues at the Stanford Arthritis Centre critized the tradi-tional process measures used in arthritis care and research, and the lack of any systematic structure for the representation of patient outcomes.[4] They set out to develop a reliable and valid set of instruments for measuring the four components of outcome mentioned above. Although the complete HAQ consists of four sections, those dealing with drug side effects and costs have not been published and have not been widely used. For this reason the remainder of this review is concerned with only the disability and pain com-ponents of the HAQ.

Potential component questions for the disability section were selected from a variety of sources, including the Barthel Index and the Index of Independence in Activities of Daily Living (pp. 43 and 48).[4,5] Sixty-two potential questions were used by a nurse assessor in interviews with patients. Areas of redundancy, imprecision, and ambiguity were identified and the questionnaire appropriately modified. The final instrument was the result of repeated applications in different settings and formats with patients suffering from rheumatoid and osteoarthritis.[5]

Description

The final version contains twenty items which cover eight categories of disability: dressing and grooming, rising, eating, walking, hygiene, reach, grip, and activities (Exhibit 8.4). The original version contained nine cate-gories but the category sex seems to have been omitted from later versions. Each item is rated and the category scored according to the item with which the respondent had most difficulty during the past week. Scores range from 0 (without any difficulty) to 3 (unable to do). Initial ratings can be modified according to whether the respondent uses any aids or is helped by another person. A disability index score is calculated by adding the scores for each category and dividing by the number of categories answered, to yield an index score in the range of 0–3.

Pain is measured on a simple visual analogue scale ranging from no pain to very severe pain. No attempt is made to specify the site of pain, its fre-quency or nature. Respondents are asked to place a mark on a 15 cm line to represent severity of pain experienced in the past week. This is also converted to a 0–3 score by simply measuring the distance from the left and multiplying by 0.2.

Since publication, the basic HAQ has remained in its original form. Minor modifications to language have been made to produce a version suitable for use in Britain.[7] A modified version has been produced which is designed to assess patients' satisfaction with their level of activity, any change in capacity over a 6 month period and need for help.[11] In order to retain a brief self-administered version for this purpose, the authors of this modified HAQ

Exhibit 8.4   Stanford Health Assessment Questionnaire as modified for use by British patients

(Reproduced, with permission, from Kirwan, J. R. and Reeback, J. S. (1986). Stanford Health Assessment Questionnaire modified to assess disability in British patients with rheumatoid arthritis. *British Journal of Rheumatology*, **25**, 206-9).

Please tick the response which best describes your usual abilities *over the past week*.

| | Are you able to: | | | |
	Without ANY difficulty	With SOME difficulty	With MUCH difficulty	Unable to do
1. Dressing & Grooming				
Dress yourself, including tying shoelaces and doing buttons?	....	....	....	....
Shampoo your hair?	....	....	....	....
2. Rising				
Stand up from an armless straight chair?	....	....	....	....
Get in and out of bed?	....	....	....	....
3. Eating				
Cut your meat?	....	....	....	....
Lift a full cup or glass to your mouth?	....	....	....	....
Open a new carton of milk (or soap powder)?	....	....	....	....
4. Walking				
Walk outdoors on flat ground?	....	....	....	....
Climb up five steps?	....	....	....	....

Please tick any *aids or devices* that you usually use for any of these activities:

.... Cane

.... Walking frame

.... Crutches

.... Wheelchair

Other (specify) ....

.... Devices used for dressing (button hook, zipper pull, long handled shoe horn, etc.)

.... Built up or special utensils

.... Special built up chair

Please tick any categories for which you usually *need help from another person*:

.... Dressing and Grooming   .... Eating

.... Rising   .... Walking

Exhibit 8.4 (continued)

Please tick the response which best describes your usual abilities *over the past week*.

	Are you able to:			
	Without ANY difficulty	With SOME difficulty	With MUCH difficulty	Unable to do
5. **Hygiene**				
Wash and dry your entire body?	....	....	....	....
Take a bath?	....	....	....	....
Get on and off the toilet?	....	....	....	....
6. **Reach**				
Reach and get down a 5 lb object (e.g. a bag of potatoes) from just above your head?	....	....	....	....
Bend down to pick up clothing from the floor?	....	....	....	....
7. **Grip**				
Open car doors?	....	....	....	....
Open jars which have been previously opened?	....	....	....	....
Turn taps on and off?	....	....	....	....
8. **Activities**				
Run errands and shop?	....	....	....	....
Get in and out of a car?	....	....	....	....
Do chores such as vacuuming, housework or light gardening?	....	....	....	....

Please tick any *aids or devices* that you usually use for any of these activities:

.... Raised toilet seat   .... Bath rail
.... Bath seat   .... Long handled appliances for reach
.... Jar opener (for jars previously opened)
        Other (specify) ....

Please tick any categories for which you usually *need help from another person*:

.... Hygiene   .... Gripping and opening things
.... Reach   .... Errands and housework

Scoring: The highest score for any component item in a category determines the score for that category. If either devices and/or help from another person is ticked for a category the score = 2, unless the score on any of the component items = 3.

reduced the number of items dealing with disability from twenty to eight, one for each category.

Administration and acceptability

The HAQ is designed for self-completion although it would also be easy for an interviewer or clinician to administer. As a self-completed instrument it takes between 5 and 10 minutes to complete. No problems have been reported in understanding or completing the questionnaire, which probably reflects the careful attention to content and format taken in the various stages of development. The modified HAQ is clearly more complex than the original but is still contained within two pages and retains a self-administered format. The British version was shown to be easier for British patients to complete than the North American version.[7]

Reliability and validity

The HAQ has been extensively tested for reliability, validity, and responsiveness to clinically significant change. Good test–retest reliability was reported when comparing interviewer-administered scores with those achieved using self-administration.[4] A more recent study also reports high test–retest reliability and high internal consistency,[6] and the modified version also achieves high levels of internal consistency for the items within each category.[11]

Initial validation of HAQ was based on direct observation of the behaviour covered in the questionnaire among a sample of 25 patients suffering from rheumatoid arthritis.[4] For individual categories, correlations between HAQ scores and observer ratings ranged from moderate to high, and for the disability index as a whole the correlation was 0.88. A variety of studies have shown good correlations between HAQ scores and scores on alternative measures of health status and disability including AIMS,[2,6] (p. 208) the Mallya and Mace index of disease activity in rheumatoid arthritis,[3] the Sickness Impact Profile (p. 133), Index of Wellbeing (p. 188) and Functional Status Index[8] (p. 56). In all cases, the HAQ shows moderate to good correlations with other measures. Whilst much of the work on validation has been with patients suffering from rheumatoid arthritis some studies have included patients suffering from osteoarthritis, and one examined its validity with diabetic patients.[6] In a study of the clinical value of HAQ, disability index scores were shown to be predictive of mortality and use of services over a three year period.[13]

In addition to the extensive evidence of validity for HAQ a great deal of attention has been paid to its sensitivity to change. One of the earliest publications,[5] focused on the ability of the HAQ to detect changes in patients suffering from both rheumatoid and osteoarthritis. All of the studies of measurement sensitivity have shown the HAQ capable of detecting change, although it does not appear to be superior to alternative instruments such as AIMS, Sickness Impact Profile (Functional Limitations Profile), or Functional Status Index.[3,8,10] In a comparison of five instruments for orthopaedic evaluation, Liang questioned the sensitivity of the HAQ mobility and global disability index for certain treatment evaluations.[10] However, Fitzpatrick and others pointed out that although the HAQ performed slightly less well than the FLP, its simpler measurement assumptions and shorter time required for administration were advantageous.[3] In comparison with one commonly employed functional classification for patients suffering from arthritis (the Steinbrocker Functional class) the HAQ was superior in detecting change.[7]

Populations/service settings

The HAQ was clearly developed for use in specialist service settings providing medical care for patients suffering from arthritis. However, it was always intended for use with patients receiving out-patient care and with normal subjects in longitudinal studies of ageing. Although most studies have utilized the HAQ in specialist rheumatology clinics, there is no reason why it should not be equally appropriate for arthritic patients in primary health care. The fact that it is self-administered, relatively easy to score, and can be completed in 5 to 10 minutes, will make it particularly useful in routine service settings. It has been used in various studies of therapeutic interventions,[1,9,10] and has been recommended for use as a routine clinical assessment of outcome following extensive use with patients suffering from rheumatoid arthritis.[13] It has been used in large scale surveys, and is currently being used extensively in AIDS research.

Comment

The Stanford HAQ is now well established as a reliable and valid outcome measure suitable for use in both research and practice with patients suffering from arthritis. Although less well established as a measure of need and/or outcome for other conditions, there may be considerable potential for extending its use. It is certainly superior to older systems of functional classification. It is not, however, superior to the AIMS or to other general measures. The choice between a number of measures has to be based on the context, the dimensions of disability of interest, the resources available, and the population to be studied. Nevertheless, a recent British paper recommended it as probably the 'best buy' currently available.[12]

References

1. Bombardier, C., Ware, J., Russell, I.J., Larson, M., Chalmers, A., and Leighton-Read, J. (1986). Auranofin therapy and quality of life in patients with rheumatoid arthritis. *American Journal of Medicine*, **81**, 565–78.
2. Brown, J.H., Kazis, L.E., Spitz, P.W., Gertman, P., Fries, J.F., and Meenan, R.F. (1984). The dimensions of health outcomes: A cross-validated examination of health status measurement. *American Journal of Public Health*, **74**, 159–61.

3. Fitzpatrick, R., Newman, S., Lamb, R., and Shipley, M. (1989). A comparison of measures of health status in rheumatoid arthritis. *British Journal of Rheumatology*, **28**, 201–6.
4. Fries, J. F., Spitz, P., Kramer, G., and Holman, H. R. (1980). Measurement of patient outcome in arthritis. *Arthritis and Rheumatism*, **23**, 137–45.
5. Fries, J. F., Spitz, P. W., and Young, D. Y. (1982). The dimensions of health outcomes: the Health Assessment Questionnaire, disability and pain scales. *Journal of Rheumatology*, **9**, 789–93.
6. Geoppinger, J., Doyle, M. A., Chorlton, S. L., and Lorig, K. (1988). A nursing perspective on the assessment of function in persons with arthritis. *Research in Nursing and Health*, **11**, 321–31.
7. Kirwan, J. R. and Reeback, J. S. (1986). Stanford Health Assessment Questionnaire modified to assess disability in British patients with rheumatoid arthritis. *British Journal of Rheumatology*, **25**, 206–9.
8. Liang, M. H., Larson, M. G., Cullen, K. E., and Schwartz, J. A. (1985). Comparative measurement efficiency and sensitivity of five health status instruments for arthritis research. *Arthritis and Rheumatism*, **28**, 542–7.
9. Liang, K., Lubeck, D., Krainer, R. G., Seleznick, M., and Holmon, H. R. (1985). Outcomes of self-help education for patients with arthritis. *Arthritis and Rheumatism*, **28**, 680–5.
10. Liang, M. H., Fossel, A. H., and Larson, M. G. (1990). Comparisons of five health status instruments for orthopaedic evaluation. *Medical Care*, **28**, 632–42.
11. Pincus, T., Summey, J. A., Soraci, S. A. Jr., Wallston, K. A., and Hummon, N. P. (1983). Assessment of patient satisfaction in activities of daily living using a modified Stanford Health Assessment Questionnaire. *Arthritis and Rheumatism*, **26**, 1346–53.
12. Thompson, P. W. (1988). Functional outcome in rheumatoid arthritis. *British Journal of Rheumatology*, **27**, Suppl 1, 37–43.
13. Wolfe, F., Kleinheksel, S. M., Cathey, M. A., Hawley, D. J., Spite, P. W., and Fries, J. F. (1988). The clinical value of the Stanford Health Assessment Questionnaire. *Journal of Rheumatology*, **15**, 1480–8.

Measures of quality of life for clinical trials (Guyatt and colleagues 1987 onwards)

Purpose

This section refers to three instruments which employ the same basic purpose and methodology for different disease groups. The Chronic Respiratory Disease Questionnaire (CRDQ), the Chronic Heart Failure Questionnaire (CHQ), and the Inflammatory Bowel Disease Questionnaire (IBDQ) are intended to assess change in disease-related dysfunction and subjective health status in clinical trials.

Background

Gordon Guyatt and his colleagues at McMaster University argued that commonly used measures of disease activity and function in chronic lung disease and inflammatory bowel disease fail to address the impact of the disease on patients' lives, including emotional and social aspects.[3,5,6] In many cases the reliability and validity of these measures is insufficiently established and, most importantly, their responsiveness to change has not been determined. They argued that existing general measures of health status or quality of life are unlikely to detect small but clinically important changes.[2] It is therefore necessary to develop disease-specific measures which should meet six key criteria:[6]

1. Items must reflect areas of function that are important to patients with the disease.
2. Summary scores should be amenable to statistical analysis.
3. Repeated administration in stable patients must yield similar results.
4. When even a small clinically important change in score has occurred, the questionnaire should reflect it (i.e. responsiveness).
5. The questionnaire should be valid.
6. The questionnaire should be relatively short and simple.

Items for inclusion in the CRDQ, CHQ, and IBDQ were selected on the basis of literature reviews, consultation with professionals, and interviews with patients suffering from the diseases. Items were then reduced on the basis of those chosen frequently and rated most important in further interviews with patients. Each instrument was then extensively tested for reliability, validity, and responsiveness to change.

This basic approach to the design of a disease-specific instrument could be used for a wide range of conditions and the researchers have set out very clearly the necessary steps in design and evaluation.[2] A similar approach has been used in the development of an arthritis-specific instrument, MACTAR, which we have not included here.[9]

Description

The CRDQ consists of 19 questions dealing with shortness of breath (dyspnoea), fatigue, emotional function, and mastery or a feeling of control over the disease during the last two weeks (Exhibit 8.5). The assessment of dyspnoea derived from questions one to four is patient specific. The researchers recognized that the activities which were associated with shortness of breath would vary greatly according to age, sex, level of disability, etc. Questions one, two, and three are therefore designed to identify those five activities which are most important to the individual and which produce

---

Exhibit 8.5   Examples from the Chronic Respiratory Disease Questionnaire

(Reproduced, with permission, from Guyatt, G. H., Berman, L. B., Townsend, M., Pugsley, S. O., and Chambers, L. W. (1987). A measure of quality of life for clinical trials in chronic lung disease. *Thorax*, **42**, 773–8)

The questionnaire begins by eliciting five activities in which the patient experiences dyspnoea during day to day activities.

1. I would like you to think of the activities that you have done during the last 2 weeks that have made you feel short of breath. These should be activities which you do frequently and which are important in your day to day life. Please list as many activities as you can that you have done during the last 2 weeks that have made you feel short of breath.

2. I will now read a list of activities which make some people with lung problems feel short of breath. I will pause after each item long enough for you to tell me if you have felt short of breath doing that activity during the last 2 weeks.

3. (a) Of the items which you have listed, which is the most important to you in your day to day life? I will read through the items and when I am finished I would like you to tell me which is the most important. (This process is continued until the five most important activities are determined).

4. I would now like you to describe how much shortness of breath you have experienced during the last 2 weeks while doing the five most important activities you have selected.

   (a) Please indicate how much shortness of breath you have had during the last 2 weeks by choosing one of the following options:
   1. Extremely short of breath
   2. Very short of breath
   3. Quite a bit short of breath
   4. Moderate shortness of breath
   5. Some shortness of breath
   6. A little shortness of breath
   7. Not at all short of breath
   (This process continues until the subject's degree of dyspnoea on all five of his/her most important activities has been determined.)

5. In general, how much of the time during the last 2 weeks have you felt frustrated or impatient?

6. How often during the past 2 weeks did you have a feeling of fear or panic when you had difficulty getting your breath?

10. How often during the last 2 weeks did you feel you had complete control of your breathing problems with shortness of breath and tiredness?

Exhibit 8.5 (continued)

14. How often during the last 2 weeks have you felt low in energy?

19. In general, how often during the last 2 weeks have you felt restless, tense, or uptight?

Response categories:
Questions 5 to 19 have seven response categories (e.g. 1. All of the time—7. None of the time).

---

breathlessness. Question four then elicits an assessment of the severity of the problem over the last two weeks. These five activities constitute the dyspnoea items for the remainder of the study, so that any change is measured against baseline assessment on these activities. The remaining fifteen questions deal with fatigue, emotional function, and mastery. All questions employ seven response categories and scores on each item within a section are summed to produce four separate scores.

The CHQ overlaps considerably with the CRDQ in content, and for this reason is not shown here. The questions dealing with dyspnoea are identical to those shown in Exhibit 8.5. The remaining eleven questions deal with fatigue (four questions) and emotional function (seven questions). Only one of these questions does not appear in identical form in the CRDQ. The main difference between the two questionnaires is that the CHQ does not address the concept of mastery.

The IBDQ consists of 32 questions dealing with gastrointestinal symptoms, symptoms not directly related to the disturbance (systemic symptoms), symptoms of emotional dysfunction, and social dysfunction (Exhibit 8.6). Unlike the CRDQ, it was not considered necessary to develop patient specific items. All questions employ seven response categories with 7 representing 'best function' and 1 representing 'worst function'. Scores on individual items are summed to produce a score for each of the four dimensions assessed.

Administration and acceptability

All three questionnaires are designed to be administered by an interviewer. Guyatt and colleagues report that the CRDQ and the IBDQ take between 15 and 25 minutes at first administration, and between 10 and 20 minutes for subsequent administrations. The CHQ being slightly shorter takes 10 to 15 minutes at first administration and 5 to 10 minutes subsequently. They report no problems of acceptability to patients, although it might be felt that the IBDQ is dealing with potentially sensitive problems. There are no published reports of any of the instruments being adapted for self-completion, but

Exhibit 8.6   Examples from the Inflammatory Bowel Disease Questionnaire

(Reproduced, with permission, from Guyatt, G. H., Mitchell, A., Irvine E. J., Singer, J., Williams, N. Goodacre, R. *et al.* (1989). A new measure of health status for clinical trials in inflammatory bowel disease. *Gastroenterology*, **96**, 804–10).

1. How frequent have your bowel movements been during the last two weeks? [B]

2. How often has the feeling of fatigue or of being tired and worn out been a problem for you during the last two weeks? [S]

4. How often during the last two weeks have you been unable to attend school or work because of your bowel problem? [SF]

8. How often during the last two weeks have you had to delay or cancel a social engagement because of your bowel problem? [SF]

10. How often during the last two weeks have you felt generally unwell? [S]

13. How often during the last two weeks have you been troubled by pain in the abdomen? [B]

14. How often during the last two weeks have you had problems getting a good night's sleep, or been troubled by waking up during the night? [S]

23. How much of the time during the last two weeks have you felt embarrassed as a result of your bowel problem? [E]

26. How much of the time during the last two weeks have you been troubled by accidental soiling of your underpants? [B]

28. To what extent has your bowel problem limited sexual activity during the last two weeks? [SF]

32. How satisfied, happy, or pleased have you been with your personal life during the past two weeks? [E]

Reponse categories: All questions employ seven response categories
(e.g. Question 1. (1) Bowel movements as or more frequent than they have ever been—
(7) Normal, no increase in frequency of bowel movements).

Categories: B—bowel symptoms; S—systemic symptoms; E—emotional function; SF—social function.

there seems no reason why this should not be possible with appropriate testing.

Reliability and validity

All three instruments have been well tested in their development. Test–retest reliability was assessed by repeat administrations to patients with stable conditions. For the CRDQ no clinically important or statistically significant trends of improvement or deterioration were found.[3] Although no systematic changes in CHQ scores were found, the coefficients of variation between test and retest were higher than for the CRDQ.[5] The IBDQ showed small improvements when administered to apparently stable subjects, but coefficients of variation were low.[6] However, in this case the definition of stable patients was based on a simple global assessment.

Validity of the CRDQ was assessed through comparisons of scores with a variety of alternative measures including forced expiratory volume, slow vital capacity, walk test, oxygen cost diagram, and various global ratings of dyspnoea, fatigue and emotional function.[3] Consensus techniques were used to generate predictions about the relationships between questionnaire dimensions and these alternative measures. Agreement between predicted and observed correlations was moderate. Construct validity of the CHQ and IBDQ was similarly assessed by testing a variety of predictions concerning correlations between scores on particular dimensions and various global ratings.[5,6]

Development work on these instruments has concentrated most on establishing responsiveness to change, since they are designed to detect significant change in clinical trials. The CRDQ was tested on patients before and after optimization of their drug treatment and before and after participation in a respiratory rehabilitation programme. The questionnaire detected statistically significant improvement in small samples on all four dimensions, and was more responsive than all alternative measures except the Transition Dyspnoea Index.[3] The CHQ was tested in a randomized controlled trial of digoxin in heart failure patients.[4] Only for the dyspnoea dimension did the difference between digoxin and placebo groups reach statistical significance. However, CHQ scores did distinguish between patients who reported improvement or deterioration and those who did not.[5] The IBDQ was tested in patients whose global rating of their condition showed improvement or deterioration. Differences in scores between baseline and follow-up were statistically significant for all four dimensions.[6] It is worth noting that assessments of physical function using the Rand general instrument did not detect any change.

In a recent paper, data from both the CRDQ and CHQ have been used to develop guidance on the interpretation of changes in scores.[8] Minimally clinically important difference was represented by a mean change in score per question of approximately 0.5. The authors also offer ranges for moderate and large changes. Although further evidence is still required to support these interpretations, it is very encouraging to see this sort of guidance on interpretation of change becoming available.

It should be noted that the design of the dyspnoea questions on the CRDQ and CHQ fails to consider activities which the respondent does not undertake because of shortness of breath. Whilst this focus is understandable in an instrument intended to measure change, it does mean that the instruments do not constitute a measure of disability. They might also fail to pick up changes in any activity not undertaken at baseline, but subsequently attempted.

An interesting methodological issue with wider implications was raised in relation to the CRDQ. The researchers examined the effects of allowing respondents to see their previous ratings when completing a follow-up questionnaire, and compared the results with those of patients who had completed the follow-up questionnaire blind.[7] The results suggest that the responsiveness of the questionnaire can be improved by allowing patients to see their previous responses.

Although the initial development and testing of both instruments has been thorough, it should be noted that further assessment of reliability, validity, and responsiveness by other investigators is essential.

Populations/service settings

The CRDQ was designed to be applicable to patients with chronic airflow limitation (chronic bronchitis and emphysema). The questionnaire would not be suitable for patients suffering from asthma, since it does not tap the episodic nature of asthma attacks. It has been used in randomized trials of bronchodilators[7] and a home exercise programme.[1] The authors are unclear about the service settings in which it was used. However, there seems no reason why it should not be appropriately used in a primary health care setting, bearing in mind the time taken to administer the questionnaire. It could of course be administered by a nurse or any other member of the primary health care team. The CHQ has been used by Guyatt and his colleagues in patients suffering from heart failure.

The IBDQ was designed for and tested on patients suffering from ulcerative colitis or Crohn's disease. Patients were recruited mainly in gastroenterology out-patient clinics, but it should be equally applicable to patients with these conditions being managed in primary health care. However, testing with respect to patients suffering from Crohn's disease was limited by the small numbers available to the researchers.[6]

Comments

Both of these questionnaires have been produced fairly recently, and require further testing by other investigators. They are, however, potentially valuable instruments in studies of specific diseases where an instrument is required which is capable of detecting change in relatively small samples of patients. The authors have focused attention on the issue of responsiveness to change and shown that it is possible to devise measures suitable for studies involving perhaps 20 or 30 patients, which is common in clinical trials. They have also elaborated a methodological approach to the development of disease-specific instruments, which could usefully be applied in other situations.

References

1. Busch, A. J., and McClements, J. D. (1988). Effects of a supervised home exercise program on patients with severe chronic obstructive pulmonary disease. *Physical Therapy*, **68**, 469–74.
2. Guyatt, G. H., Bombardier, G., and Tugwell, P. X. (1986). Measuring disease-specific quality of life in clinical trials. *Canadian Medical Association Journal*, **134**, 889–95.
3. Guyatt, G. H., Berman, L. H., Townsend, M., Pugsley, S. O., and Chambers, L. W. (1987). A measure of quality of life for clinical trials in chronic lung disease. *Thorax*, **42**, 773–8.
4. Guyatt, G. H., Sullivan, M. J. J., Fallen, E. L., Tihal, H., Rideout, E., Halcrow, S., *et al.* (1988). A controlled trial of digoxin in heart failure. *American Journal of Cardiology*, **61**, 371–5.
5. Guyatt, G. H., Nogradi, S., Halcrow, S., Singer, J., Sullivan, M. J., and Fallen, E. L. (1989). Development and testing of a new measure of health status for clinical trials in heart failure. *Journal of General and Internal Medicine*, **4**, 101–7.
6. Guyatt, G., Mitchell, A., Irvine, E. J., Singer, J., Williams, N., Goodacre, R., and Tompkins, C. (1989). A new measure of health status for clinical trials in inflammatory bowel disease. *Gastroenterology*, **96**, 804–10.
7. Guyatt, G. H., Townsend, M., Keller, J. L., and Singer, J. (1989). Should study subjects see their previous responses: data from a randomised controlled trial. *Journal of Clinical Epidemiology*, **49**, 913–20.
8. Jaeschke, R., Singer, J., and Guyatt, G. H. (1989). Measurement of health status. *Controlled Clinical Trials*, **10**, 407–15.
9. Tugwell, P., Bombardier, C., Buchanan, W. W., Goldsmith, C. H., Grace, E., and Hanna, B. (1987). The MACTAR patient preference disability questionnaires: an individualised functional priority approach for assessment of improvement in physical disability in clinical trials in rheumatoid arthritis. *Journal of Rheumatology*, **14**, 446–51.

Conclusions

The disease-specific measures included in this chapter were chosen because they deal with commonly occurring chronic conditions in primary health care, or they have the potential for wider application than the particular condition for which they were originally intended. The choice between a disease-specific and a generic measure will depend very much on the particular purpose for which it is required and the practical circumstances. For many research applications a combination of both might be required, but for clinical practice in primary health care, many disease-specific measures are likely to be too cumbersome. The variety of conditions seen, even major chronic conditions, would make it impractical to employ different measures for each condition.

To the extent that disease-specific information is required in order to make a comprehensive assessment of needs or to evaluate outcomes of treatment, one promising development is of disease-specific supplements to generic measures. These have the considerable advantage of enhancing compatibility across conditions by retaining the core elements, whilst allowing for the collection of important information not covered in generic measures. From a practical point of view they go some way towards overcoming the problem of having to transfer from one measure to another. As yet, few of these have been adequately tested, but there are a number of promising developments. The Outcomes Management System (p. 196) is probably the most advanced in this field. The central, generic measure, the SF-36, is supplemented by condition-specific measures which incorporate basic clinical and therapeutic data as well as quality of life and functional status measures relevant to the condition being assessed. As an example, catarract patients are asked about vision-related restrictions on reading and driving. Sixteen instruments are now available for further field testing by registered OMS users, and others are planned. Whilst many are more appropriate to specialty settings, others, including asthma, depression, diabetes, low back pain, osteo- and rheumatoid arthritis have more general applicability.

There seems little doubt that the number of disease-specific instruments will grow in the future. It would be most helpful for primary health care if these were to be compatible with the better generic measures.

9 Measures of patient satisfaction

Introduction

The decision about whether to include measures of patient satisfaction in a book devoted to the assessment of need and outcome was difficult to make. Satisfaction represents a complex mixture of perceived need, expectations of care, and the experience of care (see Chapter 2). It is a wholly subjective assessment of the quality of health care and, as such, is not a measure of final outcome. However, evidence has accumulated that care which is less satisfactory to the patient is also less effective, because dissatisfaction is associated with non-compliance with treatment instructions, delay in seeking further care, and poor understanding and retention of medical information. It has also been shown that patients' reported levels of satisfaction do reflect doctors' technical competence as judged by independent, professional assessors. Satisfaction or dissatisfaction is thus an intermediate outcome which may reflect a failure to answer patients' needs, meet their expectations, or provide an acceptable standard of service. Patient satisfaction is a legitimate goal for medical care, and we have therefore included instruments designed to measure it.

There are two main approaches to the measurement of patient satisfaction. The 'direct' approach seeks patients' views on their own doctors and their personal experiences of seeking and obtaining care. The 'indirect' approach, which produces lower levels of reported satisfaction, seeks opinions on doctors and health services in general. Advocates of the indirect approach believe that patients' answers are based on their personal experiences, and that the impersonal style of questions or statements simply enables them to express negative views more readily. Dissenters believe that the two styles actually measure different things. Only one of the measures we have selected has a totally indirect format; four use direct questions or statements and one combines the two styles.

Substantial research efforts have been made to identify the characteristics of providers and services which influence patient judgements. At least six major areas of patient concern have emerged. Unfortunately different studies have not always identified the same elements, grouped them into the same dimensions, or applied the same labels. The Client Satisfaction Questionnaire (CSQ) is based on the belief that satisfaction is unidimensional, although nine different aspects of care contribute to it. At the other end of the spectrum, the Patient Satisfaction Questionnaire (PSQ) contains seven separate dimensions. The other measures included are also multidimensional, but cover between three and six dimensions.

The majority of measures consist of a series of statements which respondents are asked to endorse or reject on a scale which allows degrees of opinion. Responses are summed to produce scores in each dimension. Only two of the measures adopt weighting systems which accord different values to items depending on their importance. The Evaluation Ranking Scale offers an original approach to the weighting of items by allowing each respondent to produce an individual weighting.

As we have noted in Chapter 2, one of the major problems associated with measuring patient satisfaction is the lack of a clear theoretical and conceptual framework on which to build. Only the PSQ has a clearly enunciated theoretical foundation. Unfortunately, although it is possibly the best developed and most extensively tested measure available, it mixes direct and indirect statements, which makes interpretation of the results more difficult.

In selecting measures for inclusion, we have avoided those which are designed for use with hospital in-patients, those which are aimed at a very limited or specialized patient population and those which have been used only once in a small-scale study. All six of the instruments we have reviewed were developed in the USA. Whilst the same is true for many of the measures included in earlier chapters, this may be more problematic for users of patient satisfaction measures since they inevitably reflect to some degree the organization of the health care system for which they were developed. This is particularly apparent in items dealing with satisfaction with financial arrangements. For this reason, anyone interested in using measures of patient satisfaction in other countries should pay particular heed to our earlier caution that evidence of reliability and validity is limited to the context in which the measure was developed. Further testing of reliability and validity of patient satisfaction measures should be undertaken before using them in other countries.

Patient Satisfaction Questionnaire (PSQ) (Ware and colleagues 1976)

Purpose

The PSQ was designed as a short self-administered measure of patient satisfaction, applicable in general population studies, which would yield data of both theoretical importance and practical relevance to the planning, administration, and evaluation of health services. It was intended to measure patient satisfaction across different systems of care in different settings and to identify major sources of satisfaction and dissatisfaction within a single system or setting. Three distinct types of application were envisaged: to measure satisfaction as an outcome of care, to provide information about the sources of satisfaction and dissatisfaction, and to be useful in studies of patient behaviour.

Background

Early versions of the PSQ were based on an indirect or non-specific concept of satisfaction. They were concerned with satisfaction with medical care in general rather than with a particular encounter or even a particular provider. This indirect approach assumes a direct relationship between the way that patients feel about their own provider(s) and the way they feel about providers in general.

The different versions of the PSQ have been developed as part of the Rand Corporation research programme over a period of 15 years. Based on literature reviews and empirical studies, the researchers developed a taxonomy of characteristics of health care providers and services that might influence patients' attitudes towards, or satisfaction with, medical care. An initial pool of 2300 items judged to be relevant to satisfaction were drawn from other instruments, a population survey, and the researchers' own experiences. Extensive reviews of all items reduced the pool to 500 and contributed to the formulation of a number of hypothesized dimensions of satisfaction. Factor analytic techniques were used to refine and delineate the content of these dimensions. The resulting 80-item PSQI underwent extensive field trials and analyses, leading to substantial revisions in content incorporated in the PSQII.[13-15] The PSQ11 consists of 68 items covering 18 sub-scales and 9 global scales. A 43-item short form was developed for use in two national surveys and was subsequently used in the Rand Health Insurance Experiment.[3] Both the PSQII and the short version have been extensively tested and used in a wide variety of empirical studies.

The most recent version, the PSQIII was developed, using the lessons learned in earlier studies, for use in the Medical Outcomes Study undertaken by the Rand Corporation.[5] Modifications were made to improve the relevance of item content across medical care settings, to increase reliability of the general satisfaction scale, to improve content validity with respect to quality of care, to improve relevance to cost containment procedures, to increase relevance to the respondents' *own* medical care experiences, and to exclude descriptive items dealing with continuity of care. The shift to respondents' own medical care experiences, rather than more general statements about doctors and care, is particularly important in the light of criticisms that earlier versions were measuring more general attitudes and even life satisfaction.[9, 10]

Description

The PSQIII contains 51 items including both indirect statements about medical care and doctors in general, and direct references to the respondents' own experiences of medical care (Exhibit 9.1). Each item is constructed as a statement of opinion and accompanied by five response categories, from strongly agree to strongly disagree. The balance between negatively and

Exhibit 9.1   Patient Satisfaction Questionnaire

(Adapted from Hays, R. D., Davies, A. R., and Ware, J. E. (1987). Scoring the Medical Outcomes Study Patient Satisfaction Questionnaire: PSQIII. *MOS memorandum* Rand Corporation, Santa Monica. (Unpublished))

Sample layout

On the following pages are some things people say about medical care. Please read each one carefully, keeping in mind the medical care you are receiving now. (If you have not received care recently, think about what you would *expect* if you needed care today.) We are interested in your feelings, *good*, and *bad*, about the medical care you have received.

How strongly do you AGREE or DISAGREE with *each* of the following statements?

(Circle one number on each line)

	Strongly Agree	Agree	Uncertain	Disagree	Strongly Disagree
1. If I need hospital care, I can get admitted without any trouble . . .	1	2	3	4	5

Questions

2. Doctors need to be more thorough in treating and examining me . . .
3. I am very satisfied with the medical care I receive . . .
4. I worry sometimes about having to pay large medical bills . . .
5. It is easy for me to get medical care in an emergency . . .
6. Doctors are good about explaining the reason for medical tests . . .
7. I am usually kept waiting for a long time when I am at the doctor's office . . .
8. I think my doctor's office has everything needed to provide complete medical care . . .
9. The doctors who treat me should give me more respect . . .
10. Sometimes it is a problem to cover my share of the cost for a medical care visit . . .
11. The medical care I have been receiving is just about perfect . . .
12. Sometimes doctors make me wonder if their diagnosis is correct . . .
13. During my medical visits, I am always allowed to say everything that I think is important . . .
14. I feel confident that I can get the medical care I need without being set back financially . . .
15. When I go for medical care, they are careful to check everything when treating and examining me . . .
16. It's hard for me to get medical care on short notice . . .
17. The doctors who treat me have a genuine interest in me as a person . . .
18. Sometimes doctors use medical terms without explaining what they mean . . .
19. Sometimes I go without the medical care I need because it is too expensive . . .
20. The office hours when I can get medical care are convenient (good) for me . . .
21. There are things about the medical system I receive my care from that need to be improved . . .

Exhibit 9.1 (continued)

22. The office where I get medical care should be open for more hours than it is . . .
23. The medical staff that treats me knows about the latest medical developments . . .
24. I have to pay for more of my medical care than I can afford . . .
25. I have easy access to the medical specialists I need . . .
26. Sometimes doctors make me feel foolish . . .
27. Regardless of the health problems I have now or develop later, I feel protected from financial hardship . . .
28. Where I get medical care, people have to wait too long for emergency treatment . . .
29. Doctors act too businesslike and impersonal toward me . . .
30. There is a crisis in health care in the United States today . . .
31. Doctors never expose me to unnecessary risk . . .
32. The amount I have to pay to cover or insure my medical care needs is reasonable . . .
33. There are some things about the medical care I receive that could be better . . .
34. My doctors treat me in a very friendly and courteous manner . . .
35. Those who provide my medical care sometimes hurry too much when they treat me . . .
36. Some of the doctors I have seen lack experience with my medical problems . . .
37. Places where I can get medical care are very conveniently located . . .
38. Doctors sometimes ignore what I tell them . . .
39. When I am receiving medical care, they should pay more attention to my privacy . . .
40. If I have a medical question, I can reach a doctor for help without any problem . . .
41. Doctors rarely give me advice about ways to avoid illness and stay healthy . . .
42. All things considered, the medical care I receive is excellent . . .
43. Doctors listen carefully to what I have to say . . .
44. I feel insured and protected financially against all possible medical problems . . .
45. I have some doubts about the ability of the doctors who treat me..................
46. Doctors usually spend plenty of time with me . . .
47. Doctors always do their best to keep me from worrying . . .
48. I find it hard to get an appointment for medical care right away . . .
49. I am dissatisfied with some things about the medical care I receive . . .
50. My doctors are very competent and well trained . . .
51. I am able to get medical care whenever I need it . . .

Sub-scales

General satisfaction	Items: 3, 33, 42, 21, 11, 49
Technical quality	Items: 15, 2, 8, 12, 23, 36, 50, 45, 31, 41
Interpersonal aspects	Items: 29, 47, 39, 17, 26, 34, 9
Communication	Items: 6, 18, 13, 38, 43
Financial aspects	Items: 14, 4, 27, 10, 44, 24, 32, 19
Time spent with doctor	Items: 46, 35
Access/availability/convenience	Items: 1, 16, 5, 22, 37, 28, 40, 48, 20, 7, 25, 51

positively worded statements is retained from earlier versions.

Scores for the PSQIII are calculated for the seven multi-item sub-scales shown in Exhibit 9.1. Each item is scored 1–5 with scoring reversed for positively worded items, so that high scores indicate greater satisfaction. The number of items in a sub-scale ranges from two to twelve, so that maximum scores range from 10 for time spent with doctor to 60 for access/availability/ convenience. Item 30 does not form part of the scoring system. Item scores are not weighted in any way.

The earlier PSQII and the 43-item short version employ exactly the same format as the PSQIII. An even shorter 18-item version has been developed, but this taps only four dimensions.[2] It also uses a modified wording in which statements refer to a particular doctor.

Administration and acceptability

All versions of the PSQ are designed for self-administration, but various methods have been used. Interviewer-supervised completion produces the best response rate but is obviously expensive. The cheapest method is a mailed version, but this produces low response rates. A personal 'drop off' and 'mail back' combination produces good response rates at relatively low cost. The PSQIII is likely to take about 10 minutes to complete, though administration times tend to be longer for disadvantaged populations. Completion times will be correspondingly shorter for abbreviated versions of the PSQ. Where response rates are relatively low there may be some systematic bias, responses being less likely from younger people, non-whites, those on low incomes, and those who are more satisfied with the quality of their care.[15]

Reliability and validity

Most of the evidence on reliability and validity relates to earlier versions of the PSQ. The latest version, however, closely resembles these earlier versions in both content and presentation. We would thus expect results for the PSQIII to be at least as good and probably an improvement on PSQII, particularly in terms of validity.

Although single-item test–retest reliability of PSQII was poor, the strength of the instrument lies in its global and sub-scale scores, which achieved satisfactory levels of test–retest reliability and internal consistency.[15] Initial field tests of PSQIII suggest that it improves on the performance of earlier versions in terms of internal consistency of the seven sub-scales.[5]

The content validity of the PSQ has been systematically examined against other satisfaction measures and against theory relating to concepts of satisfaction.[14] This review identified a number of omissions which the PSQIII attempts to rectify. One which remains is the standard of premises, which could be important in comparisons of different providers. Factor analyses support the construct validity of sub-scales in so far as they appear to assess distinct dimensions of satisfaction which accord with the initial hypotheses.[15] Nevertheless, inter-item and inter-scale correlations are high enough in many instances to suggest that the distinction between different dimensions may not be very clear cut. Ware *et al.* cite a number of studies which have provided evidence of convergent and discriminant validity by testing the PSQ against a variety of other methods of measuring satisfaction with care.[15] However, Pascoe, Roberts and colleagues have suggested that the indirect approach of the PSQII is measuring more generalised attitudes about health services as well as aspects of life satisfaction, rather than opinions about a specific service setting, and have shown that the PSQ produces a different pattern of responses from more direct measures.[9, 10] Other studies have shown links between PSQ scores and health care experiences, behavioural intentions, and actual behaviour.[12] Scores were shown to be predictive of subsequent changes in medical care providers and disenrolments from pre-paid health care plans.

Populations/service settings

The PSQ is suitable for use with any adult population, regardless of whether they have recently consulted a doctor. It has been used in general population surveys, with chronically ill patients, with disabled children, with low income groups, and with ethnically mixed groups.[1, 3, 4, 6, 8, 11, 12] It has also been used in studies designed to examine differences in patients' satisfaction with different types of physician.[2, 7] The items are designed specifically for primary health care and should be applicable across health care systems with only minor revisions. However, items in the sub-scale 'financial aspects' will clearly not be appropriate in socialized health care systems.

Comments

The PSQ is certainly one of the most thoroughly researched measures of patient satisfaction. It has a sound theoretical basis and great care has been taken in establishing reliability and validity. It has also been used in a wide variety of empirical studies which provide a valuable comparative data base. Unlike many other measures, this means that population norms can be used to assist in the interpretation of results from specific applications. However, there are some serious weaknesses in earlier versions. We believe that the PSQIII is a considerable improvement, although formal evidence of validity is not yet available. Despite these improvements the PSQ remains a fairly general and indirect measure. The user seeking more precise focus of experiences may need to consider consultation-specific measures, or those using more direct questioning about a specific health centre or other provider.

References

1. Breslau, N. and Mortimer, E.A. (1981). Seeing the same doctor: determinants of satisfaction with specialty care for disabled children. *Medical Care*, **19** (7), 741–50.
2. Cherkin, D.C., Gart, L.G., and Rosenblatt, R.A. (1988). Patient satisfaction with family physicians and general internists: is there a difference. *Journal of Family Practice*, **26**, 543–51.
3. Davies, A.R., Ware, J.E., Brook, R.H. *et al*. (1986). Consumer acceptance of prepaid and fee-for-service medical care: results from a randomised controlled trial. *Health Services Research*, **21**, 429–52.
4. Doyle, B.J. and Ware, J.E. (1977). Physician conduct and other factors that affect consumer satisfaction with medical care. *Journal of Medical Education*, **52**, 793–801.
5. Hays, R.D., Davies, A.R., and Ware, J.E. (1987). Scoring the Medical Outcomes Study Patient Satisfaction Questionnaire: PSQ-III. Unpublished Rand Corporation MOS Memorandum.
6. Linn, L.S. and Greenfield, S. (1982). Patient suffering and patient satisfaction among the chronically ill. *Medical Care*, **20** (4), 425–31.
7. Macmillan, R.W., Quigley, C.B., Werblun, M.N., Sumbureru, D., and Shear, C.L. (1986). Satisfaction of continuity patients in a family medicine residency – validation of a measurement tool. *Family Practice Research Journal*, **5**, 167–76.
8. Marquis, M.S., Davies, A.R., and Ware, J.E. (1983). Patient satisfaction and change in medical care provider: a longitudinal study. *Medical Care*, **21** (8), 821–9.
9. Pascoe, G.C., Attkisson, C.C., and Roberts, R.E. (1983). Comparison of indirect and direct approaches to measuring patient satisfaction. *Evaluation and Program Planning*, **6**, 359–71.
10. Roberts, R.E., Pascoe, G.C., and Attkisson, C.C. (1983). Relationship of service satisfaction to life satisfaction and perceived wellbeing. *Evaluation and Program Planning*, **6**, 373–83.
11. Ware, J.E. (1978). Effects of acquiescent response set on patient satisfaction ratings. *Medical Care*, **16** (4), 327–36.
12. Ware, J.E. and Davies, A.R. (1983). Behavioural consequences of consumer dissatisfaction with medical care. *Evaluation and Program Planning*, **6**, 291–7.
13. Ware, J.E., Snyder, M.K., and Wright, W.R. (1976). *Development and validation of scales to measure patient satisfaction with medical care services. Vol. I, part A: review of literature, overview of methods and results regarding construction of scales*. (NTIS Publication No. PB 288–329), National Technical Information Service, Springfield, Virginia.
14. Ware, J.E., Snyder, M.K., and Wright, W.R. (1976). *Development and validation of scales to measure patient satisfaction with medical care services. Vol. I, part B: Results regarding scales constructed from the Patient Satisfaction Questionnaire and measures of other health care perceptions*. (NTIS Publication No. PB 288–330), National Technical Information Service, Springfield, Virginia.
15. Ware, J.E., Snyder, M.K., Wright, W.R., and Davies, A.R. (1983). Defining

and measuring patient satisfaction with medical care. *Evaluation and Program Planning*, **6**, 247–63.

Scale for the Measurement of Satisfaction with Medical Care (Hulka and colleagues 1970, revised 1974)

Purpose

The scale developed by Hulka and her colleagues is an attempt to use attitude scaling techniques to measure satisfaction with medical care to aid in empirical research devoted to increasing knowledge about utilization and assessment of ambulatory medical care. It was intended for use in a community setting to explore the relationships between satisfaction and demographic variables and to identify sub-groups whose needs were apparently not being met.

Background

Recognizing the tendency of patients to respond positively to direct questioning (i.e. questions about the patient's own doctor), the authors adopted an indirect approach, so that statements referred to doctors in general. They observed that patients were more willing to express negative attitudes about doctors is general than about their own doctor. To the extent that one is concerned to measure attitudes towards patients' actual experiences of care, the indirect approach assumes that responses will be based on experience rather than more general views about doctors and medical care (see introductory discussion to this chapter). The scale was designed for use in a major study by the American Academy of Family Physicians and the University of North Carolina into the organization, utilization, and assessment of primary medical care.[2] It was initially developed using an adaptation of Thurstone's 'method of equal appearing intervals' (see Chapter 3). A review of lay and scientific literature yielded 300 statements in the areas of professional competence, personal qualities, and cost/convenience. These were reduced to 149 and submitted to judges (physicians, women's club members, social workers, and black college students) for rating and two parallel scales were developed for testing.[4] This original version employed dichotomous agree/disagree response categories.

The scale was revised in 1974 to overcome some of the problems experienced in use. The items were revised and the response categories expanded using Likert-type scaling. In this version, which has been used in a variety of empirical studies, the scoring procedure is a hybrid of the Thurstone and Likert methods.[13] No further modifications have been made by the authors, but other researchers have experimented with rephrasing the items to elicit views on patients' own doctors.[11]

Description

The revised version consists of 42 items concerning doctors and medical care in general without reference to the patient's own doctor (Exhibit 9.2). However, the instructions indicate that responses should be based on personal experience as far as possible. The items are equally divided between three sections representing different dimensions of satisfaction. There are 22 positive statements and 20 negative statements to which patients are asked to respond on a five-point scale from strongly agree to strongly disagree.

Scoring in the original version simply required the summing of item weights for all items with which the respondent agreed. In the revised version,

---

Exhibit 9.2   Items in the Scale for the Measurement of Satisfaction with Medical Care, showing modified item weights

(Reproduced, with permission, from Zyznski, J., Hulka, B. S., and Cassel, J. C. (1974). Scale for the measurement of 'satisfaction' with medical care: modifications in content format and scoring. *Medical Care*, **12**, 611–20)

Modified item weights		Affect of item
	I. Professional competence	
2.26	1. People do not know how many mistakes doctors really make.	Neg
3.32	2. Today's doctors are better trained than ever before.	Pos
1.77	3. Doctors rely on drugs and pills too much.	Neg
1.01	4. Given a choice between using an old reliable drug and a new experimental one, many doctors will choose the new one.	Neg
1.96	5. No two doctors will agree on what is wrong with a person.	Neg
2.85	6. Doctors will not admit when they do not know what is wrong with you.	Neg
1.14	7. When doctors do not cure mildly ill patients, it is because the patients do not cooperate.	Pos
3.04	8. Doctors will do everything they can to keep from making a mistake.	Pos
3.30	9. Many doctors just do not know what they are doing.	Neg
0.56	10. Doctors spend more time trying to cure an illness you already have than preventing one from developing.	Neg
0.21	11. Doctors are put in the position of needing to know more than they possibly could.	Pos

Exhibit 9.2 (continued)

1.92	12. Even if a doctor cannot cure you right away, he can make you more comfortable.	Pos
2.59	13. Doctors can help you both in health and in sickness.	Pos
1.38	14. Doctors sometimes fail because patients do not call them in time.	Pos

II. Personal qualities

1.21	1. You cannot expect any one doctor to be perfect.	Pos
1.77	2. Doctors make you feel like everything will be all right.	Pos
0.70	3. A doctor's job is to make people feel better.	Pos
1.63	4. Too many doctors think you cannot understand the medical explanation of your illness, so they do not bother explaining.	Neg
2.52	5. Doctors act like they are doing you a favour by treating you.	Neg
2.29	6. A lot of doctors do not care whether or not they hurt you during the examination.	Neg
2.03	7. Many doctors treat the disease but have no feeling for the patient.	Neg
1.04	8. Doctors should be a little more friendly than they are.	Neg
2.34	9. Most doctors let you talk out your problems.	Pos
2.13	10. Doctors do their best to keep you from worrying.	Pos
3.68	11. Doctors are devoted to their patients.	Pos
0.08	12. With so many patients to see, doctors cannot get to know them all.	Pos
3.11	13. Most doctors have no feeling for their patients.	Neg
3.28	14. Most doctors take a real interest in their patients.	Pos

III. Cost/convenience

2.21	1. Nowadays you really cannot get a doctor to come out during the night.	Neg
1.86	2. You may have to wait a little, but you can always get a doctor.	Pos
1.93	3. It is easier to go to the drugstore for medicine than to bother with a doctor.	Neg
2.81	4. The more money you have the easier it is to see the doctor.	Neg
1.11	5. A doctor has a right to charge what he does since he struggled years to become a doctor.	Pos
2.96	6. In an emergency, you can always get a doctor.	Pos
0.04	7. There just are not enough doctors to go around.	Pos
1.59	8. Doctors try to have their offices and clinics in convenient locations.	Pos
1.42	9. More and more doctors are refusing to make house calls.	Neg
0.57	10. People complain too much about how hard it is to see a doctor.	Pos
0.90	11. It is hard to get a quick appointment to see a doctor.	Pos
0.39	12. Doctors should have evening office hours for working people.	Neg
2.91	13. Most doctors are willing to treat patients with low incomes.	Pos
3.63	14. A doctor's main interest is in making as much money as he can.	Neg

modified item weights are used in conjunction with Likert scale responses using a technique known as Scale Product scoring.[13] The item weights shown in Exhibit 9.2 are multiplied by the scores ranging from 2 (strongly agree) to −2 (strongly disagree) for positive items. The scoring is reversed for negative items. Scores for each dimension and the total scale are calculated by summing item scores and dividing by the number of items completed. This scoring procedure gives equal weight to positive and negative responses, thus assuming a simple linear relationship between positive and negative affect.

Zastowny and Roghman produced a 14-item general satisfaction with medical care scale derived from the version shown in Exhibit 9.2.[8, 12] They have used this in conjunction with a 12-item specific satisfaction scale which refers to experiences with a specific provider.

Administration and acceptability

Although the instrument appears to be designed for self-administration, the authors have mainly employed it in conjunction with interviewer-administered schedules. Some studies have used self-administration with a researcher present to deal with any queries. One study used the instrument in a telephone survey. In principle, it should also be possible to adapt it for use in a postal survey. However, the user should be aware that apparently minor differences in method of administration or wording can produce substantial differences in the pattern of responses. Any changes would require careful evaluation in terms of their effects on reliability, validity and comparisons with data from other studies.

No information is provided on the length of time taken to complete the scale, but we would estimate it to take about 10 minutes. Similarly, there is no direct evidence concerning its acceptability to respondents. Response rates of between 60 and 80 per cent for home interviews have been achieved, but rates will depend to a large extent on the method of administration.

Reliability and validity

Hulka and her colleagues have concentrated on increasing the reliability of the scale and have given less attention to validity, since it is difficult to assess the validity of an attitude measure, and since reliability has a limiting effect on validity.[13] Even so, evidence of reliability remains somewhat limited. Correlations between judges' ratings in the initial development procedures were good, but a test of parallel form reliability produced only modest results.[4] For the 1974 version, split-half reliability was reported, showing that the scale product scoring method was most reliable, but it was not used to test the items themselves.[13] Perhaps the best evidence of reliability comes from comparisons of the distribution of scores across a variety of studies which show excellent consistency.[10,11] Evidence of internal consistency is limited and there is no evidence of test–retest or inter-rater reliability.

The original authors have presented limited evidence of content validity and of construct validity based on the relationships between scale scores and various demographic variables.[13] However, Stamps and Finkelstein questioned the validity of the scale on the basis of evidence from analyses of data from three separate studies.[10] They subjected their data to an item analysis, Guttman scalogram analysis, and factor analysis, and concluded that these did not support the validity of the scale. They questioned whether the items actually measure three distinct dimensions of satisfaction rather than a single dimension. Hulka and Zyzanski have argued that these criticisms are not justified, on the grounds that the methods employed were inappropriate, but questions must remain as to the validity of the scale, and more research is necessary.[3]

A comparison of direct versus indirect wording of both individual items and general instructions, showed that the indirect method does indeed yield lower levels of satisfaction as suggested.[11] The preferred wording was as recommended by Hulka; indirect items preceded by instructions which ask respondents to answer in the light of their own experiences. The authors argue that the evidence is at least compatible with the contention that an indirect measure of this sort provides the most valid assessment of patient satisfaction. However, in this study none of the variants used showed statistically significant associations with better outcomes or with higher scores on process of care. There is thus no evidence concerning the responsiveness of the scale to changes in the quality or amount of care provided, or to variations in outcome.

Populations/service settings

The measure is designed for use with any adult population and has been used in both community/population surveys and studies of patients attending primary health care. It has also been used in studies of particular patient groups: low income and paediatric patients and sufferers from congestive heart failure and multiple sclerosis.[1,2,5-7,9] Whilst it may have some applications for the purposes of research in primary health care, its main value is likely to be in large-scale surveys.

Comments

The Scale for the Measurement of Satisfaction with Medical Care has been used in quite a wide range of empirical studies and it is well established. However, we feel that the evidence concerning its reliability and validity remains equivocal, and that more evidence is needed. The problem of the relationship between direct and indirect measures of satisfaction remains important. This is perhaps best overcome by measuring separately both general satisfaction with medical care and specific satisfaction with a particular provider. Roughmann and Zastowny's use of a short version of the Hulka instrument alongside a specific satisfaction scale seems to offer the best solution.[8]

References

1. Counte, M. A. (1979). An examination of the convergent validity of three measures of patient satisfaction in an outpatient treatment center. *Journal of Chronic Disease*, **32**, 583–8.
2. Hulka, B. S., and Cassel, J. C. (1973). The AAFP–UNC study of the organization, utilization and assessment of primary medical care. *American Journal of Public Health*, **63** (6), 494–501.
3. Hulka, B. S. and Zyzanski, S. J. (1982). Validation of a patient satisfaction scale: theory, methods and practice. *Medical Care*, **20** (6), 649–53.
4. Hulka, B. S., Zyzanski, S. J., Cassel, J. C., and Thompson, S. J. (1970). Scale for the measurement of attitudes toward physicians and primary medical care. *Medical Care*, **8** (5), 429–35.
5. Hulka, B. S., Zyzanski, S. J., Cassel, J. C., and Thompson, S. J. (1971). Satisfaction with medical care in a low income population. *Journal of Chronic Disease*, **24**, 661–73.
6. Hulka, B. S., Kupper, L. L., Daly, M. B., Cassel, J. C., and Schoen, F. (1975). Correlates of satisfaction and dissatisfaction with medical care: a community perspective. *Medical Care*, **13** (8), 648–58.
7. Liptak, G. S., Hulka, B. S., and Cassel, J. C. (1977). Effectiveness of physician–mother interactions during infancy. *Paediatrics*, **60**, 186–92.
8. Roghmann, K. J., Hengst, A., and Zastowny, T. R. (1979). Satisfaction with medical care: its measurement and relation to utilization. *Medical Care*, **17**, 461.
9. Romm, F. J., Hulka, B. S., and Mayo, F. (1976). Correlates of outcomes in patients with congestive heart failure. *Medical Care*, **14** (9), 765–76.
10. Stamps, P. L. and Finkelstein, J. B. (1981). Statistical analysis of an attitude scale to measure patient satisfaction with medical care. *Medical Care*, **9** (11), 1108–35.
11. Stewart, M. A. and Wanklin, J. (1978). Direct and indirect measures of patient satisfaction with physicians' services. *Journal of Community Health*, **3** (3), 195–204.
12. Zastowny, T. R., Roghmann, K. H., and Hengst, A. (1983). Satisfaction with medical care: replications and theoretic re-evaluation. *Medical Care*, **21** (6), 211.
13. Zyzanski, S. J., Hulka, B. S., and Cassel, J. C. (1974). Scale for the measurement of 'satisfaction' with medical care: modifications in content, format and scoring. *Medical Care*, **12** (7), 611–20.

Evaluation Ranking Scale (ERS) (Pascoe and Attkisson 1983)

Purpose

The authors set out to develop a measure of patient satisfaction for evaluating health care delivery within practices and comparing performance between practices. The requirements of the measure were that it should be: capable of registering satisfaction with specific aspects of health care delivery; resistant to response biases and other artefacts; and brief and easily administered.

Background

Development of the ERS was a response to the inadequacies of existing measures. In particular, the authors criticized other measures of satisfaction because they failed to differentiate patient responses, both in terms of the different dimensions of care provision and in terms of the distribution of scores. It is a common observation that most attempts to measure satisfaction produce uniformly positive responses.

The literature on evaluation theory and dimensions of health care was reviewed to yield eight potentially key characteristics. These were discussed with clinicians, administrators, and patients before further revision which produced the final ERS items. Apart from the separation of different dimensions of care the ERS employs two novel features. Firstly, it attempts to attach differential weights to different aspects of care by assessing both perceived importance and satisfaction. Instead of employing standard weights derived from population averages, this approach is designed to allow weights to be defined by each individual respondent. Secondly, it uses a visual analogue scale, which allows the respondent to rate items anywhere on the scale.

Description

Unlike most other measures of satisfaction the ERS is not a pencil and paper check-list. Patients are handed six cards, each of which labels and describes an aspect of health care delivery (Exhibit 9.3). There are two stages in the rating procedure. First, the patient is asked to sort the cards in order of their importance in judging a service, regardless of the patient's positive or negative feelings about the particular service being evaluated. When this task has been completed, the patient is asked to rate the absolute and relative quality of the service on each dimension by placing the cards on a chart. The chart consists of a single long vertical line calibrated 0–100, with 0 representing the worst possible health centre, and 100 the best possible. Cards may

---

Exhibit 9.3   Dimensions of the Evaluation Ranking Scale

(Reproduced, with permission, from Attkisson, C. C., Roberts, R. E., and Pascoe, G. C. (1983). The Evaluation Ranking Scale: clarification of methodological and procedural issues. *Evaluation and Program Planning*, **6**, 349–58)

Clinic location and appointments
  Location
  Parking
  Hours of operation
  Obtaining appointment(s)
Clinic building, offices, and
  waiting time
  Amount of waiting time
  Appearance of building, offices, and
    waiting areas
  Comfort of offices and waiting areas
  Appearance and clarity of signs,
    posted instructions/announcements
Clinic assistants and helpers
  Courtesy and helpfulness of:
    Telephone operators
    Receptionists
    Aides and volunteers

Nurses and doctors
  Skillfulness
  Friendliness
  Clarity of information/advice
  Thoroughness
  Amount of time spent
Health services offered
  Received the services I wanted
  Saw the nurse or doctor I wanted
Service results
  Success of services
  Speed of results
  Value of services
  Usefulness of information/advice

---

be overlapped and the gaps between cards are completely at the patient's discretion.

Satisfaction scores are calculated by weighting individual items according to the importance attached to them. Each item score is multiplied by its rank in stage one, the most important being given a weight of six and the least important a weight of one. Thus, for example, if the most important item was rated at 90, this would yield a score of 540 (90×6). A mean score is derived by dividing scores by the sum of the weighting applied. This permits weighted scores to be calculated for each item and for the scale as a whole.

Administration and acceptability

The relative complexity of the task compared with pencil and paper check-lists means that it has to be administered by a rater. Differences in scores related to rater characteristics and the information given to patients about who will use the data have been noted. Care should therefore be exercised and training may be necessary. The need for a competent rater to assist each patient individually means that the ERS is unsuitable for use in routine practice settings.

Acceptability to patients was assessed in terms of four indicators: amount of missing data, instances of refusal to complete the measure, frequency of failure to understand the procedure, and estimated average time for completion.[1] No ERS data were missing and no participants refused to complete the procedure, but around 4 per cent were confused about the task. The average completion time was 5 to 7 minutes, but the total time taken with each respondent was about 10 minutes.

Reliability and validity

Evidence of reliability is limited to a comparison of two study populations in the same health centre.[1] There is no direct evidence of test–retest reliability, and no evidence of internal consistency. Neither is there any systematic evidence of inter-rater reliability, although it is suggested that care should be taken to standardize instructions and the procedures used by different raters.

The issue of content validity is not specifically addressed, although the development procedures were designed to ensure good content validity. Nevertheless, the combinations of descriptions are sometimes unusual (e.g. clinic location with ease of obtaining appointments, and physical environment with waiting times). The main evidence of validity derives from comparisons with the Client Satisfaction Questionnaire (CSQ), the Patient Satisfaction Questionnaire (PSQ), and a single global measure of satisfaction. In a comparison with the eight-item version of the CSQ the authors showed that the ERS produced lower overall levels of satisfaction, as a consequence of its ability to discriminate between different components of care, and a more normal distribution of scores.[2] However, in a comparison with the 18-item CSQ, both measures were good predictors of global satisfaction, and both possessed similar psychometric properties.[3] In this study the CSQ produced a more normal distribution and slightly lower scores than the ERS.

A weakness of the ERS seems to be that, although the conceptual distinction between importance and satisfaction may be justified, results appear to suggest that respondents do not make the distinction. Patients' ranking of importance closely parallels their rating of their own health centre. Although the authors have tested a variety of alternative approaches to ranking, the problem does not appear to have been resolved. It is maintained that the ranking procedure is an essential part of the process and helps to familiarize patients with the dimensions to be rated, thereby yielding greater potential discriminative capacity. Whilst this may be true, the evidence to date seems to throw some doubt on the validity of the scoring procedure. If respondents are undertaking the same process in both ranking and rating exercises, it seems inappropriate to use the rankings to apply weights to rating scores. Although the authors recommend using the ranking procedure and weighted scores,[1] in another paper they use unweighted scores, since these proved a better predictor of global satisfaction.[3]

Populations/service settings

The ERS was developed for use with adults consulting in a primary health care setting. It is not, however, a visit-specific measure and could, therefore, be used with non-consulters.

Comments

The authors of the ERS have attempted to overcome some of the problems experienced in the design of patient satisfaction measures. They have concentrated on the need to differentiate, both in terms of aspects of health care and in terms of the range of scores. Whilst the method adopted has clearly gone some way towards overcoming these problems, the ERS does not offer a complete solution. Apart from its relatively costly method of administration, evidence of reliability and validity is inadequate. In particular, we do not feel that the authors have established the validity of the distinction between the importance of an aspect of provision and the rating given to it. This is fundamental to the ERS scoring system. Indeed the authors' own evidence seems to call into question the method of weighting rating responses by the rankings awarded in an assessment of importance.

Despite these reservations, we feel that the methods adopted by Pascoe and his colleagues are a useful contribution to the measurement of patient satisfaction. We should like to see further development of this approach to develop a reliable, valid, and economical measure of satisfaction. The ERS certainly offers a different approach to a difficult problem.

References

1. Attkisson, C. C., Roberts, R. E., and Pascoe, G. C. (1983). The Evaluation Ranking Scale: clarification of methodological and procedural issues. *Evaluation and Program Planning*, **6**, 349–58.
2. Pascoe, G. C. and Attkisson, C. C. (1983). The Evaluation Ranking Scale: a new methodology for assessing satisfaction. *Evaluation and Program Planning*, **6**, 335–47.
3. Pascoe, G. C., Attkisson, C. C., and Roberts, R. E. (1983). Comparison of indirect and direct approaches to measuring patient satisfaction. *Evaluation and Program Planning*, **6**, 359–71.

Client Satisfaction Questionnaire (CSQ) (Attkisson and colleagues 1979)

Purpose

The CSQ was developed as a simple measure of overall satisfaction that could be used in a wide variety of settings. Although originally developed for use in a clinic programme providing mental health therapy, it was intended to have more general application.

Background

The authors identified a number of key problems with using satisfaction data in evaluations of human services: high rates of reported satisfaction, lack of meaningful comparison bases, and difficulties in obtaining unbiased samples. They observed that the tendency of investigators to invent their own questionnaires or to modify existing scales to measure satisfaction gave rise to a lack of standardized measures.[2] A series of studies of patient satisfaction carried out over a period of six years at the University of California provided the opportunity to develop and refine the CSQ. The research was designed to construct and assess a simple client satisfaction scale that possessed sound construct validity, a coherent structure, and stable psychometric properties. The research also attempted to identify the relationships between client satisfaction and mental health outcome, and to identify variables which need to be controlled in any attempts to standardize a scale.[4]

Despite the authors' concern with methodological issues, there is no clear account of the conceptual basis of the CSQ. From existing literature on client satisfaction, they identified nine dimensions of service delivery that could be targets of satisfaction ratings: physical surroundings, support staff, type of service, treatment staff, quality of service, amount of service, outcome of service, general satisfaction, and procedures. Nine items were created for each and submitted to panels of experts, reducing the number of items to 31. This original version of the CSQ was field tested with mental health patients, and a short eight item version produced (CSQ-8).[2] Subsequent studies have resulted in two 18-item versions (CSQ-18A, CSQ-18B).[3] The original scale was clearly developed for use in community mental health care settings, but the shorter versions have been field tested in primary health care.

Description

The CSQ consists of between 8 and 31 direct questions about a specific programme of services, rather than a single encounter or continuous general care. Exhibit 9.4 shows the CSQ-18B, which also includes all of the items found in the CSQ-8. Although items reflect the nine categories of service delivery mentioned above, they are all held to contribute to a single general dimension of satisfaction. Responses are classified on a four-point Likert-type scale. The order of response categories is varied to avoid the danger of respondents ticking the same category throughout, and the absence of a mid-category avoids neutral responses. Scores are calculated by simply adding

Exhibit 9.4   Client Satisfaction Questionnaire

(Adapted, with permission, from Nguyen, T. D., Attkisson, C., and Stegner, B. L. (1983). Assessment of patient satisfaction: development and refinement of a service evaluation questionnaire. *Evaluation and Program Planning*, **6**, 299-314)

Please help us improve our programme by answering some questions about the services you have received. We are interested in your honest opinions, whether they are positive or negative. *Please answer all of the questions.* We also welcome your comments and suggestions. Thank you very much, we really appreciate your help.

Circle Your Answers

1. When you first came to our program, were you seen as promplty as you felt necessary?
   4) Yes, very promptly; 3) Yes, promptly; 2) No, there was some delay; 1) No, it seemed to take forever.
2. In general, how satisfied are you with the comfort and attractiveness of our facility?
   1) Quite dissatisfied; 2) Indifferent or mildly dissatisfied; 3) Mostly satisfied; 4) Very satisfied.
3. Did the characteristics of our building detract from the services you have received?
   1) Yes, they detracted very much; 2) Yes they detracted somewhat; 3) No, they did not detract much; 4) No, they did not detract at all.
4. How satisfied are you with the amount of help you have received?
   1) Quite dissatisfied; 2) Indifferent or mildly dissatisfied; 3) Mostly satisfied; 4) Very satisfied.
5. Considering your particular needs, how appropriate are the services you have received?
   4) Highly appropriate; 3) Generally appropriate; 2) Generally inappropriate; 1) Highly inappropriate.
6. Have the services you received helped you to deal more effectively with your problems?
   4) Yes, they helped a great deal; 3) Yes, they helped somewhat; 2) No, they really didn't help; 1) No, they seemed to make things worse.
7. When you talked to the person with whom you have worked most closely, how closely did he or she listen to you?
   1) Not at all closely; 2) Not too closely; 3) Fairly closely; 4) Very closely.
8. Did you get the kind of service you wanted?
   1) No, definitely not; 2) No, not really; 3) Yes, generally; 4) Yes, definitely.
9. Are there other services you need but have not received?
   1) Yes, there definitely were; 2) Yes, I think there were; 3) No, I don't think there were; 4) No, there definitely were not.
10. How clearly did the person with whom you worked most closely understand your problem and how you felt about it?
    4) Very clearly; 3) Clearly; 2) Somewhat unclearly; 1) Very unclearly.
11. How competent and knowledgeable was the person with whom you have worked closely?

Exhibit 9.4 (continued)

1) Poor abilities at best; 2) Only of average ability;
3) Competent and knowledgeable; 4) Highly competent and knowledgeable.

12. How would you rate the quality of the service you have received?
4) Excellent; 3) Good; 2) Fair, 1) Poor.

13. In an overall, general sense, how satisfied are you with the service you have received?
4) Very satisfied; 3) Mostly satisfied; 2) Indifferent or mildly dissatisfied;
1) Quite dissatisfied.

14. If a friend were in need of similar help, would you recommend our program to him or her?
1) No, definitely not; 2) No, I don't think so; 3) Yes, I think so; 4) Yes, definitely.

15. Have the people in our program generally understood the kind of help you wanted?
1) No, they misunderstood almost completely; 2) No, they seemed to misunderstand; 3) Yes, they seemed to generally understand; 4) Yes, they understood almost perfectly.

16. To what extent has our program met your needs?
4) Almost all of my needs have been met; 3) Most of my needs have been met; 2) Only a few of my needs have been met; 1) None of my needs have been met.

17. Have your rights as an individual been respected?
1) No, almost never respected; 2) No, sometimes not respected;
3) Yes, generally respected; 4) Yes, almost always respected.

18. If you were to seek help again, would you come back to our program?
1) No, definitely not; 2) No, I don't think so; 3) Yes, I think so; 4) Yes, definitely.

scores on each item. No weighting is applied. Thus total scores for the 18 item versions range between 18 and 72, and for the eight item version between 8 and 32, higher scores indicating greater satisfaction.

Administration and acceptability

All versions of the CSQ are designed to be self-administered, and CSQ-8 takes between 3 and 8 minutes to complete. It is usual, but not essential, to have someone present to answer queries. An experiment which compared written and oral administration showed that whilst the oral method produced fewer unanswered questions, it also produced a higher overall level of satisfaction.[3] The content of CSQ items appears to be acceptable to most respondents, but some problems have been experienced with the longer versions, because patients have failed to complete all of the items.

Reliability and validity

The authors of the CSQ have carried out extensive tests of reliability and validity. The two 18-item versions were produced to test split-half reliability in a study of clients of a community mental health day treatment programme. Mean scores were not significantly different and there was a high correlation between scores.[3] The CSQ-8 also had high internal consistency.[2]

Although the procedures used in development of the CSQ seem to have been intended to ensure content validity, the lack of a clear definition of satisfaction makes it difficult to assess how far this was achieved. The CSQ-8, which is referred to as the final version, was derived from a factor analysis of the full CSQ. This indicated that all items were tapping a general satisfaction dimension. The eight items with the highest loading on this factor were selected for the CSQ-8.[2] Evidence of construct and predictive validity is provided in a number of studies comparing the CSQ with other measures of satisfaction and with patient outcomes. CSQ-8 and CSQ-18B have been compared with the Patient Satisfaction Questionnaire and the Evaluation Ranking Scale.[5-7] CSQ scores were more closely related to a measure of global service satisfaction than PSQ scores, which seemed to reflect more generalized attitudes to health services and life satisfaction of respondents. CSQ-18B and CSQ-8 scores were correlated with both service utilization and psychotherapy outcome measures in a study of patients attending a community mental health centre.[1]

Although evidence of construct validity and predictive validity is quite good, the CSQ does not seem to have overcome the problem of detecting dissatisfaction. As with other scales, scores remain heavily skewed. It was for this reason that Attkisson and his colleagues went on to develop the Evaluation Ranking Scale. Of the different versions, CSQ-18B seems to produce a wider range of scores and a more normal distribution of scores than CSQ-8.[5,6] However, in this somewhat confusing array of studies, there seems to be no evidence of the sensitivity of diffferent versions of the CSQ to changes in service delivery.

Populations/service settings

It should be emphasized that the CSQ was originally developed to assess the satisfaction of patients attending mental health programmes. The authors have subsequently reported good results using the CSQ-8 and CSQ-18B with people attending an urban public health centre,[6,7] but it is our view that the content of the items reflects the original purpose of the measure. Questions such as: Have the services you received helped you to deal more effectively with your problem? may be difficult to understand for patients who have consulted only for acute physical illness. Also the questions seem to presuppose a specific episode of care for a particular problem, rather than continuing care for a variety of problems over a considerable period of time.

Comments

The CSQ has been used in a number of published studies. The majority of these have been mounted by the original authors and their collaborators, and many have been concerned primarily with development and testing. It is worthy of consideration, particularly in studies concerned with client evaluation of community mental health services. The number of versions is somewhat confusing, but the authors seem to have used the CSQ-8 and CSQ-18B most often. Further work to assess the validity and sensitivity of these two versions would be desirable, and an exploration of the weights attached to different items by respondents might increase the precision of the measure.

References

1. Attkisson, C. C. and Zwick, R. (1982). The Client Satisfaction Questionnaire: psychometric properties and correlations with service utilization and psychotherapy outcome. *Evaluation and Program Planning,* **5**, 233–7.
2. Larsen, D. L., Attkisson, C. C., Hargreaves, W. A., and Nguyen, T. D. (1979). Assessment of client/patient satisfaction: development of a general scale. *Evaluation and Program Planning,* **2**, 197–207.
3. Levois, M., Nguyen, T. D., and Attkisson, C. C. (1981). Artefact in client satisfaction assessment: experience in community mental health settings. *Evaluation and Program Planning,* **4**, 139–50.
4. Nguyen, T. D., Attkisson, C. C., and Stegner, B. L. (1983). Assessment of patient satisfaction: development and refinement of a service evaluation questionnaire. *Evaluation and Program Planning,* **6**, 299–314.
5. Pascoe, G. C. and Attkisson, C. C. (1983). The Evaluation Ranking Scale: An alternative methodology for assessing satisfaction. *Evaluation and Program Planning,* **6**, 335–47.
6. Pascoe, G. C., Attkisson, C. C., and Roberts, R. E. (1983). Comparison of indirect and direct approaches to measuring patient satisfaction. *Evaluation and Program Planning,* **6**, 359–71.
7. Roberts, R. E., Pascoe, G. C., and Attkisson, C. C. (1983). Relationship of service satisfaction to life satisfaction and perceived wellbeing. *Evaluation and Program Planning,* **6**, 373–83.

Medical Interview Satisfaction Scale (MISS) (Wolf 1978, revised 1981)

Purpose

The MISS is designed to measure satisfaction with a particular provider or consultation rather than more general attitudes to medical care. It is intended to be responsive to variations in the style and content of the consultation rather than the structural setting in which care is provided. As well as research applications, it is designed to be useful in clinical practice and teaching by identifying dissatisfied patients, providing evidence of the effect of changes in personnel or style, and evaluating the consultation skills of trainees.

Background

It was felt that existing measures of patient satisfaction were mostly inappropriate for the assessment of satisfaction with an individual provider or with a specific consultation. Those measures which did address patients' feelings about the consultation showed little evidence of reliability or validity.

Wolf and his colleagues[3] generated a pool of 63 statements concerning the quality of patient–provider interactions from interviews with patients, observations of consultations, and a literature review. These were progressively reduced in three separate field trials involving a total of 150 patients, by selecting those items which discriminate best in terms of three clinically relevant dimensions of satisfaction with patient–provider interaction: cognitive, affective, and behavioural. Cognitive items referred to the doctor's giving explanations and information, and the patient's understanding. Affective items referred to the patient's perception of the treatment relationship. Behavioural items referred to the patient's evaluation of physician behaviour. The final version contained 26 items. The original MISS has subsequently been revised in order to overcome the problem of high intercorrelations between sub-scales.[2] A further field trial of an extended 44-item version and factor analysis of the results produced a 29-item measure.

An offshoot of the MISS has been the development of a parental satisfaction measure (P-MISS) for use with parents accompanying their children.[1] Using the same approach as for the MISS, the authors developed a 27-item P-MISS.

Description

Exhibit 9.5 shows the final 29-item version of the MISS with the assignment to sub-scales. The sub-scales used in this latest version differ from those employed in earlier versions. Four partially independent sub-scales were identified: distress relief, communication and comfort, rapport, and compliance intent. Each item is scored on a Likert type seven point scale ranging from very strongly agree to very strongly disagree. Scores on positively worded items have to be recoded so that high scores indicate greater satisfaction. Sub-scale and total scale scores are calculated by simply adding all item scores without weighting.

Exhibit 9.5   Medical Interview
Satisfaction Scale (MISS)

(Adapted, with permission, from Wolf, M. H. and Stiles, W. B. (1981). Further development of the Medical Interview Satisfaction Scale. Paper presented to the *American Psychological Association Meeting*)

Item no./order	Sub-scale assignment
1. The doctor gave a poor explanation of my illness.	DR
2. The doctor told me just what my trouble is.	DR
3. After talking with the doctor, I know just how serious my illness is.	DR
4. The doctor told me all I wanted to know about my illness.	DR
5. I am not really certain about how to follow the doctor's advice.	CC
6. After talking with the doctor, I have a good idea of how long it will be before I am well again.	DR
7. The doctor seemed interested in me as a person.	R
8. The doctor seemed warm and friendly to me.	R
9. I felt that this doctor did not treat me as an equal.	R
10. The doctor seemed to take my problems seriously.	R
11. I felt embarrassed while talking with the doctor.	CC
12. I felt free to talk to this doctor about private matters.	R
13. The doctor gave me a chance to say what was really on my mind.	R
14. I really felt understood by my doctor.	R
15. The doctor did not allow me to say everything I had wanted about my problems.	CC
16. The doctor did not really understand my main reason for coming.	CC
17. This is a doctor I would trust with my life.	R
18. I would hesitate to recommend this doctor to my friends.	R
19. The doctor seemed to know that (s)he was doing.	R
20. After talking with the doctor, I feel much better about my problems.	DR
21. The doctor has relieved my worries about my illness.	DR
22. Talking with the doctor has not at all helped my worries about my illness.	DR
23. The doctor has come up with a good plan for helping me.	DR
24. This doctor visit has not at all helped me.	DR
25. The doctor seemed to know just what to do for my problem.	DR
26. I expect that it will be easy for me to follow the doctor's advice.	CI
27. I intend to follow the doctor's instructions.	CI
28. It may be difficult for me to do exactly what the doctor told me to do.	CI
29. I'm not sure the doctor's treatment will be worth the trouble it will take.	CI

Sub-scales

DR = distress relief; CC = communication comfort; R = rapport; CI = compliance intent.

Administration and acceptability

The scale is self-administered, but where it is used in an office setting its administration can be supervised. Although systematic evidence on response rates is not available, we would not anticipate any major difficulties in completing the scale. However, it is worth remembering that it is frequently difficult to interview patients after a consultation when they are in a hurry to leave.

Reliability and validity

Evidence of both reliability and validity for the MISS is extremely limited. The earlier version showed reasonable internal consistency, although the intercorrelations between sub-scales provided some cause for concern.[3] Although it would be difficult to mount a satisfactory study of test–retest reliability because of the problem of recall, it should not be impossible. The original research did not include a systematic assessment of validity, and work on the validity of the most recent version remains unpublished. Correlations of MISS scores with patients' reported attitudes and beliefs are cited as evidence of construct validity,[2] but there is a clear need for more careful validation. The most recent version is claimed to be more sensitive than earlier versions since it produces a pattern of responses less skewed towards satisfaction, but there is no evidence of how responsive the scale is to changes in the content of the consultation or the behaviour of the doctor. Such evidence seems essential for a measure which claims to be useful in clinical practice.

Populations/service settings

The MISS is suitable for use with all adults consulting in primary care or outpatient care. The fact that it is consultation specific means that its most likely use will be with patients who have just completed a consultation.

Comments

The MISS is included in this guide because it is one of the few consultation-specific measures available. We cannot, however, recommend its use on the basis of the information currently available. Considerably more evidence of reliability, and particularly validity, seems essential. Nevertheless, the MISS does provide an approach to the important problem of measuring satisfaction with individual consultations. We believe that there is a need for satisfaction measures which are suitable for clinical and teaching applications as well as for research.

References

1. Lewis, C. C., Scott, D. E., Pantell, R. H., and Wolf, M. H. (1986). Parent satisfaction with children's medical care: development, field test and validation of a questionnaire. *Medical Care*, **24** (3), 209–15.
2. Wolf, M. H. and Stiles, W. B. (1981). Further development of the Medical Interview Satisfaction Scale. Paper presented to the American Psychological Association Meeting.
3. Wolf, M. H., Putnam, S. M., James, S. A., and Stiles, W. B. (1978). The Medical Interview Satisfaction Scale: development of a scale to measure patient perceptions of physician behaviour. *Journal of Behavioural Medicine,* **1** (4), 391–401.

Patient Satisfaction Scale (PSS) (Dimatteo 1980)

Purpose

The PSS was developed to assess the relative contributions of doctors' communication skills, affective behaviour, and technical competence on patients' overall satisfaction. It can be used either as a general measure of satisfaction with a particular doctor or to assess satisfaction with each of the components mentioned.

Background

Little information is provided by the authors concerning the reasons for developing the PSS or the methods used. Some of the items were written specifically for the PSS, but others were drawn from the Medical Interview Satisfaction Scale (MISS). The scale was originally developed for use in a study of patients attending a family practice clinic in California.[1] The construction of sub-scales was based on an a priori theoretical grouping of items drawing on previous work in the area of patient satisfaction. No attempt was made to test reliability or validity of the PSS prior to its use in an empirical study and there have been no subsequent modifications to the scale.

Description

The PSS consists of 25 items divided into four categories: general satisfaction with and commitment to doctor (five items), satisfaction with communication (eight items), satisfaction with doctor's manner of 'affective care' (nine items) and perceptions of technical competence. Exhibit 9.6 shows the item wording. Thirteen of the items are positively worded and the remainder are negatively worded, in order to avoid the danger of an acquiescent response set. Responses are scored on a five-point Likert scale ranging from strongly agree to strongly disagree. Two additional items deal with the doctor's

---

Exhibit 9.6   Items in the Patient Satisfaction Scale (PSS), their categories, and scoring

(Adapted, with permission, from: DiMatteo, M. R. and Hays, R. (1980). The significance of patients' perceptions of physician conduct: a study of patient satisfaction in a family practice center. *Journal of Community Health*, 6, 18–34)

	Category
*1. I feel this doctor does not spend enough time with me	Affective
2. This doctor explains perfectly to me everything I could ever want to know about my medical condition	Communication
*3. I have some doubts about the ability of this doctor	Technical
4. This doctor really cares about me as a person. I'm not just part of his/her job	Affective
*5. I don't think I would recommend this doctor to a friend	General
*6. This doctor acts like I don't have any feelings	Affective
7. This doctor always gives me suggestions on what I can do to stay healthy	Communication
8. This doctor always treats me with a great deal of respect and never 'talks down' to me	Affective
9. This doctor always relieves my worries about my medical condition	Affective
*10. During the examination, this doctor hardly ever tells me what he or she is doing	Communication
11. I really like this doctor a great deal	General
12. I don't like this doctor very much as a person	General
13. This doctor is the nicest person I have ever known	General
*14. This doctor doesn't give me a chance to say what is on my mind	Communication
*15. This doctor doesn't act like I'm important as a person	Affective
16. This doctor always seems to know what he/she is doing	Technical
17. I wish I could stay with this doctor and never have to change to another one	General
18. I have a great deal of confidence in this doctor	Technical
*19. I feel this doctor does not take my problems very seriously	Affective
20. This doctor always listens to everything I have to say	Communication
*21. This doctor doesn't tell me very much about his/her plans to take care of me	Communication
22. This doctor is always very kind and very considerate of my feelings	Affective
*23 When this doctor gives me medicines, he/she does not tell me as much as I would like to know about them	Communication
*24. This doctor usually does not try to make me feel better when I am upset or worried	Affective
25. This doctor always explains the reason for examination procedures or medical tests	Communication

Note: Asterisked item — scoring reversed.

interest in the patient's family and job. These are not, however, incorporated into the measure of satisfaction and are therefore excluded from Exhibit 9.6. Scores on individual items range between 1 and 5 and sub-scale scores are calculated by simply adding item scores. Scores for negatively worded items should be reversed.

Administration and acceptability

The instrument can be self-completed in a few minutes, and is therefore suitable for use with patients attending the doctor. Response rates have varied from 30 per cent in a postal survey to 82 per cent where an interviewer was available to answer questions and supervise completion. However, it should be noted that 13 per cent of patients failed to complete at least one item even when an interviewer was present. Although there are no obviously sensitive or difficult items, the relatively poor response rate for the postal version and the failure to complete all items are causes for concern.

Reliability and validity

Limited evidence of reliability is available but the only indication of validity is from the use of the PSS in empirical studies, rather than any systematic attempt to establish validity. Internal consistency was high and test–retest reliability, although considerably lower, was acceptable.[1] However, it should be noted that the test–retest results were based on only 24 respondents. Intercorrelations between the sub-scales were uniformly high, suggesting that the PSS is in fact measuring a single dimension of satisfaction with the doctor, rather than the four dimensions proposed by the authors. There is some evidence that the PSS discriminates between patients from different socio-economic groups,[1] but this was not confirmed in another study.[3] The scale seems to have little value as a means of predicting appointment keeping behaviour or demand for consultations. Lastly, it should be noted that the distribution of item scores is heavily skewed. Average item scores exceeded 4 in all cases and on 16 items exceeded 4.5.[1]

Populations/service settings

The PSS was originally developed for use in a family practice clinic. It is suitable for use with adults who have recently consulted a general practitioner. Since it is not consultation specific, it does not need to be administered immediately following a consultation, but it does require that the patient have sufficient knowledge of the doctor to form a judgement. It may therefore be inappropriate for new patients or for those who have not consulted recently.

Comments

The PSS is an interesting attempt to develop a non-consultation-specific measure of satisfaction suitable for use in primary health care. Unfortunately, its development is limited and evidence of validity is woefully inadequate. It has been used in only three studies that we have been able to trace in the literature.[1-3] We cannot therefore recommend its use without further work. However, we do feel that further work, particularly on validation, would be worthwhile and that this might also explore modifications, particularly with respect to response categories. Alternative wording of response categories might produce a wider spread of responses.

References

1. Dimatteo, M. R. and Hays, R. (1980). The significance of patients' perceptions of physician conduct: a study of patient satisfaction in a family practice center. *Journal of Community Health,* **6** (1), 18–34.
2. Dimatteo, M. R., Hays, R. D., and Prince, L. M. (1986). Relationship of physicians' non-verbal communication skill to patient satisfaction, appointment non-compliance and physician workload. *Health Psychology*, **5** (6), 581–94.
3. Murphy-Cullen, C. L. and Larsen, L. C. (1984). Interaction between the socio-demographic variables of physicians and their patients: its impact upon patient satisfaction. *Social Science and Medicine,* **19** (2), 163–6.

Conclusions

A fundamental problem in selecting measures for inclusion in this chapter was that there are almost as many instruments as there are studies of patient satisfaction. Most are not published and many have no evidence of reliability or validity. The six measures we have reviewed here represent a range of different approaches to the problem of measuring satisfaction and all have some evidence of reliability and validity. Nevertheless, they all suffer from weaknesses of one kind or another. We believe that too little attention has been paid to the theoretical and conceptual problems raised in Chapter 2. We do not yet understand enough about how patients make evaluations in order to be able to comprehend their meaning. Evidence of reliability and validity is in most cases very limited and considerably more work needs to be done on this. In the meantime we believe that a careful appraisal of the different approaches adopted by these six instruments will help in the design of satisfaction studies, even where none of these is considered suitable.

Of all the aspects of outcomes of health care dealt with in this book, satisfaction is the least developed. There is therefore considerable scope for the development of new and modified versions of satisfaction measures. In particular there is a need for visit-specific measures which address patients' evaluations of particular consultations. The MISS instrument is designed to do this, but it is relatively long and has poor evidence of reliability and validity. A much shorter nine item visit specific measure has been developed and tested by John Ware and his colleagues for use in the Medical Outcomes Study.[2] This instrument had not been published at the time of writing, although we anticipate that it will appear in the near future, along with evidence of reliability and validity. Although most measures to date have been designed for general use, there may be a case for developing measures which tap the different concerns of particular groups. One recent measure has addressed the particular concerns of older patients.[1]

In conclusion, we want to emphasize the importance of patient satisfaction in the evaluation of health care. However, we believe that the same attention should be paid to conceptual, theoretical, and methodological issues as is the case for other dimensions of health care outcomes.

References

1. Cryns, A. G., Nichols, R. C., Katz, L. A., and Calkins, E. (1989). The hierarchical structure of geriatric patient satisfaction: An older patient satisfaction scale designed for HMOs. *Medical Care,* **27**, 802–16.
2. Ware, J. E. and Hays, R. D. (1988). Methods for measuring patient satisfaction with specific medical encounters. *Medical Care,* **26**, 393–402.

10   Miscellaneous measures

Introduction

It was almost inevitable that having developed an apparently comprehensive system for grouping and presenting instruments for the measurement of need and outcome in health care, there would be some which failed to fit the system. We could have forced these into earlier chapters, but we felt it was better to recognize the fact that they did not fit into any obvious category and to create a 'miscellaneous' chapter. The three entries included in this chapter have no common theme, but all are potentially important in considering the measurement of needs and outcomes in primary health care.

The Health Perceptions Questionnaire, another product of the RAND Health Insurance Studies, is concerned with how patients see their own present assessment of health state. It is the only instrument available at present which is designed to tap perceptions. We believe this is a particularly important topic for primary health care since it addresses an important outcome of health care interventions that is not covered by measures of function or health status. One of the tasks of the primary care physician is to reliably exclude serious illness, or to provide appropriate reassurance. Whilst patients receiving such reassurance will have benefited from their contact, there is unlikely to be any measurable improvement in health status. They may, however, exhibit less anxiety and a more positive perception of their health. If we are to measure the full range of outcomes of primary health care interventions, it is essential that health perceptions should be included. The RAND measure might perhaps be seen as a starting point for the development of instruments in this area.

The McGill Pain Questionnaire is included as a representative of pain measurement, for which there are a few well validated instruments. However, most of these are best suited to specialist settings and would be unlikely to find applications in primary health care. Nevertheless, the alleviation of pain is an important component in the treatment of many chronic conditions. For this reason many of the multidimensional and disease-specific measures dealt with in earlier chapters include assessments of pain. However, there may be situations in which these instruments provide insufficient detail and lack the necessary responsiveness to change to be adequate measures. The McGill Pain Questionnaire is one of the most commonly used pain measures. It has established reliability and validity, and a shortened version is available.

The final entry in this chapter covers a variety of single-item measures. It is common in both clinical practice and survey research to employ global questions which rate either particular aspects of health or overall health/quality of life. In this entry we have reviewed four different methods of constructing single-item measures which have some claims to reliability and validity. Whilst the use of global assessments is sometimes attractive, the user must be aware of the price paid in terms of reliability, validity, and responsiveness to change. However, there will be situations in which single-item measures are necessary, and they are often used in conjunction with multi-item instruments.

Health Perceptions Questionnaire (HPQ) (Davies and Ware 1976, 1981)

Purpose

The HPQ is a measure of people's perceptions of their own health intended for use in evaluations of medical care, explaining health and illness behaviour, studies of the relationships among health constructs, and population assessments of general health status.[5]

Background

John Ware and colleagues at the Rand Corporation in Santa Monica considered that self-ratings of general health status differed from other methods of measuring health status in a number of important ways.[7] They ask about personal 'health' as opposed to descriptions of function, behaviour, or feelings. They seek an integrated perception rather than separating physical and mental dimensions. They are intentionally subjective in seeking individuals' own evaluations of their health rather than objective descriptions. The researchers pointed out that most attempts to measure health perceptions were based on single items, there was little or no evidence of reliability and little attention to the problems of scaling. Whilst existing literature was deficient in these respects, the consistent associations between general health-related constructs suggested that such ratings do reflect an underlying health construct.

Initial development work on the first version of the HPQ was reported in 1976.[6] Items included were drawn from questionnaire items used in previous research and comments obtained in consumer surveys. The items stressed 'general health' and 'feeling' states rather than particular components of health. Six hypothesized constructs were measured: perceptions of past, present, and future health (health outlook), resistance or susceptibility to illness, sickness orientation (tendency to accept illness as a part of life), and health worries/concern.[7] Thirty items were selected and grouped on the basis of factor analysis. These were then further evaluated using Likert and multi-trait scaling and further factor analysis. Four items failed to satisfy the scaling criteria and were thus rejected. Six additional items dealt with rejection of the sick role and attitude toward going to the doctor. In the final development three single-item measures were incorporated and used in the questionnaires for the Rand Health Insurance experiment (HIE).[3] Data from the HIE were used to test the hypothesized major health perceptions constructs.

Description

The final version of the HPQ contains 29 items that assess general health perceptions (Exhibit 10.1). Twenty-six of these are statements rated on a five-point true/false scale and three are single-item measures similar to those used

---

Exhibit 10.1   Health Perceptions Questionnaire

(Adapted from Davies, A. R. and Ware, J. E. (1981). *Measuring health perceptions in the Health Insurance Experiment*, Rand Publication No. R-2711-HHS. Rand Corporation, Santa Monica)

Single item measures of general health

A.   In general, would you say your health is excellent, good, fair, or poor?
(Responses: 1. Excellent; 2. Good; 3. Fair; 4. Poor)

B.   During the *past 3 months*, how much pain have you had?
(Responses: 1. A great deal of pain; 2. Some pain; 3. A little pain; 4. No pain at all)

C.   During the *past 3 months*, how much has your health worried or concerned you?
(Responses: 1. A great deal; 2. Somewhat; 3. A little; 4. Not at all)

Health perceptions

Please read each of the following statements, and then circle one of the numbers *on each line* to indicate whether the statement is true or false *for you*.

THERE ARE NO RIGHT OR WRONG ANSWERS

SOME OF THE STATEMENTS MAY LOOK OR SEEM LIKE OTHERS. BUT EACH STATEMENT IS DIFFERENT, AND SHOULD BE RATED BY ITSELF.

D.   According to the doctors I've seen, my health is now excellent.
E.   I seem to get sick a little easier than other people.

Exhibit 10.1 (continued)

F. I feel better now than I ever have before.
G. I will probably be sick a lot in the future.
H. I never worry about my health.
I. Most people get sick a little easier than I do.
J. I am somewhat ill.
K. In the future, I expect to have better health than other people I know.
L. I was so sick once I thought I might die.
M. I'm not as healthy now as I used to be.
N. I worry about my health more than other people worry about their health.
O. My body seems to resist illness very well.
P. Getting sick once in a while is a part of my life.
Q. I'm as healthy as anybody I know.
R. I think my health will be worse in the future than it is now.
S. I've never had an illness that lasted a long period of time.
T. Others seem more concerned about their health than I am about mine.
U. My health is excellent.
V. I expect to have a very healthy life.
W. My health is a concern in my life.
X. I accept that sometimes I'm just going to be sick.
Y. I have been feeling bad lately.
Z. I have never been seriously ill.
AA. When there is something going around, I usually catch it.
BB. Doctors say that I am now in poor health.
CC. I feel about as good now as I ever have.

(*Responses:* 5. Definitely true; 4. Mostly true; 3. Don't know; 2. Mostly false; 1. Definitely false)

---

elsewhere. The six constructs are measured by grouping the items as shown in Exhibit 10.2. The single-item measure of 'worry' is incorporated with the other items dealing with health worries and concerns, but the remaining two single items (pain and overall health state) are treated independently. In addition to the construct scores, a global General Health Rating Index can be calculated using 22 of these items. The authors recommend using this entire 22-item index in other studies, but they also offer a variety of options for reducing the total number of items depending on the constructs which the researchers want to measure and constraints on length.

A short form version of the current health scale utilizing only four items has been developed and incorporated in the MOS short-form measure (see p. 153).

Administration and acceptability

The HPQ is designed for self-administration and can be completed in 5 to 10 minutes.[2] No problems have been reported in getting patients to complete the questionnaires and response rates seem to be high.

Exhibit 10.2   Scoring rules for Health Perceptions Questionnaire

(Adapted from Davies, A. R. and Ware, J. E. (1981). *Measuring health perceptions in the Health Insurance Experiment*, Rand Publication No. R-2711-HHS. Rand Corporation, Santa Monica)

Health perception scales

Item Scoring

General Health:	Item A: 1 = 40, 2 = 34, 3 = 25, 4 = 15
	Item B: 1 = 5, 2 = 4, 3 = 3, 4 = 2, 5 = 1
Health Perceptions:	Items: E,G,H,J,L,M,R,T,Y,AA,BB;
	1 = 5; 2 = 4; 3 = 3; 4 = 2; 5 = 1

All other items are scored as coded.

Scale Scoring

Current health	D + F + J + M + Q + U + Y + BB + CC
Prior health	J + S + Z
Health outlook	G + K + R + V
Resistance to illness	E + I + O + AA
Health worry/concern	C + H + N + T + Y
Sickness orientation	P + X

General health rating index

Item Scoring

Items:	E,G,J,L,M,N,R,Y,AA,BB:	1 = 5; 2 = 4; 3 = 3; 4 = 2; 5 = 1

All other items scored as coded.

Index Scoring

D + E + F + G + H + I + J + K + L + M + N + O + Q + R + S + U + V + Y + Z + AA + BB + CC

Reliability and Validity

As with the other instruments developed for the Rand HIE, careful attention has been paid to the reliability and validity of the HPQ. All of the evidence currently available is drawn from the HIE and is discussed in detail in reports from the Rand Corporation.[3,7]

Estimates of reliability based on internal consistency indicate that the multi-item measures are sufficiently reliable for group comparisons, equalling or exceeding the minimum 0.5 standard for group comparisons. The 'current health' scale and the General Health Ratings Index achieved the highest levels of internal consistency. Test–retest reliability or stability over time was assessed by comparing scores obtained at a one-year interval. Stability coefficients indicated that the measures reflect change over time, but are stable enough to warrant their use in repeated measures designs. The most stable scores were for prior health and sickness orientation, which suggests that the latter assesses more of a personal trait than a perception of current health, which might be expected to change over time.

Content validity is claimed for the measures, which well represent the range of items covered in published studies. Construct validity is demonstrated in extensive analyses of the relationships between the measures and a variety of health-related variables, including measures of physical function and mental health. However, the sickness orientation scale is not recommended to test hypotheses concerning health status, since the evidence suggests that it assesses a health-related personality trait. Regression analysis of longitudinal data indicates that the measures predict use of medical care over and above that predicted by measures of physical and mental health. This finding has been confirmed in a more recent study which looked at the health perceptions of primary care patients.[5] Patients with low health perceptions made more office visits, more telephone calls to the physician, and incurred more charges than patients with higher scores. Health perceptions accounted for 5 per cent of the variance in office visits after allowing for differences in physical health.

Although the HPQ is recommended by its authors for use in repeated measures designs, they have not directly assessed its responsiveness to change. There is good evidence that scores vary over time, and that the measures discriminate between groups, but how sensitive it is to small but significant changes in patients' health perceptions has not yet been established.

Populations/service settings

The HPQ was designed for use in large-scale population surveys. It is likely to be of particular value in research in primary care settings where subjective evaluation of health status is an important component in both decisions to consult and satisfaction with care received. Apart from the HIE studies, its use has also been reported in two studies undertaken in primary health care[2,4] and in patients suffering from chronic illness.[1] The relative ease of administration suggests that it could be incorporated into normal routine with little or no disruption.

Comments

Measures of health perceptions are likely to be particularly relevant to primary health care. However, apart from the widely used single-item measures which ask respondents to rate their health from excellent to poor, there are very few instruments available. The HPQ is far superior to these single-item measures in terms of the range of constructs measured, the reliability of the scales, and their validity. Nevertheless, there is a need for considerably more research in this area. In order to assess the outcomes of primary health care interventions, instruments are required which measure the effects of reassurance resulting from the exclusion of serious illness. The HPQ is one of the only instruments which touches on this issue, although it was not designed for that purpose.

References

1. Bobo, L., Miller, S. T., Smith, W. R., Elam, J. T., Rosmorin, P. C., and Lancaster, D. J. (1989). Health perceptions and medical care opinions of inner city adults with sickle cell disease or asthma compared with those of their siblings. *Southern Medical Journal*, **82**, 9–12.
2. Connelly, J. E., Philbrick, J. T., Smith, G. R., Kaiser, D. L., and Wymer, A. (1989). Health perceptions of primary care patients and the influence of health care utilisation. *Medical Care*, **27** Suppl, S99–S109.
3. Davies, A. R. and Ware, J. E. Jr. (1981). *Measuring health perceptions in the Health Insurance Experiment*, Rand: Publication No. R-2711-HHS. Rand Corporation Santa Monica.
4. Hall, J., Hall, N., Fisher, E., and Killer, D. (1987). Measurement of outcomes of general practice: comparison of three health status measures. *Family Practice*, **4**, 117–22.
5. Ware J. E. Jr. (1976). Scales for measuring general health perceptions. *Health Services Research*, **11**, 396–415.
6. Ware, J. E. Jr. and Karmos, A. H. (1976). *Development and validation of scales to measure perceived health and patient role propensity: Vol II of a final report.* Southern Illinois University School of Medicine, Carbondale, Illinois.
7. Ware, J. E. Jr., Davies-Avery, A., and Donald, C. A. (1978). *Conceptualisation and measurement of health for adults in the Health Insurance Study: vol V general health perceptions.* Rand: Publication No. R-1978/5-HEW. Rand Corporation Santa Monica.

McGill Pain Questionnaire (MPQ) (Melzack 1975)

Purpose

The MPQ was designed to provide quantitative measures of clinical pain that could be treated statistically.[8] It was originally intended to provide a means of detecting differences among different methods of relieving pain, but it has also been used for diagnostic differentiation. It has been widely used in both research and clinical practice.

Background

In designing the MPQ, Ronald Melzack was responding to the absence of any measures which adequately tapped the subjective experience òf pain. Measures in use at that time treated pain as though it were a specific sensory quality that varied only in intensity.[8] He pointed out that the word 'pain' refers to an endless variety of qualities that are categorized under a single heading, rather than to a single sensation which varies only in intensity. Thus to describe pain solely in terms of intensity is like describing the visual world only in terms of light flux, without regard to pattern, colour, texture, etc.

Melzack and Torgerson used existing literature to identify 102 words relating to pain which were then classified into three major classes; words that describe sensory qualities, words that describe affective qualities, and evaluative words.[10] These classes were then divided into subclasses which were qualitatively similar. Groups of doctors, patients, and students were asked to assign intensity values to each word using a numerical scale from least to worst. After deleting words on which there was disagreement between judges, the remainder were included in a questionnaire which, although considered only a rough instrument which would require further revision, has become the established MPQ.

Description

There arc at least five versions of the MPQ including a comprehensive version (MCPQ)[12] and a short version (SF-MPQ).[9] All versions incorporate lists of pain descriptors. Exhibit 10.3 shows the original version and Exhibit 10.4 the short-form. In the standard version the respondent is asked to select one word which best describes his or her pain at that time. If none of the words in a subclass is appropriate, that item is left blank. In addition to the 20 word selection items, there is a present pain intensity item ranging from 'no pain' to 'excruciating'. The short form consists of 15 descriptive words selected because they were used by at least one third of respondents to the standard version.[9] The descriptions represent the sensory dimension (items 1–11) and the affective dimension (12–15). Respondents are asked to rate the intensity of each particular quality of pain. The present pain intensity item is also used along with a visual analogue assessment of present pain.

In the first version of the MPQ, respondents were asked to base their answers on the pain they were experiencing at that time. Other instructions such as 'average pain' or how the pain 'typically feels' have also been tried.[1,7] The relevant time period for the short form is not clearly specified.[9]

A variety of additional questions is included in different versions of the standard MPQ, although these do not figure in the scoring system. Respondents are asked to indicate the location of their pain on a body outline. The original version also includes questions concerning drugs,

Exhibit 10.3   McGill Pain Questionnaire

(Reproduced, with permission, from Melzack, R. (1983). The McGill Pain Questionnaire. In *Pain measurement and assessment* (ed. R. Melzack), pp. 41-7. Raven Press, New York)

The descriptors fall into four major groups: sensory, 1 to 10; affective, 11 to 15; evaluative, 16; and miscellaneous, 17 to 20. The rank value for each descriptor is based on its position in the word set. The sum of the rank values is the pain rating index (PRI). The present pain intensity (PPI) is based on a scale of 0 to 5.

Patient's Name _____ Date _____ Time_____ am/pm

PRI: S_____ A_____ E_____ M_____ PRI(T)_____ PPI____
   (1-10)   (11-15)   (16)   (17-20)   (1-20)

1 FLICKERING	11 TIRING
QUIVERING	EXHAUSTING
PULSING	
THROBBING	12 SICKENING
BEATING	SUFFOCATING
POUNDING	
	13 FEARFUL
2 JUMPING	FRIGHTFUL
FLASHING	TERRIFYING
SHOOTING	14 PUNISHING
	GRUELLING
3 PRICKING	CRUEL
BORING	VICIOUS
DRILLING	KILLING
STABBING	
LANCINATING	15 WRETCHED
	BLINDING
4 SHARP	
CUTTING	16 ANNOYING
LACERATING	TROUBLESOME
	MISERABLE
5 PINCHING	INTENSE
PRESSING	UNBEARABLE
GNAWING	
CRAMPING	17 SPREADING
CRUSHING	RADIATING
	PENETRATING
6 TUGGING	PIERCING
PULLING	
WRENCHING	18 TIGHT
	NUMB
7 HOT	DRAWING
BURNING	SQUEEZING
SCALDING	TEARING
SEARING	
	19 COOL
8 TINGLING	COLD
ITCHY	FREEZING
SMARTING	
STINGING	20 NAGGING
	NAUSEATING
9 DULL	AGONIZING
SORE	DREADFUL
HURTING	TORTURING
ACHING	
HEAVY	PPI
	0 NO PAIN
10 TENDER	1 MILD
TAUT	2 DISCOMFORTING
RASPING	3 DISTRESSING
SPLITTING	4 HORRIBLE
	5 EXCRUCIATING

BRIEF	RHYTHMIC	CONTINUOUS
MOMENTARY	PERIODIC	STEADY
TRANSIENT	INTERMITTENT	CONSTANT

E = EXTERNAL
I = INTERNAL

COMMENTS:

Exhibit 10.4   Short-form McGill Pain Questionnaire

(Reproduced, with permission, from Melzack, R. (1987). The short-form McGill Pain Questionnaire. *Pain* 30 191–7)

Descriptors 1–11 represents the sensory dimension of pain experience and 12–15 represent the affective dimension.

Each descriptor is ranked on an intensity scale of 0 = none, 1 = mild, 2 = moderate, 3 = severe. The present pain

intensity (PPI) of the standard long-form McGill Pain Questionnaire (Exhibit 10.3) and the visual analogue (VAS)

are also included to provide overall intensity scores.

Patients Name:_____   Date: _____

	NONE	MILD	MODERATE	SEVERE
THROBBING	0) ____	1) ____	2) ____	3) ____
SHOOTING	0) ____	1) ____	2) ____	3) ____
STABBING	0) ____	1) ____	2) ____	3) ____
SHARP	0) ____	1) ____	2) ____	3) ____
CRAMPING	0) ____	1) ____	2) ____	3) ____
GNAWING	0) ____	1) ____	2) ____	3) ____
HOT-BURNING	0) ____	1) ____	2) ____	3) ____
ACHING	0) ____	1) ____	2) ____	3) ____
HEAVY	0) ____	1) ____	2) ____	3) ____
TENDER	0) ____	1) ____	2) ____	3) ____
SPLITTING	0) ____	1) ____	2) ____	3) ____
TIRING-EXHAUSTING	0) ____	1) ____	2) ____	3) ____
SICKENING	0) ____	1) ____	2) ____	3) ____
FEARFUL	0) ____	1) ____	2) ____	3) ____
PUNISHING-CRUEL	0) ____	1) ____	2) ____	3) ____

NO |_____| WORSE
PAIN   POSSIBLE
                                                  PAIN

PPI

0 NO PAIN	_____
1 MILD	_____
2 DISCOMFORTING	_____
3 DISTRESSING	_____
4 HORRIBLE	_____
5 EXCRUCIATING	_____

medical history, pain pattern, aggravating and alleviating factors, and influence of pain on aspects of life.[8]

The standard MPQ produces six pain quality scores and one pain intensity score. Each of the 78 description words is ranked within its group so that 'flickering' is ranked 1 and 'pounding' is ranked 5. For the 10 sensory, 5 affective, and 4 miscellaneous word groups, the rank values of words chosen are summed to produce pain rating indexes (PRIs). The PRI-sensory has a range of 0–42, the PRI-affective 0–14, the PRI-miscellaneous 0–17, and the PRI-evaluative 0–5. A total PRI score is calculated by summing the four subscores. A sixth quality score can be calculated by simply counting the total number of words chosen (range 0–20). The ranks are based on weights derived from the original work by Melzack and Torgerson.[10] As an alternative to ranks, the weights can be used to generate scores and a weighted rank score can be calculated.[11] Short-form scores are calculated by summing the intensity scores for sensory, affective, and all items.[9]

Administration and acceptability

Melzack recommends verbal administration of the questionnaire,[8] but other investigators have tested it in a self-completed form.[3,5] The standard MPQ takes 15 to 20 minutes to complete on the first occasion, but only 5 to 10 minutes in subsequent applications. It was because of this relatively long administration time that the short form was developed. The short form can be administered in 2 to 5 minutes. Verbal administration of either version could be undertaken by any member of the primary health care team with appropriate training.

Whilst no problems with understanding or acceptability to patients have been reported in the literature, we consider that it would be desirable to investigate the effects of differences in vocabulary, since some of the descriptors are terms which might not constitute part of the commonly employed vocabulary of many respondents. There is also a need to investigate the appropriateness of the terms to different cultural and ethnic groups. A number of foreign language versions of the MPQ have been developed and these have usually returned to Melzack's original methodology for developing pain descriptors. However, there is also a need to examine differences in language among subcultural groups in English-speaking countries, where differences in vocabulary and use may be important.

Reliability and validity

Good test–retest reliability was demonstrated in the original development of the MPQ, but the exercise was conducted on only ten patients.[8] Subsequent studies have, however, confirmed the stability of scores in unchanged respondents.[3,4,15] Alternate forms reliability has also been demonstrated.[5,17] The reliability of the short-form MPQ has not yet been reported.

There is considerable evidence to support the concurrent and predictive validity of the MPQ as a measure of pain quality and pain intensity.[2,16,20] Other studies have provided good evidence of construct validity,[6,18,19] both in terms of the differentiation of sensory, affective, and evaluative components, and in terms of the relationship between MPQ scores and psychological state. In a comprehensive appraisal of the MPQ, Reading also cites evidence of its ability to distinguish between patient groups.[15] The short-form MPQ has been validated only in terms of its correlation with the standard version.[12]

In the extensive literature on the MPQ a recurring theme is the factor structure of the instrument. Other investigators have questioned whether Melzack's selection and grouping of descriptors does in fact reflect the three dimensions he proposed. Although there is evidence that groups which might be expected to differ in their scores on the sensory and affective components do so,[15] one study concluded that the scales were highly intercorrelated and did not display adequate discriminative validity.[19] Factor analyses have suggested that there may be four or even five factors in the MPQ as opposed to the three proposed by Melzack.[14]

There is evidence from one study of patients suffering from arthritis that one third of patients volunteered affective words not included in the MPQ.[13] The same study also highlighted the failure of the MPQ to detect differences in pain experience in individual joints and on movement.

Whilst much attention has focused on the validity and factor structure of the MPQ, relatively little attention has been given to its responsiveness to change. However, Melzack's initial validation of both standard and short forms provides clear evidence that both are sufficiently sensitive to demonstrate differences due to treatment in a variety of patient groups,[8,12] Also, the fact that it is widely used in clinical trials indicates that other investigators consider it sufficiently sensitive to detect treatment effects.

Populations/service settings

The standard MPQ has been used in a wide variety of patient groups including those suffering from low back pain, arthritis, headache/migraine, cancer, and post-operative pain. A survey of published papers over the past three years showed that the MPQ was being used in epidemiological studies to determine the prevalence and severity of pain, in studies designed to differentiate pain resulting from different causes, in psychological research explaining the dimensions and correlates of the experience of pain, and in outcome studies to assess the relative benefits of alternative therapies. Whilst much of the research using the MPQ has originated in hospital specialist settings, most of the studies have involved out-patients and the MPQ has been administered in a wide variety of settings. We consider that it is potentially useful in research, audit, and clinical practice among a wide variety of patients suffering moderate or severe pain. For routine use with larger numbers of patients, the short-form MPQ might be a more practical proposition in primary health care than the longer standard version.

Most studies using the MPQ are relatively small scale. They do not, therefore, provide adequate data from which to construct norms for particular categories of patient. However, a recent paper describes a meta-analysis of results from many different studies which drew on assessments of more than 3000 subjects to construct population norms.[21]

Comments

Although there are a number of alternative pain measures available, the MPQ is the most widely used instrument. It is preferable to simpler measures of pain intensity because it recognizes the complexity of the experience of pain and is based on a clear theoretical formulation of this. However, there remain some doubts as to whether the different dimensions adequately reflect Melzack's theoretical model and how far they are independent of each other. There must also be doubts about how well the MPQ captures patients' perceptions of pain where these vary according to site and situation, as in arthritis. Further research and development of the MPQ is therefore needed, but it is at present one of the best available measures of pain resulting from a wide variety of conditions.

References

1. Crockett, D.J., Pokachin, K.M., and Craig, K.D. (1977). Factors of the language of pain in patient and volunteer groups. *Pain*, **4**, 175–82.
2. Duboisson, D. and Melzack, R. (1976). Classification of clinical pain descriptors by multiple group discriminant analysis. *Experimental Neurology*, **51**, 480–7.
3. Graham, C., Band, S.S., Gerkovich, M.M., and Cook, M.R. (1980). Use of the McGill Pain Questionnaire in the assessment of cancer pain: replicability and consistency. *Pain*, **8**, 377–87.
4. Hunter, M., Philips, C., and Rachman, S. (1979). Memory for pain. *Pain*, **6**, 35–46.
5. Klepac, R.K., Dowling, J., Rokke, P., Dodge, L., and Schafer, L. (1981). Interview vs paper and pencil administration of the McGill Pain Questionnaire. *Pain*, **11**, 241–6.
6. Kremer, E. and Atkinson, J.H. (1981). Pain measurement: construct validity of the affective dimension of the McGill Pain Questionnaire with chronic benign patients. *Pain*, **11**, 93–100.
7. Leavitt, F., Garron, D.C., Whisper W.W., and Sheinkop, M.B. (1978). Affective and sensory dimensions of back pain. *Pain*, **4**, 273–81.
8. Melzack, R. (1975). The McGill Pain Questionnaire: major properties and scoring methods. *Pain*, **1**, 277–99.
9. Melzack, R. (1987). The short-form McGill Pain Questionnaire. *Pain*, **30**, 191–7.
10. Melzack, R. and Torgerson, W.S. (1971). On the language of pain. *Anesthesiology*, **34**, 50–9.
11. Melzack, R., Katz, J., and Jeans, M.E. (1985). The role of compensation in chronic pain: analysis using a new method of scoring the McGill Pain Questionnaire. *Pain*, **23**, 101–12.
12. Monks, R. and Taeuzer, P. (1983). A comprehensive pain questionnaire. In: *Pain*

measurement and assessment (ed. R. Melzack), pp. 233–7. Raven, New York.

13. Papageorgiou, A. C. and Badley, E. M. (1989). The quality of pain in arthritis: the word patients use to describe overall pain and pain in individual joints at rest and on movement. *Journal of Rheumatology*, **16**, 106–12.

14. Prieto, E. J. and Geisinger, K. F. (1983). Factor analytic studies of the McGill Pain Questionnaire. In *Pain measurement and assessment* (ed. R. Melzack), pp. 63–70. Raven New York.

15. Reading A. E. (1983). The McGill Pain Questionnaire: an appraisal. In *Pain measurement and assessment* (ed. R. Melzack), pp. 55–61. Raven, New York.

16. Reading, A. E., Everett, B, S., and Sledmere, C. M. (1982). The McGill Pain Questionnaire: a replication of its construction. *British Journal of Clinical Psychology*, **21**, 339–49.

17. Reading, A. E., Hand, D. J., and Sledmere, C. M. (1983). A comparison of response profiles obtained on the McGill Pain Questionnaire and an adjective checklist. *Pain*, **16**, 375–83.

18. Toomey, T. C., Gover, V. F., and Jones B. N. (1983). Spatial distribution of pain: a descriptive characteristic of chronic pain. *Pain*, **17**, 289–300.

19. Turk, D. C., Rudy, T. E., and Salovey, P. (1985). The McGill Pain Questionnaire reconsidered: confirming the factor structure and examining appropriate uses. *Pain*, **21**, 385–97.

20. Wagstaff, S., Smith, O. V., and Wood, P. H. N. (1985). Verbal pain descriptors used by patients with arthritis. *Annals of Rheumatic Disease*, **44**, 262–5.

21. Wilkie, D. J., Savedra, M. C., Holzemer, W. L., Terler, M. D., and Paul, S. M. (1990). Use of the McGill Pain Questionnaire to measure pain: a meta-analysis. *Nursing Research*, **39**, 36–41.

Single-item measures (various authors)

Purpose

In this entry we deal with a selection of commonly used single-item measures of health, quality of life, satisfaction, etc. They can all be used to measure global constructs on a single scale. They are frequently used in situations where, for one reason or another, multi-item measures are impractical.

Background

Single-item measures of health, quality of life, satisfaction, etc. have a long history of use in population surveys whose main purpose is something other than the measurement of these particular variables. Thus, for example, the British General Household Survey is an annual survey which covers a wide range of topics such as housing, income, expenditure, leisure, and transport.[11] Health is therefore only one among many issues which have to be covered in a reasonably short interview. In such circumstances it is only practicable to include two or three items which tap aspects of health status.

Because single items necessarily require a global assessment of the aspect of health under consideration, they are essentially subjective evaluations on the part of respondents. They make no attempt to describe behaviour or experience, only to tap the evaluative component. It is arguable therefore, that what they are measuring is perceptions of health rather than health status. This is not, however, a criticism, since the evaluative component is an essential aspect of health status. As far as quality of life is concerned, it is arguable that the individual's evaluation of objective conditions is fundamental to the concept.

Description

We have selected for inclusion here four different methods of constructing single item measures which have been commonly used and which have been shown to have some claims to reliability and validity.

Category labels

Probably the most common method of constructing single item global measures is to ask the respondent to evaluate his or her health, quality of life, satisfaction, etc. according to a list of descriptive words. Exhibit 10.5 shows a common form of general health question. The number of response categories used varies from three to seven and the labelling of response categories varies slightly. Although responses are variously treated as nominal, ordinal or interval level data, it is safest to assume that it is only ordinal (i.e. responses are rank ordered, but the distance between categories is unknown and may be unequal).

Faces scales

A visual approach to the measurement of feelings can be achieved through the use of stylized faces as shown in Exhibit 10.5. Andrews and Withey employed seven faces for this purpose,[2] although the same approach used to assess patient mood used 20 faces.[9] Because the faces scale does not use descriptive terms, it has a stronger claim to interval level scaling.

Ladder scales

The ladder scale offers a method of allowing the respondent to situate his or her response according to personal experience and expectations. It is for this reason often referred to as a self-anchoring scale.[4] It achieves interval level measurement since each of the points on the ladder can be assumed to be equidistant from its neighbours.

Visual analogue scales

The visual analogue scale is a further extension of the principal employed in the ladder scale, in that the end points are identified but no categories or even

Exhibit 10.5 Single-item measures

(Faces scale and ladder scale reproduced, with permission, from Andrews, F. M. and Withey, S. B. (1976). *Social indicators of well-being: Americans' perceptions of quality of life.* Plenum, New York)

Category Labels

Over the last 12 months, would you say your health has on the whole been good, fairly good, or not good?

Good ☐   Fairly Good ☐   Not Good ☐

Faces Scale

Here are some faces expressing various feelings. Which face comes closest to expressing how you feel about your physical health?

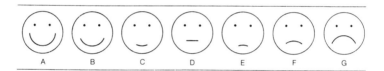

Ladder Scale

Here is a picture of a ladder. At the bottom of this ladder is the worst situation you might reasonably expect to have. At the top is the best you might expect to have. The other rungs are in between. Where on the ladder would you put your quality of life over the past four weeks? On which rung would you put it.

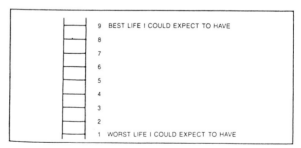

Visual Analogue Scale

Here is a line which represents the severity of pain. Please place a cross on the line at the point which represents the severity of pain you are experiencing now.

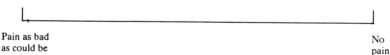

Pain as bad   No
as could be   pain

points in between are provided. It is simply a straight line, the ends of which are taken to be the minimum and maximum extremes of the variable to be rated. The respondent is simply required to mark the line at a point which represents his or her perception or evaluation. The length of the line is not crucial, but a 10 cm line is normally used. End points should be marked with a stop as in Exhibit 10.5, and care should be taken in formulating the anchoring phrases at the end points.[7]

Variations on the visual analogue scale include vertical lines and the graphical rating scale, which simply includes additional descriptive phrases located along the line.[6] All versions are scored either by measuring the distance between one end point and the respondent's marks, or by placing a template over the line and categorizing the response.

Administration and acceptability

All of these single-item measures are easy to administer and can be completed very quickly. The non-verbal approach of the faces scale might make it particularly suitable for use with respondents who have difficulty reading.

Reliability and validity

Evidence of reliability and validity is variable. The most comprehensive evaluation of global single-item indicators was undertaken by Andrews and Withey in a study in which they examined a total of 68 variants of global measures.[2] They reported satisfactory test–retest reliability over varying time periods, from only a few hours to two years. Rodgers and Converse also reported moderately high stability coefficients for a wide range of single item measures over a period of eight months.[12] However, many surveys using global assessments of health have made little attempt to establish test retest reliability. More systematic evidence for the reliability of visual analogue scales is available, and correlation coefficients as high as 0.99 have been achieved between successive measurements of pain.[14]

It is almost impossible to summarize evidence concerning the validity of single-item measured, since this depends on the concept being measured and the phrasing employed. Although general questions concerning health or quality of life are frequently employed in surveys without any attempt to validate them, there is evidence from more systematic study that single item measures can provide valid measurements of global health perceptions[5] or quality of life.[1] However, care should be taken to define what is being measured. Although global assessments of health will correlate with health profiles or index scores, the evaluative component will mean that correlation is far from perfect,[8] and that responses may vary systematically according to age, gender, ethnicity, etc.[3] As for reliability, visual analogue scales seem to have been subject to more systematic assessment of validity, particularly in the measurement of pain. Good correlations have been reported with verbal rating scales.[6]

Although on the whole single item measures would not be recommended for repeated measurement studies, claims have been made for the responsiveness of visual analogue scales. Nevertheless, the inherent instability and lack of precision in single item measures makes them unsuitable as measures of clinically significant change.

Populations/service settings

The sorts of single-item measures illustrated in this review are widely used with many different groups and in many different service settings. Their main role in health care research will be as adjuncts to other measurements, rather than as sufficient in themselves. One particular attraction of visual scales such as the faces scale, ladder scale, or visual analogue is that they may be used with children and others who might have difficulty completing a questionnaire.

Comments

A number of the measures reviewed elsewhere in this book employ single item measures within more comprehensive instruments (e.g. Dartmouth Coop Charts, McGill Pain Questionnaire, Rand Health Perceptions Questionnaire).

They are a valuable means of incorporating an evaluative component into research. They are, however, generally less precise, less reliable, and less valid than multi-item scales.[10] They may be useful in research or clinical situations where speed is essential, but the user should bear in mind the subjective evaluative nature of such measures and the price paid in reliability, validity, and precision.

References

1. Andrews, F.M. and Crondall R. (1976). The validity of measures of self reported well-being. *Social Indicators Research*, **3**, 1–19.
2. Andrews, F.M. and Withey, S.B. (1976). *Social indicators of well-being: Americans' perceptions of life quality*, Plenum, New York.
3. Blaster, M. (1985). Self definitions of health status and consulting rates in primary care. *Quarterly Journal of Social Affairs*, **92**, 131–71.
4. Cantril, H. (1965). *The pattern of human concerns*. Rutger University Press, New Brunswick.
5. Davies, A.R. and Ware, J.E. (1981). *Measuring health perceptions in the Health Insurance Experiment*. Rand: Publication No. R-2711-HHS. Rand Corporation, Santa Monica.
6. Huskisson, E.C. (1974). Measurement of pain. *Lancet*, **2**, 1127–31.

7. Huskisson, E. C. (1983). Visual analogue scales. In *Pain measurement and assessment*, (ed. R. Melzack), pp. 33-7. Raven, New York.

8. Leavey, R. and Wilkin, D. (1988). A comparison of two survey measures of health status. *Social Science and Medicine*, **27**, 269-75.

9. Lorish, C. D. and Maisiak, R. (1986). The face scale: a brief non-verbal method for assessing patient mood. *Arthritis and Rheumatism*, **29**, 906-9.

10. Manning, W. G., Newhouse, J. P., and Ware J. E. (1982). The status of health in demand estimation: or beyond excellent, good, fair and poor. In *Economic aspects of health* (ed. V. R. Fuchs). University of Chicago Press, Chicago.

11. Office of Population Censuses and Surveys (1986). *The General Household Survey 1984*. HMSO, London.

12. Rodgers, W. L. and Converse, P. E. (1975). Measures of the perceived overall quality of life. *Social Indicators Research*, **2**, 127-52.

13. Scott, J. and Huskisson, E. C. (1976). Graphic representation of pain. *Pain*, **2**, 175-84.

14. Scott J. and Huskisson E. C. (1979). Vertical or horizontal visual analogue scales. *Annals of Rheumatic Disease*, **38**, 560.

11   Final comments

We believe that the reviews of instruments contained in previous chapters demonstrate a healthy state of development in the measurement of needs for, and outcomes of, health care. There is a plethora of instruments available, only a selection of which have been included in the present review. They serve a wide variety of purposes and are of varying degrees of sophistication and quality. Development under different subject headings (function, mental health, satisfaction, etc.) is patchy. In some areas we had a large number of measures from which to choose, and could thus afford to apply fairly stringent criteria of appropriateness to primary health care and quality. In others we have had little or no choice, including measures of poorer quality and which are less obviously applicable to primary health care. Nevertheless, the overall message to both researchers and practitioners in primary health care who want to employ measures of need and outcome should be one of encouragement. There are already reliable and valid instruments in many areas, and future development and testing is likely to extend their applicability to primary health care.

There are no overall conclusions or recommendations to be drawn from a review such as this, but there are a number of general comments and observations which we think should be kept in mind by those engaged in the development of measures and potential users.

Documentation of measures

The authors of many of the instruments included in this review could do much more to ensure adequate documentation of their instruments. Users' manuals, where they exist, provide a summary of the development and testing of an instrument, practical instructions for administering and scoring it, a definitive copy of the schedule, and any variants. Unfortunately, they are only available for a minority of instruments and some of them are not easily obtainable. In many cases copies of the schedules and instructions are provided only as appendices to lengthy research reports. Subsequent amendments to the original or the development of shortened versions or variants are rarely incorporated into a single document. It thus becomes difficult for the user to track down a definitive version with adequate documentation of development, testing, and uses.

We recognize that it would be impossible for the authors of widely used instruments to provide a comprehensive and up-to-date summary of all uses, but we believe it should be possible to make basic information more readily available to potential users. Where users have developed a modified version of a particular instrument it is also essential that this should be published and clearly labelled in such a way as to distinguish it from the original. Lastly, the editors of journals could assist in this process by ensuring that papers describing new measures or variants of existing measures should include a copy of the instrument, including relevant instructions, or at least a clear indication of where to obtain this information.

Reliability and validity

We have stressed the importance of reliability and validity throughout. Evidence with regard to individual measures is extremely variable, but even in the best examples further evidence is desirable. It is worth reiterating here that evidence of reliability and validity is frequently limited to particular categories of patients, service settings, and uses. The potential user should carefully evaluate existing evidence to assess how relevant this is to the purpose for which the measure is required and the circumstances in which it will be used. In many instances further testing, particularly of reliability, will be required, and it will often be possible to add to existing evidence of validity by incorporating new tests in substantive research or clinical practice.

Responsiveness

Perhaps the most important criterion for the selection of a measure to evaluate patient outcomes is whether it is responsive to changes which would be considered significant by patients and/or practitioners. It should be recognized that the usual methods of establishing reliability and validity will not indicate how responsive a measure is to change. Indeed they may militate against responsiveness by excluding items which fail to discriminate between individuals, but which are nevertheless sensitive to change within individuals. Few of the measures reviewed in previous chapters have been adequately evaluated in terms of their responsiveness to change. It will be important for users who wish to apply these instruments to measure outcomes over time in the same individuals to examine their responsiveness. This can be done by testing a measure on patients receiving treatment of known efficacy to ensure that it is capable of detecting treatment effects.

Directions for future development

It is difficult to generalize concerning the need for further development of instruments, because of the varying stages of development in different areas.

In areas such as social well-being and patient satisfaction there is scope for new instruments which need to be carefully developed and tested to meet particular needs. In most areas, however, further proliferation of new measures may be counter-productive. The researcher or clinician who requires a measure for a particular application will rarely have the resources to embark on the development and testing of a new instrument. Too often new instruments are developed with inadequate attention to their reliability and validity, when existing measures would serve perfectly well. There is little point in reinventing the wheel, and even less in inventing an inferior version of the wheel.

We believe that the most useful developments in coming years will arise from work which builds on existing instruments. There is considerable scope in many cases for refinement of content, improved weighting and scoring systems, and adaptations to particular situations. One of the most important aspects of development for users in Britain and other European countries is the translation and/or adaptation of content in instruments developed and tested in the USA. The development and testing of the Functional Limitations Profile (see Chapter 7) is an excellent example of this sort of work. The other major area of development is likely to be in the area of disease-specific measures. Where generic measures are insufficiently responsive to clinically significant change, a disease-specific measure will often be necessary. However, even in this area it should be possible to build on existing instruments rather than starting afresh. In particular, we would like to see an increasing use of disease-specific supplements to generic measures. In this way it is possible to retain comparability with other research and across disease groups.

Choosing an appropriate instrument

We have carefully avoided offering advice on 'best buys', since the most appropriate choice of instrument for any particular application will depend on a wide variety of considerations. It will be evident from our comments on individual measure that we are more critical of some than of others. Nevertheless, all of those that we have included have potential applications for researchers and/or practitioners in primary health care. The decision as to which measures best meets the needs of a particular application will have to be taken by the user. However, we should emphasize that our reviews provide only sufficient information to make a preliminary selection. It is essential that, having made such a selection, the intending user should obtain further information by following up the references provided at the end of each chapter.

Research versus clinical use

Most measures of need and outcome in health care have been developed primarily for use in research, although a minority have arisen out of clinical practice and a few have been developed in a research programme for use in clinical practice. One of the consequences of this is that most of the evidence of reliability and validity relates to research applications. However, we expect that clinicians and other health care professionals will increasingly want to make use of a variety of instruments to assess needs for care and to monitor the outcomes of treatment in routine clinical practice. For such purposes the criteria for selecting an appropriate instrument will be rather different from those commonly employed in selecting a measure for research purposes. For clinical use instruments must be short, easily administered, easily interpreted, and suitable for repeat administration. Most important of all, they must be responsive to clinically significant change.

Applications in primary health care

Measures of need and outcome have been less extensively used in primary health care than in other specialties. However, despite the fact that most existing measures have been developed for uses other than in primary health care, we have illustrated in previous chapters a wide variety of instruments which we consider to have a place in either research or practice at the primary care level. Nevertheless, it is important to recognize the particular circumstances of primary health care and the bearing which these will have on the selection of suitable instruments. Firstly, the very wide range of problems presented and varying degrees of severity make it almost impossible to think in terms of universally applicable measures. Multidimensional measures are likely to be of most general relevance, but these are unlikely to include sufficient detail to evaluate the care of certain major chronic conditions (e.g. arthritis, bronchitis, diabetes). Thus, disease-specific measures or disease-specific supplements will be essential. Secondly, the continuing nature of much primary medical care and the inability to be able to define clear start and end points in treatment mean that for outcome purposes measures should be easy to administer repeatedly. Thirdly, although the problem of intervening variables affects all research into the outcomes of treatment, it is particularly serious in primary care. This provides a further rationale for using multidimensional instruments which incorporate measures of areas of functioning and resources which may not be considered directly relevant to the care provided. It also means that it will usually be necessary to assess other inputs (e.g. other services, social support, environment, economic circumstances) as well as focusing on needs for, and outcomes of, medical care.

Measurement requires resources

To many doctors, nurses, and other health professionals unfamiliar with measurement techniques in the field of health services evaluation, the cost of measurement may appear excessive. We have deliberately excluded instruments which require administration by a specialist and have included as many simple self-completed instruments as possible. Nevertheless, whatever measure is used will require resources to be devoted to printing, administration, and analysis, and for many measures these costs can be considerable. We believe, however, that it is a worthwhile investment. Doctors working in primary health care are used to making extensive use of laboratory investigations and X-rays. Measures of health status and patient satisfaction should be seen as complementary to these diagnostic tests in clinical practice. If we want to achieve more effective and efficient medical care it is essential to see expenditure on measurement as an investment.

Final remarks

Measures of health, illness, and patient satisfaction are essential to the establishment of needs for and outcomes of health care. They can be as precise and as useful as many accepted clinical measures, but they are as yet relatively unfamiliar in primary health care. There is increasing attention in all complex health care systems to the need to maximize effectiveness and efficiency. Monitoring needs for, and outcomes of, care is essential to this process. One of the results of this trend is an increasing use of audit as a means of monitoring care. However, much medical audit, particularly in primary care, stops short of recording information on the extent to which patients' needs are met and desirable outcomes achieved. Measures such as those reviewed here provide a method of systematically evaluating both individual treatments in primary health care and patterns of service delivery. They thus have a vital role to play in the development of medical audit.

Index

Page numbers in **bold** denote main sections in the text.

Names of instruments have been listed as sub-headings under entries for which they have been mentioned in the text. Appropriate measures can therefore be selected:

- by purpose (e.g. clinical practice; research; surveys);

- by type of administration (e.g. interviewer administration; postal surveys; self-report measures);

- by population served (e.g. elderly people; groups; outpatients);

- by service setting (e.g. community care; hospital settings; primary health care);

- by disease category (e.g. arthritis; cancer; heart disease);

- by broader health/illness status (e.g. disability; function; mental health and illness).